10 3 60

D1159639

CANCER

A COLOUR ATLAS

A slide atlas of *Cancer: A Colour Atlas*, based on the contents of this book, is available. In the slide atlas format, the material is split into volumes, each of which is presented in a binder together with numbered 35mm slides of each illustration. Each slide atlas volume also contains a list of abbreviated slide captions for easy reference when using the slides. Further information can be obtained from:

Gower Medical Publishing
Middlesex House
34–42 Cleveland Street
London W1P 5FB

Gower Medical Publishing
101 5th Avenue
New York, NY 10003
USA

Igaku Shoin Ltd
Tokyo International
P.O. Box 5063, Tokyo, Japan

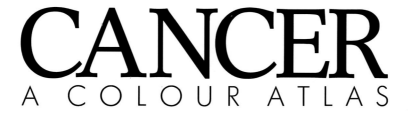

CANCER
A COLOUR ATLAS

Dr Jeffrey S Tobias
MA (Cantab), MD, FRCP, FRCR

Consultant in Radiotherapy and Oncology
Department of Radiotherapy and Oncology
University College Hospital
Gower Street
London

Honorary Clinical Senior Lecturer
University College and Middlesex School of Medicine
Gower Street
London

Dr Christopher J Williams
DM, FRCP

Senior Lecturer in Medical Oncology and Honorary
Consultant Physician
University of Southampton
Southampton General Hospital
Southampton

J B Lippincott Company PHILADELPHIA
Gower Medical Publishing LONDON · NEW YORK

Distributed in USA and Canada by:
J.B. Lippincott Company
East Washington Square
Philadelphia, PA 19105
USA

Gower Medical Publishing
101 5th Avenue
New York, NY 10003
USA

Distributed in UK, Europe and rest of World by:
Gower Medical Publishing Ltd
Middlesex House
34–42 Cleveland Street
London W1P 5FB
UKq

Distributed in Japan by:
Igaku Shoin Ltd
Tokyo International
P.O. Box 5063
Tokyo, Japan

Project editors:	Claire Hooper
	Stephen McGrath
Design:	Judith Gauge
Illustration:	Lee Smith
	Balvir Koura
Paste-up:	Olgun Hassan
	Lee Riches
	Ruth Miles
	Mike Smith
	Patrizia Cavaliere

British Library Cataloguing in Publication Data:
Tobias, Jeffrey S.
Cancer: A Colour Atlas
1. Man. Cancer.
I. Title. II. Williams C.J.H.
616.994

Library of Congress Cataloging-in-Publication Data
Tobias, Jeffrey S.
Cancer: A Colour Atlas/Jeffrey S. Tobias,
Christopher J. Williams.
Includes index.
1. Cancer. I. Williams, C.J.H. (Christopher John Hacon). II. Title.
[DNLM: 1. Neoplasms. 2. Neoplasms—atlases. QZ 200 T629c.]
RC261. T63 1990
616.99'4-dc20

ISBN 0-397-44585-7

Originated in Hong Kong by Bright Arts
Typesetting by M to N Typesetters, London
Text set in Rotation; captions set in Futura
Produced by Mandarin Offset
Printed in Hong Kong

Preface

On an international scale, the prevention, treatment and control of cancer represents one of the most formidable medical challenges in the World today. Cancer is a vast medical problem with a high mortality, second in the Western World only to cardiovascular disease, and has become increasingly the focus of worldwide medical research. Both in the United States and Europe, co-ordinated efforts to reduce cancer mortality by the year 2000 have attracted major government support and funding, yet the present methods of treatment with surgery, radiotherapy, chemotherapy and hormone therapy still lack precision, and our best efforts at treatment still fail far too often. In the cancer sciences, on the other hand, there has in the past decade been an explosion of understanding of biological mechanisms, of the importance of oncogenes in the subcellular evolution of cancer, and in the potential of cytokines and other growth factors both in the development of cancer and possibly as a further means of therapy.

This book provides an illustrated overview of all aspects of cancer, for non-specialists who are interested in the management of cancer, for trainee and practising oncologists and physicians in related specialties. In addition, we hope the book may be of interest to medical students who wish to know more about a critically important part of medicine which is often neglected in undergraduate courses. Whilst this is a clinical book which does not attempt to discuss the mechanisms and genetics of cancers, we have attempted to provide a cohesive account of the major clinical problems occurring within each site, together with adequate illustration of the complications that may arise and wherever possible, brief details of current therapy and outcome. Cancer medicine has become a very rapidly moving specialty, indeed in the last 20 years there have been spectacular advances in a number of areas.

We now expect regularly to cure almost all patients with testicular tumours, even when widely metastatic, and successful management of Hodgkin's disease and many non-Hodgkin's lymphomas has been a reality for more than 20 years now. Adjuvant therapy of cancer has also become firmly established, particularly in the treatment of breast cancer, a disease whose management has altered remarkably over this same period. In recent years, much more attention has also been paid to the supportive and continuing care of patients whose cancers cannot be cured. The hospice movement has taught us a great deal about the proper principles of treatment in patients where the cancer is likely to be fatal, emphasizing the many possibilities for improved quality of life that can be achieved by expert attention to the many problems of management.

All these areas are explored and discussed in some detail in this book. We have attempted to give a working knowledge of the diagnosis, staging and management of the important tumours, with emphasis on the interplay between different types of treatment, and wherever possible, an indication of some of the present controversies in management. Although no bibliography is supplied, we have tried to include some of the more important recent advances as part of the text or by illustration.

Finally, this is not intended to be a handbook of cancer management since there are very large specialist texts available which concentrate on the details of current therapy. Although no two people can be expert in all branches of cancer, we hope that this volume will provide adequate insight for doctors who wish to learn more about malignant disease, and we trust that the many illustrations will offer a greater degree of understanding than can be achieved by words alone.

Jeffrey S. Tobias
Christopher J. Williams

Acknowledgements

We are indebted to Judith Gauge for expert artwork and design; to Claire Hooper and Stephen McGrath for their many hours of patient editing work; to Lee Smith for illustrations; to Elizabeth Johnston and Hilary Webster for typing and re-typing the text; and finally to Fiona Foley whose enthusiasm has carried us through many difficulties. Without this remarkable team from Gower Medical, this book could never have been successfully completed.

Dedication

For our children:
Joanna, Sarah, Kate, Ben and Max.

Contents

Cancer: An International Problem

1

Introduction

Cancer is a universal problem and is a leading cause of death in many different parts of the world. The most intriguing aspect of the study of geographical variations is that the incidence of some malignant tumours varies so much (100-fold or more) from one part of the world to another. These observations have led to the development of the science of epidemiology. The frequency of disease in peoples living in different conditions in different parts of the globe gives useful clues as to its cause.

Variations in Incidence

Data on the yearly incidence of new cases and death rates for individual tumours have been collected in various countries for a considerable period of time (Fig. 1.1). These crude data (corrected for each population according to its age distribution) yield some startling variations in the incidence of particular tumours. For instance, skin cancer is 200 times more common in Queensland, Australia than in Bombay, India. This finding is probably a result of both environmental and genetic factors (Fig. 1.2) –

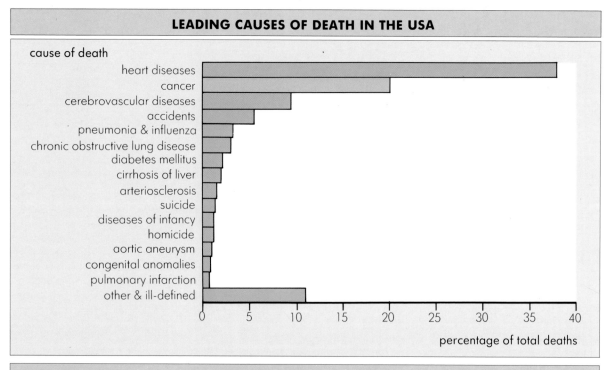

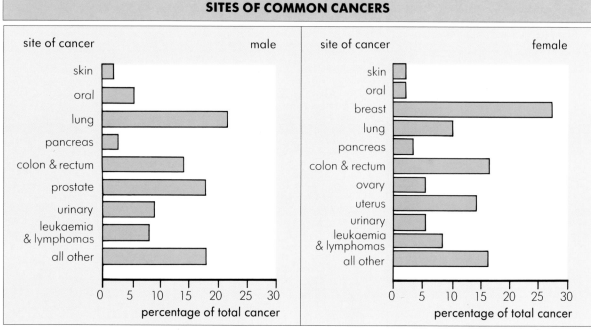

Fig. 1.1 Causes of death in the Western world.
(Top) Cancer is the second leading cause of death in the USA. [Modified from *Vital Statistics of the United* *States* (1978).] (Bottom) Histogram showing the frequencies of various cancers in men and women in the USA.

the pigmentation and inherent resistance of Indian skin to the carcinogenic properties of UV light, compared with fair Caucasian skin exposed to strong sunlight in Queensland.

In contrast, cancer of the oesophagus is common in certain parts of the Middle and Far East – in northern Iran the incidence is 300 times that in Nigeria – and these differences are likely to be environmental in origin. A variety of potential cancer-causing factors have been identified, some apparently operating in a number of different parts of the world. Some well-documented examples include the following:

- excessive alcohol (especially high alcohol content and Bantu Kaffir beer);
- tobacco usage (cigarette, pipe, cigar and chewing tobacco);
- benign stricture secondary to ingestion of caustics;
- deficiency of vitamin A and other nutrients;
- diet deficient in vegetables and fruit;
- diet including Bracken fern (Japan);
- diet high in nitrosamines and low in vitamins (northern China);
- ingestion of the juices of *Croton flavens*.

Even though cancer is important all around the world with a relatively small overall variation in incidence (threefold), some tumours which are a major problem in one country may be rare in another. Although overall incidence rates are generally higher in Western countries, this does not apply to all types of cancer. For instance, England and Wales have one of the highest incidences of lung cancer but are at the bottom of the world league table for primary cancers of the liver and nasopharynx.

In order to try to decide the causes for these geographical variations in cancer incidence the data have been studied in various special situations.

The Influence of Population Migration

A well-defined population which has moved from one country to another provides a natural cohort, allowing the relative effects of environmental and genetic factors to be assessed. The requirements are:
- a large, well-defined population group;
- a move to a very different environment;
- little or no intermarriage with the surrounding population;
- good data collection and long-term follow-up.

The best example of such a group is the Japanese who left Japan late in the last century and in the early years of the 20th century. Many moved to Hawaii, and they have been extensively studied. This is an excellent model, since native Japanese have a

UV EXPOSURE, GENETIC FACTORS AND MALIGNANT MELANOMA

Geographical groups with a high incidence of malignant melanoma

Long-term European residents in Israel
Fair-skinned Australians (especially of Scottish descent)
Caucasians in the Sun Belt in the USA

Overall, the risk increases with decreasing latitude

Racial groups at low risk of developing melanoma

Negroes
Oriental peoples

When non-Caucasians develop melanoma they tend to do so in less pigmented parts of the body (sole of foot, palms, mouth, anus, vagina)

Sites of melanoma

	Arms	Trunk	Legs	Head & Neck	Other
Men	17%	38%	14%	23%	8%
Women	37%	22%	17%	19%	5%

Incidence of melanoma is higher on sun-exposed parts of the body

Incidence and mortality with time

Malignant melanoma has risen nearly threefold over the last forty years at a time when increased sun exposure has been fashionable

Fig. 1.2 Malignant melanoma. A number of observations support the idea that both UV exposure and genetic factors are important in the causation of this cancer.

very different pattern of cancer from Caucasian Americans and, as a racial group, they have inter-married very little. Data for ten common tumours (Fig. 1.3) show that in every case there has been a change in the incidence of the tumour away from the Japanese pattern, towards the pattern seen in Caucasian Hawaiians. So, while cancer of the endometrium is rare in Japan, it has increased in incidence

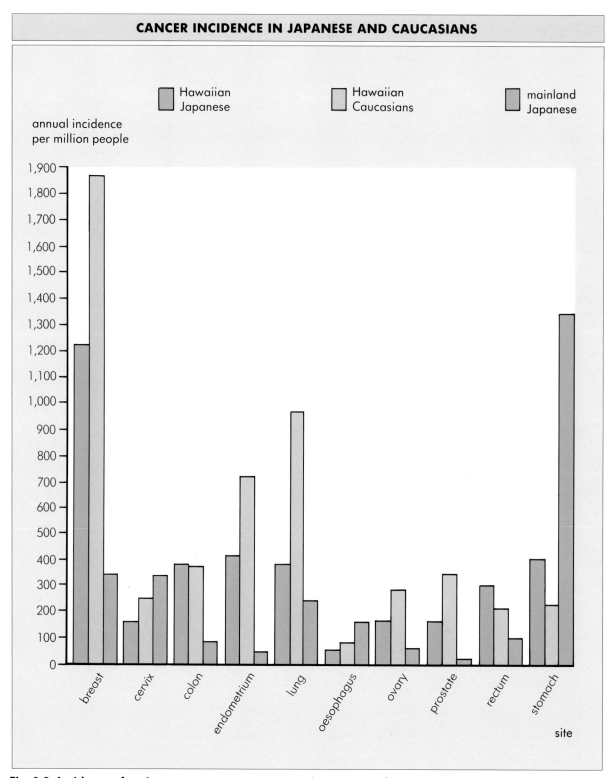

Fig. 1.3 Incidence of various common cancers among Japanese and Caucasians in Hawaii. The incidence in Hawaiian Japanese is closer to that of Hawaiian Caucasians than it is to mainland Japanese. Assuming no intermarriage, this strongly suggests that environmental factors are of major importance.

13-fold in Japanese in Hawaii and approaches that found in Caucasians. In contrast, cancers of the oesophagus and stomach were diagnosed significantly more often in mainland Japanese than in Hawaiians. These data, and others from around the world (Fig. 1.4), strongly suggest that environmental factors play a primary role in the causation of many types of cancer.

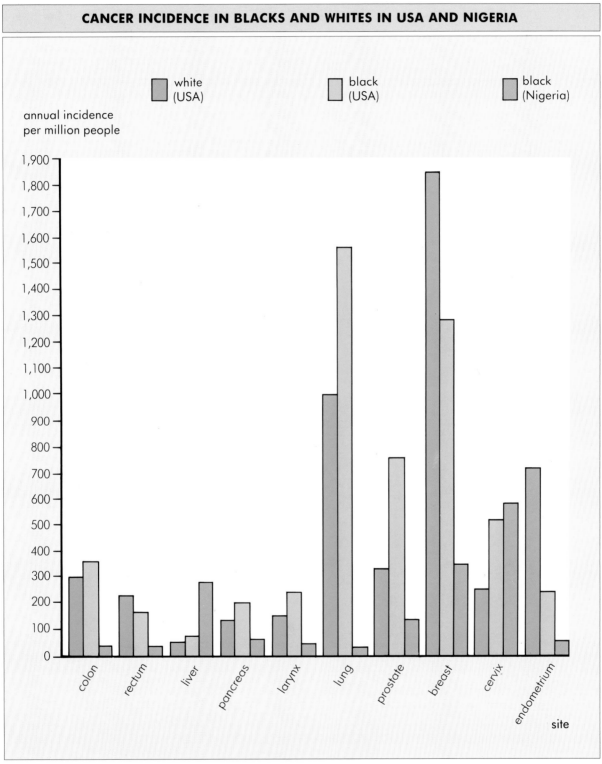

CANCER INCIDENCE IN BLACKS AND WHITES IN USA AND NIGERIA

Fig. 1.4 Incidence of various common cancers in Nigerian blacks compared with blacks and whites in the USA. In general, blacks in the USA show a closer relationship to American Caucasians than to Nigerian blacks. These data are not so 'clean' as those for Japanese immigrants (Fig. 1.3), since the black slaves transported to North America were from various racial groups and intermarriage has occurred. However, the data are consistent with an environmental origin.

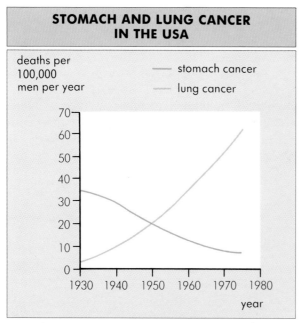

This has been extensively studied. Major variations of incidence with time are most likely to be environmental, since genetic changes in a population could not occur so quickly. Accuracy of data collection over long periods is a potential problem but useful data is available from a number of countries. Stomach and lung cancer provide the best examples of a change in the incidence of individual types of malignant tumour. While there has been a dramatic increase in the incidence of lung cancer in the USA this century, there has been a steady decline in the incidence of carcinoma of the stomach (Fig. 1.5). These changes are not confined to North America; similar data have been reported in many industrial countries (Fig. 1.6).

Another striking example of change in incidence with time is the increasing frequency of testicular cancer. This has been particularly well studied in Denmark where there has been a threefold increase in incidence between 1940 and 1980. At the same time mortality has decreased because of marked improvements in treatment (Fig. 1.7).

Fig. 1.5 Changes in the incidence of stomach and lung cancers in the USA this century. There has been a dramatic increase in the incidence of lung cancer and a gradual decrease in the number of cases of stomach cancer.

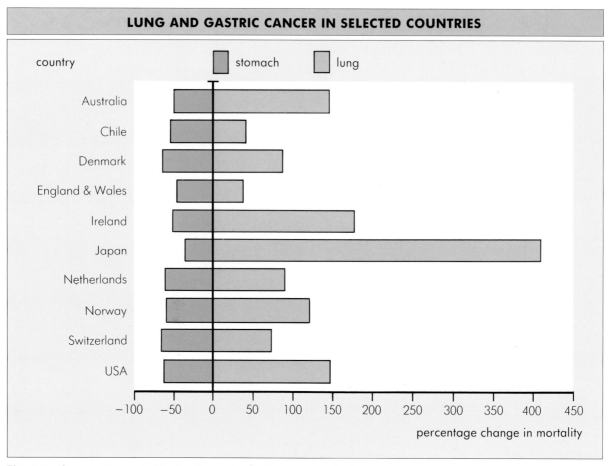

Fig. 1.6 Changes in mortality for stomach and lung cancer between 1950 and 1975 in selected countries. There has been a consistent increase in lung cancer and decrease in stomach cancer in all of these countries. This suggests that environmental factors are of major importance. Note that, for these cancers, mortality is similar to incidence, since 90% of patients who develop such tumours die of their cancer.

TESTICULAR CANCER IN DENMARK

age-standardized
incidence per 100,000

— incidence
— mortality

(graph with y-axis 0–8, x-axis years 1943–47, 1948–52, 1953–57, 1958–62, 1963–67, 1968–72, 1973–77, 1978–82; year)

Fig. 1.7 Incidence and mortality rates of testicular cancer in Denmark between 1943 and 1982. There has been a steady increase in incidence, while mortality rates have fallen as a result of major improvements in therapy.

Identifying Environmental Causes

Basic epidemiological data overwhelmingly suggest that environmental factors are important and much effort has been expended in trying to pin these factors down. The pioneering work of Percival Pott, who in 1775 identified organic products in soot as causative agents in cancer of the scrotum, led to the development of the study of cancers caused by exposure to carcinogens in the workplace (Fig. 1.8). Although this work has been very important, only a minority of cancers appear to be caused by occupational exposure (Fig. 1.9).

Non-workplace environmental factors have, in fact, proved to be the more important. Cigarette smoking is an extremely important cause of cancers of the respiratory and upper digestive systems. The onset of lung cancer can be dated back to the introduction of cigarettes mild enough to be inhaled, at the end of the last century. At the turn of the century a medical student would be lucky if he saw a single case of lung cancer during his training – indeed there were even arguments as to whether carcinoma of the lung should be included in a classification of

ESTABLISHED CARCINOGENIC AGENTS WHICH ARE AN OCCUPATIONAL HAZARD

Agent	Site of cancer
Aromatic amines	Bladder
Arsenic	Skin, lung
Asbestos	Lung, pleura, peritoneum
Benzene	Bone marrow
Bis (chloromethyl) ether	Lung
Cadmium	Prostate
Chromium	Lung
Ionizing irradiation	Bone marrow and all other sites
Isopropyl alcohol manufacture	Nasal sinuses
Leather goods manufacture	Nasal sinuses
Mustard gas	Larynx, lung
Nickel	Nasal sinuses, lung
Polycyclic hydrocarbons	Skin, lung
UV light	Skin, lip
Vinyl chloride	Liver
Wood dust	Nasal sinuses

Fig. 1.8 Occupational hazards. This table shows those carcinogenic chemicals which are known to be occupational hazards and the type of cancer with which they are associated.

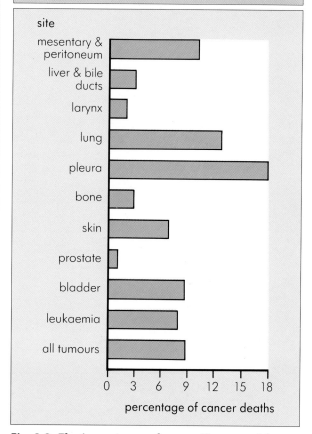

CANCERS BY OCCUPATIONAL EXPOSURE

site
mesentary & peritoneum
liver & bile ducts
larynx
lung
pleura
bone
skin
prostate
bladder
leukaemia
all tumours

0 3 6 9 12 15 18

percentage of cancer deaths

Fig. 1.9 The importance of occupation as a risk factor at various sites on the body. Overall, it has been estimated that occupation plays an important role in causing about 10% of all tumours.

diseases of the respiratory system (Fig. 1.10). The increases in smoking that occurred with both World Wars (Fig. 1.11) were a stimulus to further rises in lung cancer incidence, after a latent interval of about 20 years. A series of epidemiological studies since the Second World War have consistently shown that smokers have an increased risk of developing lung cancer (Fig. 1.12). This risk is directly related to

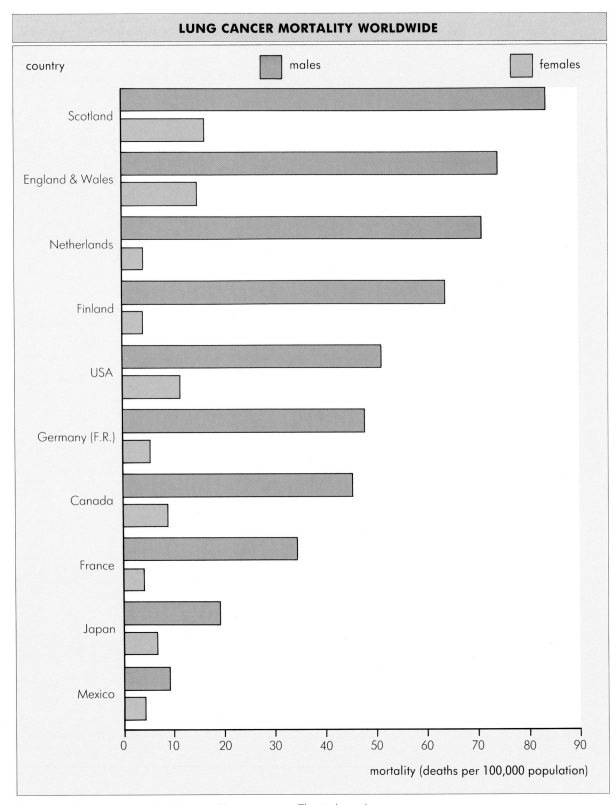

Fig. 1.10 The increasing incidence of lung cancer. 'This is the only case of lung cancer which I have ever met with; so that I presume that the disease rarely attacks this organ in Scotland' (John Hughes Bennet, Edinburgh, 1849). This quote contrasts grimly with current data, which show Scotland to have the highest lung cancer mortality rate in the world.

TOBACCO CONSUMPTION AND LUNG CANCER

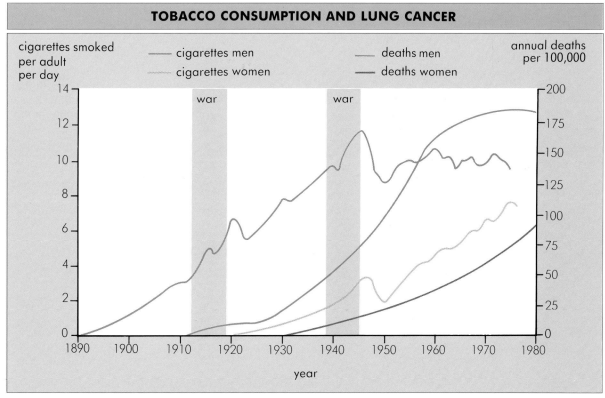

Fig. 1.11 Tobacco consumption and lung cancer mortality 1890–1980.
The two World Wars each mark large increases in tobacco consumption.
The increase in lung cancer mortality has followed the increase in
consumption with a lag of about twenty years.

THE INCREASED RISKS RUN BY SMOKERS

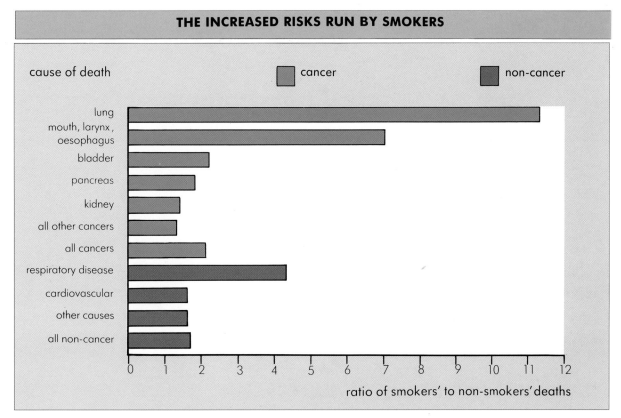

Fig. 1.12 Causes of death in smokers and in non-smokers. This shows
the ratio of smokers' to non-smokers' deaths in various disease categories.

the number of cigarettes smoked per day, the way the cigarette is smoked, its tar content and use of filter tips. More importantly, the risk reduces when smokers stop (Fig. 1.13).

Alcohol consumption is clearly related to cancers of the upper airways and digestive tracts. This appears to be interlinked to tobacco use; at any given level of tobacco intake, the risk of oesophageal cancer increases with increasing alcohol intake. Recently it has also been claimed that breast cancer risk increases with increasing use of alcohol.

Diet is likely to play a major part in the causation of a wide variety of cancers, though current data are undoubtedly incomplete. Some specific links have been found – aflatoxin for instance, a fungal contaminant of food in some tropical countries, is implicated in the development of liver cancer. Similarly, consumption of Bracken ferns in Japan increases the risk of oesophageal cancer. A number of cancers (breast, endometrium, gall bladder, ovary) are more common in obese individuals; a direct link with fat consumption, although suspected (Fig. 1.14), has not been fully substantiated. The link between obesity and cancer is likely to be an altered sex hormone metabolism. This is probably particularly true for endometrial cancer.

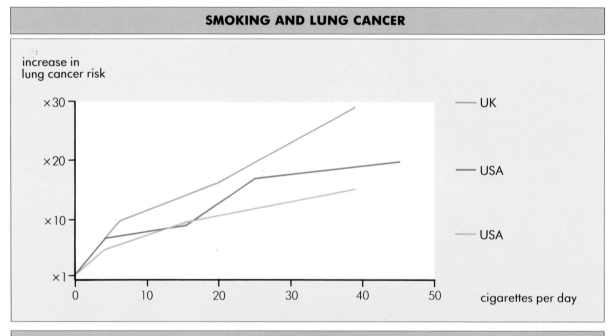

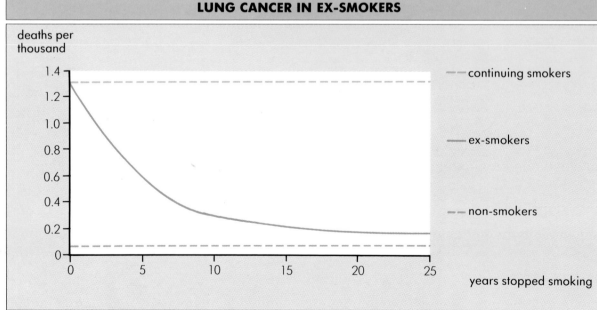

Fig. 1.13 Cigarettes and lung cancer. (Top) These three prospective studies, which looked at the relationship between the number of cigarettes smoked and the risk of death from lung cancer, showed that those smoking 40 cigarettes a day increase the risk of lung cancer 20-fold. (Bottom) Lung cancer mortality declines steadily over the years among ex-smokers.

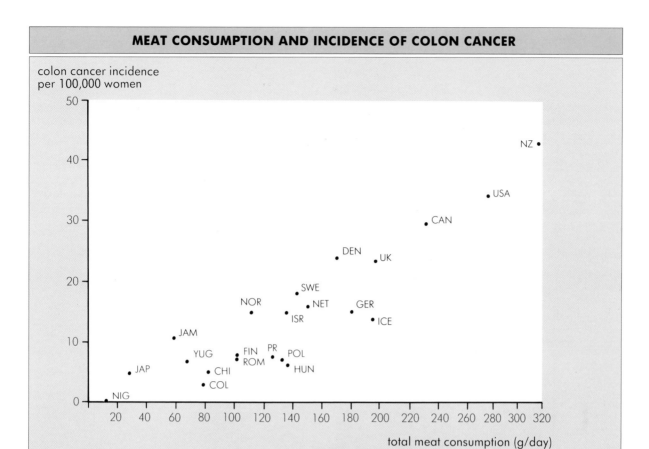

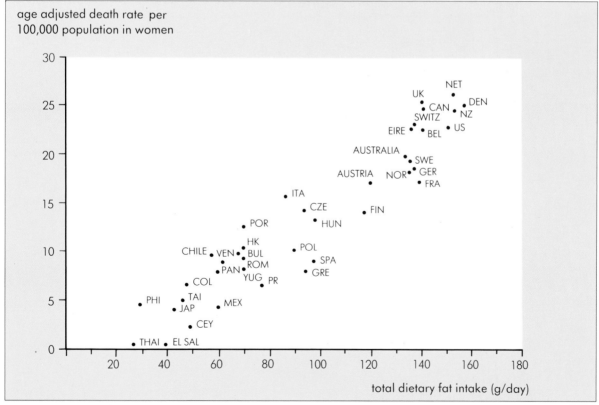

Fig. 1.14 The relationship between diet and cancer. The results of several studies suggest that diet does play some part in the causation of a number of cancers. (Top) The relationship between the incidence of cancer of the colon and meat consumption in 23 countries. [Modified from Armstrong & Doll (1975) *Int J Cancer*, **15**, 617–631.] (Bottom) Breast cancer mortality and fat consumption in 44 countries. [Modified from Carrol (1975) *Cancer Res*, **35**, 3574–3583.]

Cancer of the large bowel has been linked to low-roughage diets, because the resulting lengthy bowel-transit time allows potentially carcinogenic substances to remain in contact with the mucosa for long periods. This apparent correlation probably conceals a more complicated mechanism and other dietary factors may be implicated. Diets high in carcinogens, such as nitrosamines, and low in certain vitamins, such as vitamin C, have been connected with an increased risk of developing certain cancers. The use of chemicals in agriculture and as food additives has attracted much interest, though the risks are as yet unquantified. Some of these chemicals may actually reduce the risk by preventing deterioration of food which may produce natural carcinogenic chemicals.

Radiation undoubtedly can cause cancer (Fig. 1.15) though the risks in a general population appear

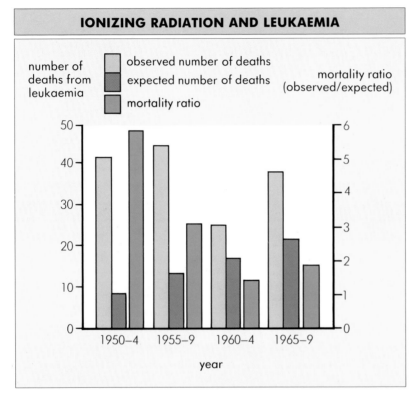

Fig. 1.15 Exposure to ionizing radiation and subsequent development of malignancy. In this study leukaemia rates in exposed populations (Hiroshima and Nagasaki survivors) were compared with rates in unexposed populations. Most excess deaths occurred within the first ten years. The excess has persisted for more than 20 years. [Modified from Jablan & Kato (1972) *Rad Res*, **50**, 649–609.]

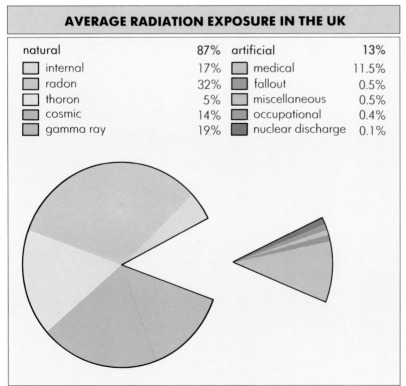

Fig. 1.16 Average radiation exposure for inhabitants of the UK. The overall effective dose from radiation (natural and artificial) is, on average, about 2mSv. Natural radiation contributes nearly 90% of this figure. [Modified from National Radiological Protection Board (1986) *Living with Radiation*. London: HMSO.]

to be relatively small. Most exposure to irradiation is 'natural'. Medical exposure far exceeds that from the nuclear industry (Fig. 1.16).

The use of powerful chemicals in medical products is unlikely to contribute greatly to the risk of developing cancer, although anticancer drugs (especially alkylating agents) are well known to induce cancer; potentially more important are the possible risks of widely used drugs such as oral contraceptives. There is currently much debate surrounding the risks associated with the use of these sex steroid hormones.

Infection is likely to play a relatively important role in the causation of cancer, though this remains to be defined. One thing that is clear, however, is that hepatitis B infection results in an increased risk of liver cancer, one of the commonest tumours in third world countries (Fig. 1.17). Another cancer that may be caused by a virus is Burkitt's lymphoma, which has been closely linked to the Epstein–Barr virus. It is wholly confined to tropical areas, though sporadic cases do occur in temperate areas (Fig. 1.18).

INCIDENCE OF HEPATOCELLULAR CARCINOMA WORLDWIDE

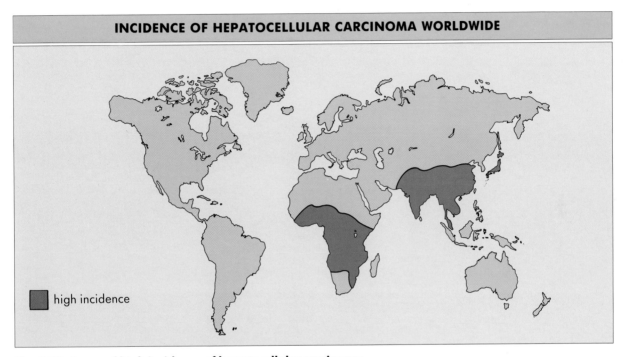

high incidence

Fig. 1.17 Areas of high incidence of hepatocellular carcinoma worldwide. Sub-Saharan Africa and Southeast Asia are areas where hepatitis is endemic.

INCIDENCE OF BURKITT'S LYMPHOMA WORLDWIDE

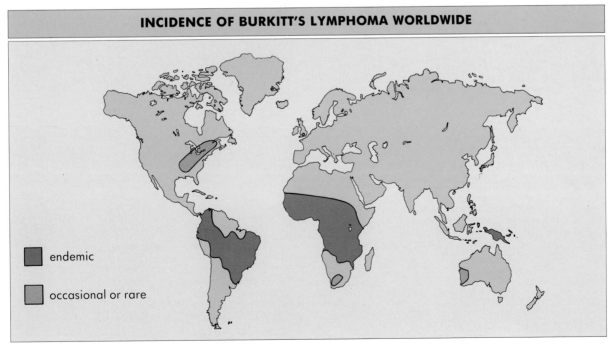

endemic

occasional or rare

Fig. 1.18 Worldwide incidence of Burkitt's lymphoma.

Doll and Peto have estimated the importance of some of the main risk factors in the causation of cancer in the USA (Fig. 1.19). Some of these are clearly amenable to change; others may become so as we learn more about them. Some cancers may be related to a number of factors working together. Breast cancer, for instance, appears to be related to hormonal changes brought about by altered nutrition, obesity, alcohol consumption and exposure to pharmacological doses of hormones. As might be expected from these data, it is a tumour of the Western world.

Conclusions

Study of the causes of cancer is important since it is likely that avoidable or manipulable factors may be found. The reduction in cigarette smoking and consequent reduction in lung cancer and respiratory and cardiovascular disease is a prime example though cigarettes remain a major cause of illness, to which the Third World is now increasingly being exposed. Any risks to life, however, have to be put into the context of those risks that we are all willing to accept every day (Fig. 1.20).

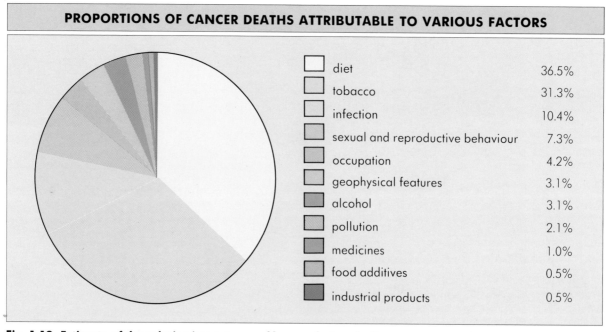

PROPORTIONS OF CANCER DEATHS ATTRIBUTABLE TO VARIOUS FACTORS

Factor	Percentage
diet	36.5%
tobacco	31.3%
infection	10.4%
sexual and reproductive behaviour	7.3%
occupation	4.2%
geophysical features	3.1%
alcohol	3.1%
pollution	2.1%
medicines	1.0%
food additives	0.5%
industrial products	0.5%

Fig. 1.19 Estimate of the relative importance of known factors in the development of cancer in the USA.

PROBABILITY OF DEATH FROM VARIOUS CAUSES

Cause	Probability per individual per year
Smoking (10 cigarettes a day)	one in 200
All natural causes, age 40	one in 850
Influenza	one in 5,000
Road accident	one in 8,000
Leukaemia	one in 12,500
Football accident	one in 25,000
Accident at home	one in 26,000
Accident at work	one in 43,500
Radiation (working in radiation industry)	one in 57,000
Homicide	one in 100,000
Railway accident	one in 500,000
Hit by lightning	one in 10,000,000

Fig. 1.20 The risks an individual runs in any one year.

Clinical Behaviour

2

Clinical Behaviour

Cancers are characterized by uncontrolled cell division of a malignant clone, generally from a single primary site. In haematological malignancies such as leukaemia, multiple myeloma and many non-Hodgkin lymphomas however, the malignant change clearly arises more widely, either from bone marrow or from the lymphatic system (see chapter 13). With some exceptions, most cancers do appear to be clonal in origin (Fig. 2.1).

Metastatic spread with wide dissemination is a common (but not invariable) feature of many cancers. Some tumours very rarely metastasize beyond the primary site, with the critical implication that local tumour control, whether by surgery, radiotherapy or a combination of the two, is likely to lead to cure. An excellent example would be the collection of tumours known as gliomas, which are the commonest form of brain tumour. Gliomas only recur locally, having very low potential for metastatic spread even when high-grade and appearing histologically to be aggressive. These tumours are, however, rarely cured and it is failure of control of the primary tumour that has proved to be the greatest stumbling block.

Other common cancers, notably squamous carcinomas of the head and neck, have a relatively low rate of blood-borne metastasis, but a marked propensity to local lymphatic involvement. Control of the primary site with adequate treatment of nodal disease is generally curative; in advanced cancers of the head and neck a cure rate of some 30% is now possible (see chapter 6). Even where a tumour has a marked predisposition for blood-borne metastasis, as does squamous carcinoma of the bronchus, the primary tumour may initially grow slowly over many months, causing few if any symptoms at the primary site, and without evident metastasis (Fig. 2.2).

Some types of cancer are associated with very rapid and widespread haematogenous dissemination. A tumour such as small-cell lung cancer is hardly ever curable by local methods such as surgery; on simple staging tests, two-thirds of all cases are found to have widespread metastases at the initial diagnosis. Even where the tumour is apparently localized and curable with surgery, nearly all patients develop recurrent disease at distant sites after excision, suggesting that metastases were initially present in nearly 100% of cases. Since these tumours appear to evolve very rapidly, the presumption must be that metastatic spread begins early. The same is clearly true in most patients with breast cancer,

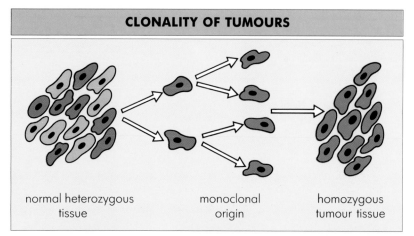

CLONALITY OF TUMOURS

normal heterozygous tissue   monoclonal origin   homozygous tumour tissue

Fig. 2.1 Clonality of tumours. X-linked enzymes have been used to study this feature of tumours. One such study looked at the two isoenzymes of glucose-6-phosphate dehydrogenase in heterozygous black females. Although normal tissue produced both isoenzymes, tumour tissue was found to express only one or the other. This observation is consistent with the hypothesis that the tumour tissue arose from a single cell.

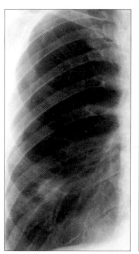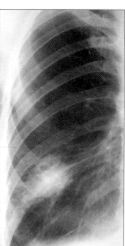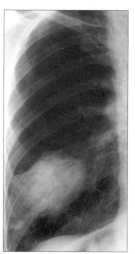

Fig. 2.2 Squamous carcinoma of the bronchus. These three X-rays of the lower lobe cover a period of eighteen months, during which the patient remained asymptomatic and received no treatment.

which is a particularly fascinating tumour due to the frequent occurrence of late relapse. This may be many years after the initial diagnosis and surgery, implying that the metastatic cells, not recognised at the initial diagnosis, have the potential to remain dormant for decades. Unless the recurrence of the cancer is entirely random, it is presumably stimulated by a hitherto unrecognized event. It has been suggested that psychological stress factors could trigger the recurrence. Much current research is being carried out in this area and recent evidence seems to give some support to the hypothesis. Other late-relapsing tumours include malignant melanoma and renal adenocarcinoma, both of which can present after a decade of apparent cure with wide dissemination to liver, lung, brain and other sites (Fig. 2.3).

At the other end of the scale, testicular teratomas are tumours of very high malignant potential but surprisingly predictable behaviour. It is very unusual for such tumours to metastasize widely without also involving abdominal lymph nodes (Fig. 2.4). It is clear that the probability of metastatic involvement can be predicted by considering a number of primary features of the tumour, such as the initial histological appearance, the height of marker levels such as AFP and the presence of tumour cells in the blood vessels surrounding the spermatic cord (on resection, the latter is generally removed together with the diseased testis).

Tumour staging using imaging and other techniques is essential for choosing optimum therapy, avoiding unnecessary postoperative treatment and accurately identifying patients requiring systemic

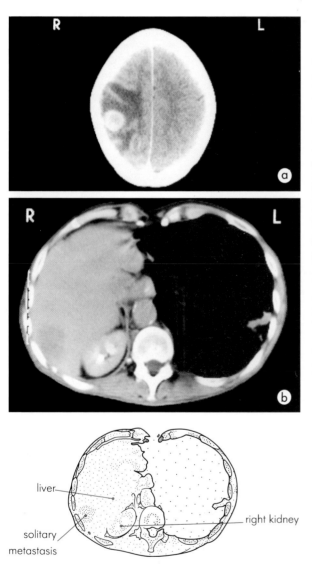

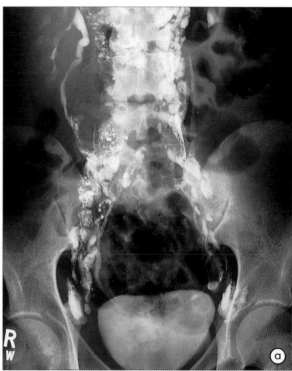

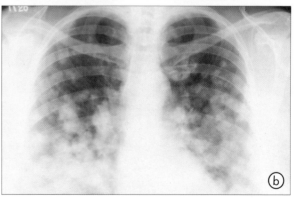

Fig. 2.3 Late systemic relapse. (a) Single cortical metastasis from breast cancer. Mastectomy was performed 5 years previously. Neurosurgical removal of the cerebral deposit was successful. (b) Liver metastasis in a melanoma patient, appearing 7 years after the primary was excised.

Fig. 2.4 Massive abdominal lymphadenopathy from testicular teratoma. (a) This IVU lymphogram clearly shows the right ureter laterally deviated by the glandular mass. (b) Chest X-ray confirming multiple pulmonary metastases in the same patient.

therapy. Accurate identification of disease sites is also important if the response of the tumour to therapy is to be adequately monitored.

The search for prognostic indicators in human cancer has become an important part of current research; the advent of intensive treatments, particularly chemotherapy, has heightened the need for careful selection of patients to undergo these potentially curative but highly unpleasant treatments. For most tumours the important prognostic factors include the histological grade, degree of spread (tumour stage), size of the primary tumour, operability and, for some tumours, specific histological features (such as the tumour's sub-type). In some types of cancer, for instance small-cell lung cancer, simple biochemical parameters such as the initial serum sodium and alkaline phosphatase levels give surprisingly helpful prognostic information. In multiple myeloma the presenting haemoglobin, serum creatinine, degree of symptomatic bone involvement and serum calcium allow for a simple system of tumour grading. Recently the $ß_2$-microglobulin level has also been used to distinguish a poor prognosis (1–2 years survival) from much more favourable cases, where survival may be prolonged to a decade or more.

Routes of Spread

The main routes of spread in human tumours are by direct local extension (Fig. 2.5), lymphatic involvement (Fig. 2.6) and haematogenous metastases. Some brain tumours seed only into the cerebrospinal fluid (CSF), so that an attempt has to be made to treat not only the primary site (often medulloblastoma and ependymoma) but also to give prophylactic treatment to the whole of the central nervous system (Fig. 2.7). Extensive spread within the abdominal cavity (trans-coelomic spread) is particularly characteristic of ovarian cancer. Although even in its most advanced forms it often spreads no further than this, it may produce kilograms of metastatic disease, almost filling the cavity before finally exhausting the patient (Fig. 2.8).

Local extension is particularly common in squamous cancers of the head and neck where, for example, a tumour primarily situated in the mouth or supraglottic larynx may reach large proportions if neglected (see Fig. 6.29). The same is true for basal cell skin cancers which may also reach a large size, usually without any evidence of dissemination to lymph nodes or more distant organs. Many of the sarcomas, whether of bony origin or from soft tissues such as

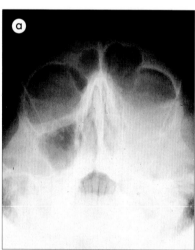
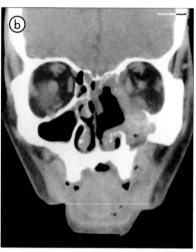
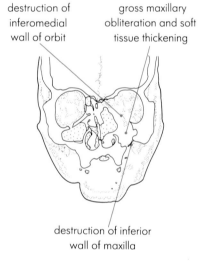

destruction of inferomedial wall of orbit

gross maxillary obliteration and soft tissue thickening

destruction of inferior wall of maxilla

Fig. 2.5 Direct extension of a large maxillary carcinoma. (a) The tumour has eroded local bone structures, notably the floor of the orbit. (b) The CT confirms bone destruction in the nasal cavity and ethmoid sinus.

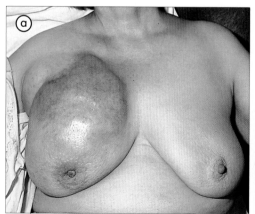
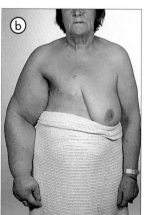

Fig. 2.6 Lymphatic involvement in breast cancer. (a) Axillary nodes clearly visible in a patient with a huge primary tumour occupying the whole right breast. (b) Late onset lymphadenopathy denoting local and axillary node infiltration.

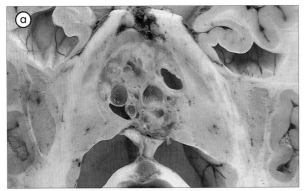

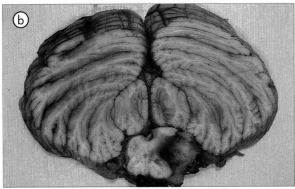

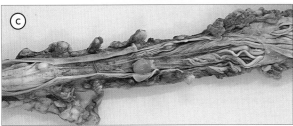

Fig. 2.7 Central nervous system involvement from a primary pineal teratoma. (a) Primary lesion at post-mortem. (b) Metastasis in the cerebello-pontine angle. (c) Spinal cord nodular seedlings.

muscle, attain a large primary size with microscopic extension well beyond the apparent clinical and radiological limits (Fig. 2.9). Again, this has important clinical implications, particularly now that internal prosthetic replacement of primary bone tumours has become established (see chapter 15).

The size and local extension of the primary tumour is rarely a barrier to surgical resection, particularly with the advent of increasingly sophisticated surgical reconstruction. However, many large primary cancers are also accompanied by local node involvement or distant spread, and this is a more critical consideration both for surgical resection and also the prospect of eventual cure. In general, local node involvement is highly predictive of outcome. In head and neck tumours, gynaecological tumours, cancer of the bladder, cancer of the breast and malignant melanoma, it is the single most important piece

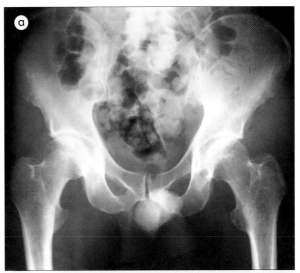

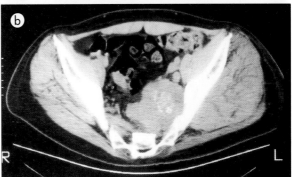

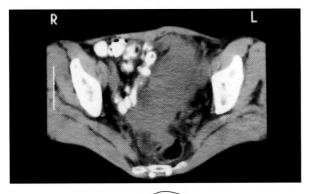

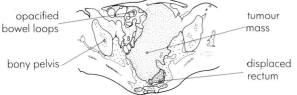

opacified bowel loops

tumour mass

bony pelvis

displaced rectum

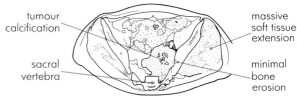

tumour calcification

massive soft tissue extension

sacral vertebra

minimal bone erosion

Fig. 2.8 CT scan in carcinoma of the ovary. This shows the tumour spreading directly throughout the pelvis and up towards the abdomen. The large tumour mass is clearly distinguishable from opacified bowel.

Fig. 2.9 Ewing's sarcoma of the pelvis (ischium and pubic region). (a) The plain X-ray is normal. This is due to the low degree of bone erosion and the inability of the X-ray to show soft tissue detail. (b) The CT scan reveals the true extent of the tumour.

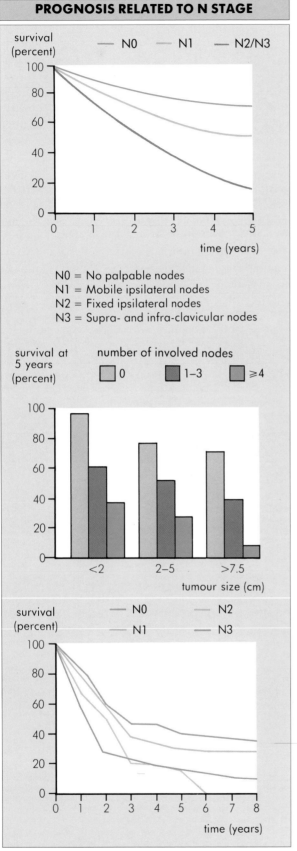

PROGNOSIS RELATED TO N STAGE

N0 = No palpable nodes
N1 = Mobile ipsilateral nodes
N2 = Fixed ipsilateral nodes
N3 = Supra- and infra-clavicular nodes

number of involved nodes: 0, 1–3, ≥4

tumour size (cm)

survival (percent) — N0, N1, N2, N3

of information one can have (Fig. 2.10). Although this partly relates to the probability of successful surgical resection, it is more likely that the presence or absence of lymph node metastases denotes a specific type of biological behaviour. In breast cancer for example, the extreme prognostic importance of axillary lymph node metastases lies not in the difficulty of resecting and controlling such regional disease, but rather in the fact that the presence of such metastases is a clear indicator that blood-borne dissemination has taken place. This is also true for malignant melanoma. In tumours which tend not to metastasize via blood-borne routes, such as squamous carcinomas of the head, neck and cervix, the importance of lymph node involvement as a prognostic feature cannot be explained in this way. Such tumours, however, do tend to be more locally aggressive and difficult to eradicate when the nodes are clearly involved. In cancer of the cervix the pattern of local recurrence has a depressing similarity from case to case, with local pelvic side-wall infiltration by uncontrolled node disease leading to a very specific group of symptoms including leg oedema, sciatic pain and hydronephrosis due to ureteric obstruction (Fig. 2.11).

Despite these features of local and nodal involvement, it is haematogenous metastasis which is the most characteristic and most feared feature of many

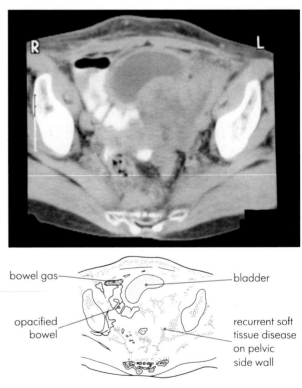

Fig. 2.11 Recurrent carcinoma of the cervix. CT scan showing massive soft tissue involvement on the left pelvic side-wall indenting the bladder postero-laterally.

Fig. 2.10 Prognosis related to N stage. (Top, middle) Prognosis for all breast cancer patients related to N stage, tumour size and number of involved nodes. (Bottom) Prognosis for head and neck cancer patients related to N stage at presentation. [Modified from SECOG Head and Neck Cancer Trial Data.]

human cancers. Involvement of distant sites is usually fatal although, as with breast cancer, the presence of metastatic disease may not become manifest for many years. In a few instances where chemotherapy is particularly effective, such as choriocarcinoma, high grade lymphoma and testicular teratoma, patients with widespread metastases can be cured.

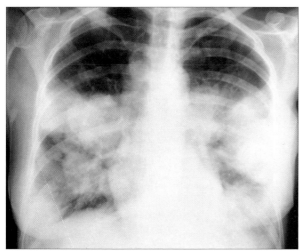

Fig. 2.12 The 'soil' phenomenon. Chest X-ray showing bilateral pulmonary metastases in a patient with breast carcinoma. The apices of the lung fields were remarkably spared. The metastases are otherwise symmetrical.

In general, however, treatment is never fully effective; widespread metastases are the commonest cause of death in most of the common cancers, such as those of the lung, breast, prostate and pancreas. Gastrointestinal cancers have the characteristic that their blood-borne spread is chiefly to the liver, with a much lower risk of distant spread to other sites. As with breast cancer and melanoma, there is a clearly increased risk of haematological spread in patients where the primary tumour is associated with local node involvement.

The reasons for widely differing patterns of blood-borne metastatic spread observed in human tumours are not well understood. Why, for example, do breast cancers metastasize so frequently to bone, liver and lungs but only rarely to the kidneys or spleen? Even within single metastatic sites, such as bone, there are clear differences in frequency of involvement. Prostatic cancer, for example, is notorious for its involvement of the lower lumbar spine and sacroiliac joints, but rarely spreads to ribs or long bones. Within the lung fields, the apices are sometimes surprisingly free of metastatic disease, even when the lungs are otherwise heavily involved (Fig. 2.12). These characteristics suggest a 'soil' phenomenon (Fig. 2.13), whereby some sites are much more receptive, presumably because of vascularity, oxygenation, local immune defences, presence

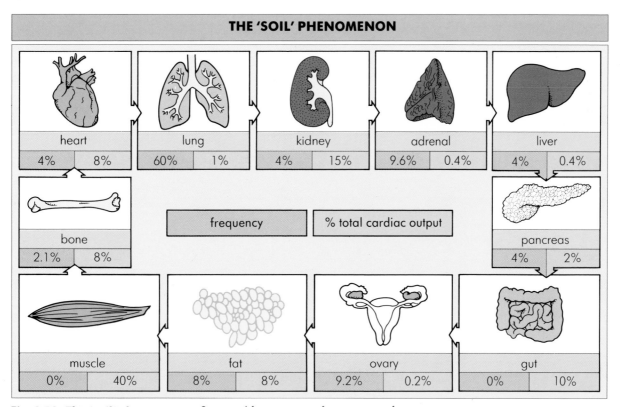

Fig. 2.13 The 'soil' phenomenon. Sites and frequencies of metastasis after intracardiac injection of breast carcinoma cells, compared with the blood distribution at those sites (expressed as a percentage of total cardiac output). It is striking that certain sites receiving a relatively small proportion of the total bloodflow have a very high incidence of metastasis. Conversely, metastasis is very uncommon in organs receiving a large proportion of cardiac output.

or absence of growth factors, or other mechanisms. Some breast cancers are widely metastatic even from a small, histologically low-grade primary, whereas others with horrendous local involvement show little if any tendency to widespread metastasis. This wide variety of clinical presentations makes accurate prognosis, particularly of survival, extremely difficult even for the specialist. The literature is full of stories of unexpected responses and miracle cures which are, in truth, mostly examples of the highly uncertain nature of the malignant process.

With such a diversity of primary sites, the signs and symptoms of cancer are equally variable (Fig. 2.14). In superficial or visible sites a discrete mass or non-healing ulcer is the commonest presenting feature and as such should always be taken seriously, particularly if it has no obvious traumatic basis. In many primary skin tumours the non-healing ulcer is painless. This may also be true of intra-oral malignant ulcers such as those of the tongue or floor of mouth, although pain is sometimes a feature, particularly where there is erosion of the underlying mandible. Rapid growth, discomfort, or bleeding within a previously pigmented part of the skin also needs to be taken seriously, particularly since the incidence of melanoma is clearly increasing.

With lung cancer, the commonest of all malignancies, patients may be aware of surprisingly few symptoms. Many are lifelong smokers, familiar with dyspnoea and cough and with frequent bouts of acute bronchitis requiring antibiotics. This may be one reason why so many lung cancers are locally advanced at presentation, with many lung cancer patients presenting in the first instance with symptoms from secondary deposits, such as bone pain or pathological fracture, or anorexia from metastases in the liver and other widespread sites. Regular screening, though occasionally detecting primary tumours, has not improved the chances of survival.

In the past some women with breast cancer similarly delayed their diagnosis, though most patients now present to their doctor promptly on discovering a mass in the breast. Although the clinical features of a breast lump often give a fair indication of the likely pathology, all lumps should be regarded as suspicious – such patients should be referred to a breast clinic or surgeon without delay. In general, younger patients with mobile firm breast lumps will prove to have benign disease, usually a fibroadenoma (see chapter 8). Middle-aged women with bilateral granularity of the breasts are usually suffering from fibroadenosis but firm, fixed, unilateral masses in middle-aged patients should be regarded with grave suspicion. Such lumps frequently prove to be carcinomas although breast cysts, almost invariably benign, may feel very similar.

It is surprising how few constitutional symptoms may be caused by a cancer. However, a patient with disseminated disease is usually unwell, with widespread discomfort, anorexia and frequently with a variety of obvious clinical signs from the metastatic lesions. Profound anorexia is particularly common with carcinomas of the oesophagus and stomach and with oropharyngeal tumours, which often make swallowing difficult. If the tumour advances with extreme rapidity as, for example, do small cell lung cancers, anorexia and lethargy can be very marked. For patients in remission of their cancer the quality of life is usually excellent, although long-term adverse effects related to treatment may result in important bodily changes (see chapter 3). Once the acute effects of treatment (such as alopecia, nausea and neuropathy) have passed, many cancer patients are able to lead perfectly normal lives.

SIGNS AND SYMPTOMS OF CANCER

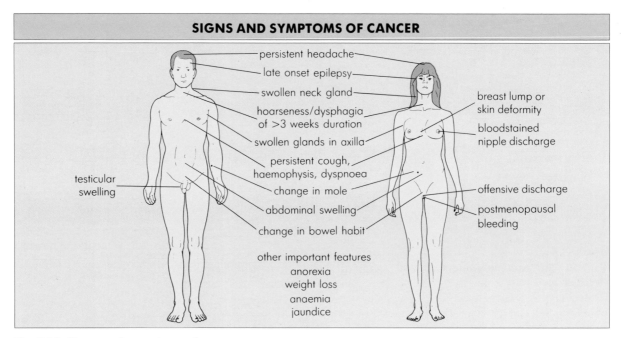

persistent headache
late onset epilepsy
swollen neck gland
hoarseness/dysphagia of >3 weeks duration
swollen glands in axilla
persistent cough, haemophysis, dyspnoea
change in mole
abdominal swelling
change in bowel habit

testicular swelling

breast lump or skin deformity
bloodstained nipple discharge
offensive discharge
postmenopausal bleeding

other important features
anorexia
weight loss
anaemia
jaundice

Fig. 2.14 Signs and symptoms of cancer.

Therapeutic Approaches

Introduction

In order to plan the management of a particular malignant tumour the clinician needs to know:
- the histological subtype and grade;
- the apparent extent of spread of the tumour;
- the natural history of the tumour type;
- the effectiveness of available treatments.

Only when this information is available can the clinician decide whether the aim of treatment is cure or palliation. Before making a final decision the patient's general health, as well as the likely toxicity of therapy, have to be taken into account together with the wishes or preferences of the patient.

All too often clinicians and patients fail to make a realistic assessment of the goals of therapy leading to potential errors in judgement (Fig. 3.1).

The main therapeutic options are:
- Surgery
- Radiotherapy
- Chemotherapy
- Hormone therapy

The importance of simple supportive care (analgesia, antiemetics, laxatives etc.) to ameliorate symptoms should not, however, be forgotten. More recently new biological therapies have been developed and some are starting to show benefit in selected tumours.

Surgery

Surgeons have a key role in cancer management – they see over 90% of patients presenting with cancer

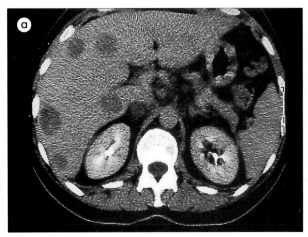 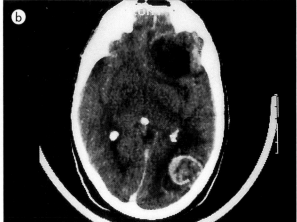

Fig. 3.1 Extensive metastatic melanoma. A 50-year old man with a history of radical excision of a malignant melanoma of the abdominal wall, presented with back pain referred to his right leg. Investigation revealed liver (a), bone and lung metastases. He then developed an intussusception caused by tumour in the bowel. He was treated with IL-2 but the disease progressed and he developed brain metastases (b). An informed decision about therapy can only be made if both the patient and the clinician acknowledge that such treatment is entirely palliative. Only if the goals of treatment are set out from the start can unnecessary toxic treatment be avoided.

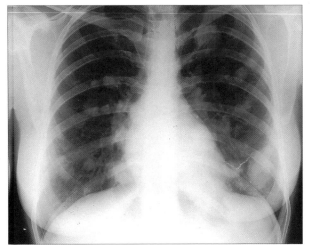 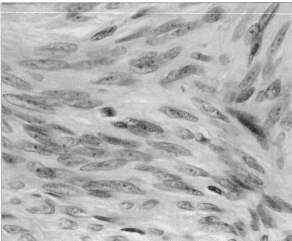

Fig. 3.2 A benign cause of multiple pulmonary masses. A 33-year old woman presented with a dry cough, but had no other evidence of disease. She had a history of hysterectomy for fibroids at age 28 years. Biopsy revealed benign leiomyomatous hamartoma, a smooth muscle tumour typically found in patients with a history of hysterectomy for fibroids at an early age. Failure to biopsy may have led to the erroneous conclusion that the patient had widely metastatic cancer.

and very often make the initial diagnosis. Making such a diagnosis relies on a good understanding of the natural history of a variety of tumours and of the usefulness of available investigative techniques. For a definitive diagnosis, however, a tissue biopsy is essential, or there is a real risk of treating a benign condition as malignant (Fig. 3.2). Because biopsy is a relatively simple procedure the operation is all too often delegated to an inexperienced member of the surgical team. This may have serious repercussions, as a small, traumatized and inadequately fixed biopsy may be difficult or even impossible to interpret.

Whenever cancer is diagnosed patients should be assessed to see if primary surgical excision is feasible and practical. In many cases there is clinical evidence of widespread metastatic disease, making this evaluation simple. In others, adequate assessment requires specific investigations, with consideration of the common patterns of spread of the cancer concerned (see Fig. 7.4). However, in some instances the natural history will suggest that surgery is inappropriate even when there is no obvious evidence of metastatic disease. Clearly current techniques are incapable of detecting small tumour burdens and many patients with micrometastases are treated by primary therapy alone. In such cases, later relapse is not surprising. This series of events is not uncommon, indeed it is the mechanism of failure of surgery in a large number of patients with a wide variety of tumours. Relapse of an apparently resectable malignancy is a risk with many solid tumours.

These data are particularly depressing as they apply only to patients with disease apparently curable by surgery. The realization that many operable patients have micrometastatic disease has led to the concept of 'adjuvant systemic therapy' (see below).

If surgery is indicated the aims of a curative operation are:

- Complete excision of the tumour with a margin of normal uninvolved tissue;
- In some instances, excision of draining lymph nodes, preferably *en-bloc*.

These principles were most clearly delineated by the American surgeon Halsted at the turn of the century. The principles underlying his operation for breast cancer were based on the hypothesis that breast cancer spreads in a predictable sequence. First, a local phase when the tumour is entirely confined to the breast. Second, a phase of regional extension when draining lymph nodes are involved in a predictable fashion. Third, a final phase when the tumour becomes widely disseminated.

It now appears that this hypothesis was incorrect, since we know from modern staging techniques that patients with small and apparently local tumours often have metastatic disease. Surgery for breast cancer was, however, largely based on Halsted's principles for most of this century. This led to increasingly extensive operations, in an attempt to improve results, until a series of randomized trials showed that conservative surgery was as effective as radical operations (see chapter 8).

Currently, the emphasis is on complete surgical excision, allowing a reduction in local recurrence rates, organ conservation and surgical reconstruction designed to improve function and cosmesis. The days of ever more radical operations to improve cure rates have passed.

Occasionally, surgery may be used to palliate symptoms or to prevent unpleasant local complications, even when the cancer is clearly incurable. Such surgery can be of real benefit to patients but the advantages and disadvantages of an operation must be weighed carefully for each individual.

An unusual form of cancer surgery involves removal of an organ at particularly high risk of

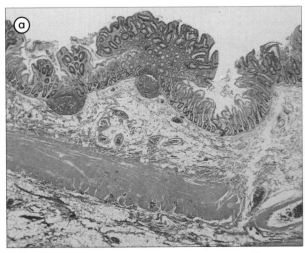
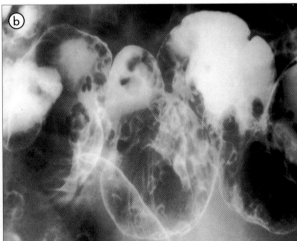

Fig. 3.3 Familial adenomatous polyposis coli (FAPC). (a) A section of colon from a patient with FAPC showing numerous polyps at different stages of development. (b) Characteristic radiographic appearance. The nature of the polyps must be confirmed histologically. Courtesy of Dr F.A. Mitros.

developing cancer. Despite the trauma of surgery and potential mutilation, such operations may be justifiable in certain well defined circumstances. Good examples of such an approach are total colectomy in sufferers of familial polyposis coli (see Fig. 3.3) and chronic ulcerative colitis (Fig. 3.4).

Radiotherapy

Wilhelm Roengten discovered X-rays in 1895. Three years later Marie and Pierre Curie isolated radium and Becquerel coined the term 'radioactivity'. Less than a year after that Villard demonstrated that gamma rays and X-rays are identical. From these early beginnings diagnostic and therapeutic radiology grew very rapidly.

At first equipment was primitive and workers in the field did not appreciate the dangers of irradiation. Unfortunately, many pioneers in the field, as well as their patients, suffered severe complications from radiation exposure and some died. However, the dangers of radiation quickly became apparent and by 1911 the first paper on the hazards of irradiation had been published.

During this century our understanding of radioactivity has advanced immeasurably, leading to improved methods of treatment for a variety of cancers. In order to understand the concept of radioactivity it is necessary to understand the electromagnetic spectrum (Fig. 3.5). The energy of an electromagnetic wave is inversely proportional to the length of the wave itself. Thus X-rays have a very high energy and extremely short wavelength – visible light falls in the middle of the spectrum. Electromagnetic waves of very short wavelengths are, by virtue of their high energy, able to ionize

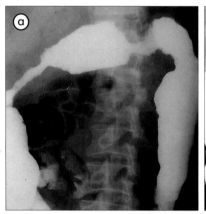
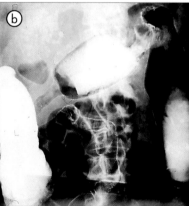

Fig. 3.4 Ulcerative colitis leading to carcinoma. (a) Barium enema showing ulcerative colitis with two strictures of the transverse colon. (b) Double contrast study of the same patient who was found to have two separate carcinomas of the large bowel.

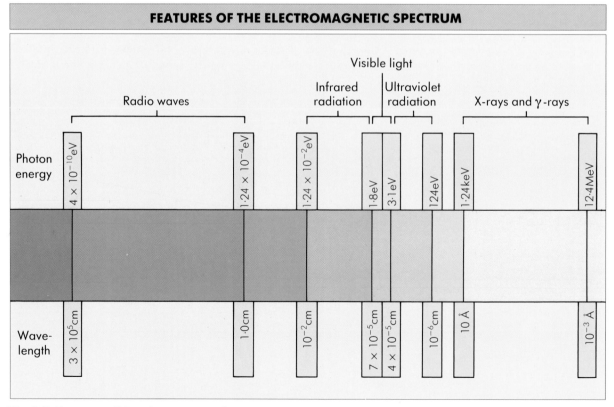

Fig. 3.5 Features of the electromagnetic spectrum.

atoms in their path by displacing an electron from its orbit around the nucleus. The ionized atom is then unstable – the free electron is usually captured by a nearby atom which in turn also becomes unstable, due to the extra negative atomic particle.

The process of interaction of ionizing radiation with biological tissues goes through several stages, the first three of which occur extremely rapidly (Fig. 3.6).

Selection of Irradiation Sources

The effects of radiation passing through living tissue vary with the type of radiation. For diagnostic imaging, waves with energies which cause short-lived and generally safe changes, and which have no long-term biological effect, are used. When the aim is therapeutic more energetic sources are used, with the intention of producing potentially lethal changes in cells within the irradiated tissues. As well as electromagnetic waves ionizing irradiations may be composed of subatomic particles (Fig. 3.7).

Many naturally occurring elements which exist in an unstable state are radioactive. Although an element is defined by the number of protons and electrons each of its atoms possesses, some atoms may exist with abnormal numbers of neutrons. These are called 'isotopes' and they are present in many substances, especially in metals. Some isotopes are particularly unstable, and as they decay to form more stable atoms, they emit electromagnetic waves.

Traditionally, radioactive emissions are discussed in terms of 'alpha' (positive), 'beta' (negative) or 'gamma' (uncharged) rays. Of these, gamma irradiation is of the greatest practical importance. For example, cobalt-60, an isotope which has been widely used therapeutically decays to a more stable

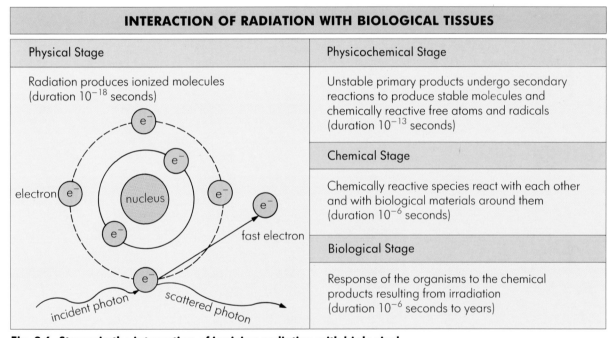

Fig. 3.6 **Stages in the interaction of ionizing radiation with biological tissues.**

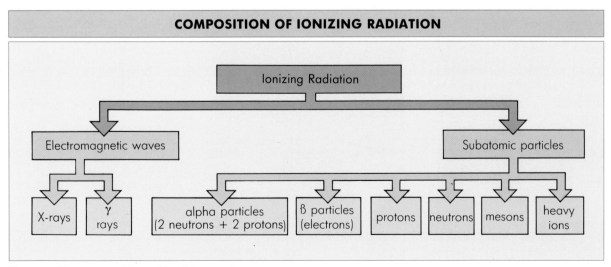

Fig. 3.7 **The composition of ionizing radiation.**

isotope, cobalt-59, by discharging a neutron together with gamma rays. Nuclear decay is exponential in nature and characteristic for any given isotope. cobalt-60 takes 5.3 years to fall to one-half its original activity and is therefore said to have a half-life of 5.3 years. The half-lives of isotopes are very varied – from a fraction of a second to thousands of years. Selection of an isotope with a suitable half-life is one element in the selection of an appropriate radioactive source.

Since the early days of radiation physics the number of radiation sources has been increased by the development of radionuclides, manufactured in nuclear reactors by bombarding appropriate materials with heavy particles. In this way, it may be possible to produce a radiation source of ideal half-life, gamma ray characteristics and intensity.

Radioactive isotopes can be used in a variety of ways some of which are outlined in Fig. 3.8.

Isotopes can also be used to deliver external beam irradiation (teletherapy). Installed in a custom-built apparatus, cobalt-60 is frequently used as a source of high-energy gamma irradiation. A radiotherapy machine is no more than a mechanism for moving the radioactive source into the correct position for treatment. By use of a variable shielding system and multibeam treatment, however, the radiation can be focussed to give therapy to a pre-determined target. The main disadvantages of teletherapy are the penumbra of radiation scatter, which affects tissues

USE OF RADIOACTIVE ISOTOPES

Isotope	Delivery	Indication
Radium-226	Intracavitary in needles	Local high doses to tumour
Iridium-192	Implanted wires	Local high dose in tumour (eg. breast, tongue)
Iodine-131	By mouth	Selective uptake by thyroid for ablation
Iodine-125	Transperineal implant	Cancer of prostate
Phosphorus-32	By IV injection	Marrow ablation
Gold-198	Intra-peritoneal colloid As gold grains	Control of ascites Intra-oral

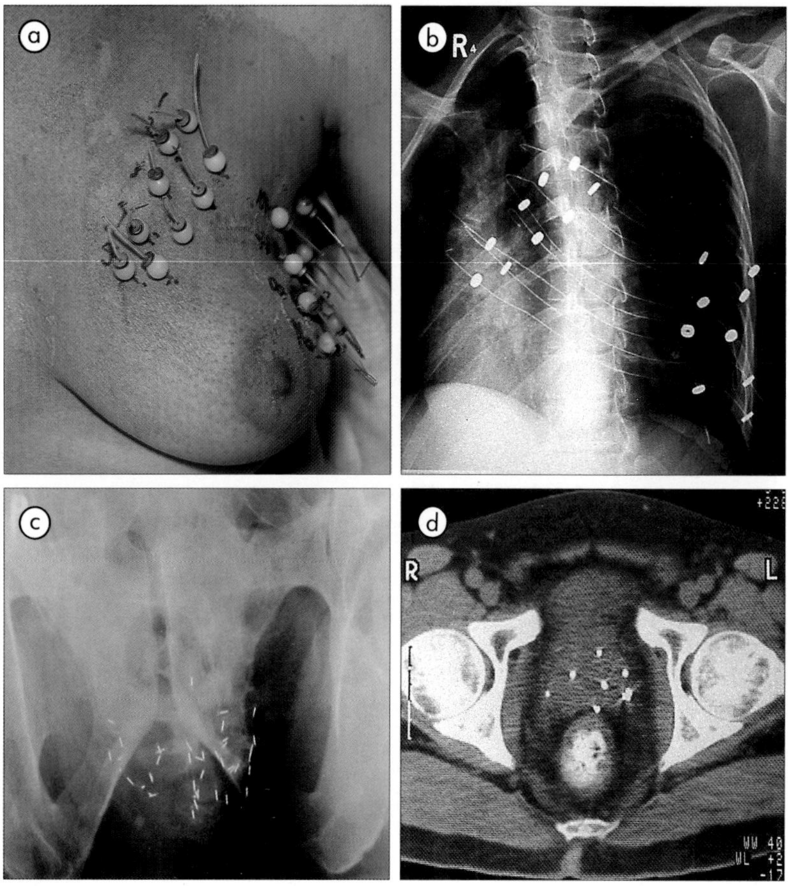

Fig. 3.8 Use of radioactive isotopes. (a) Iridium-192 implant for boosting the tumour bed after excision of breast carcinoma and postoperative external radiation. (b) X-ray confirms excellent geometry of this implant. (c) Transperineal iodine-125 implant for prostatic carcinoma. (d) CT scan shows seeds well positioned within the prostate. This technique has been facilitated by the advent of transrectal ultrasonography, allowing excellent imaging of this organ. In this patient with locally advanced disease, the alternative would have been a radical course of external beam radiotherapy or radical surgical excision.

outside the target area, and the relatively long treatment times. Advantages are its reasonable cost and the fact that the source needs to be replaced only every 3–4 years. Treatment times will of course increase as the source decays and frequent recalibration is required.

Generation of X-rays and Particles

Roentgen produced X-rays by placing a high voltage across an almost evacuated glass vacuum tube. This caused an acceleration of electrons (from residual gas in the tube) which, in the vacuum, bombarded a target at the other end of the tube. This in turn produced characteristic rays which could fog a photographic plate – so called X-rays. It soon became clear that X-rays were fundamentally the same as gamma rays. The great advantage of this method of producing X-rays is that their characteristics can be altered simply by varying the voltage input to the cathodes of the X-ray tube.

When used therapeutically, the radiotherapist must be able to deliver an effective dose of irradiation to a deeply situated tumour. To achieve this, high-energy machines and multi-field techniques are required. Electrons are streamed almost at the speed of light down a 'wave guide' to bombard a target; this results in a beam of high-intensity radiation which is capable of greater depth dose and much less scatter than cobalt-60 machines. Such megavoltage equipment makes planning easier and reduces normal tissue damage from penumbra. In addition, treatment times are shorter since the dose rate is higher. Disadvantages are a very high initial cost and lower reliability than cobalt-60 machines. The therapeutic advantages of these 'linear accelerators', however, make them ideal as treatment units for most deeply-seated tumours.

Other types of therapeutic radiation developed in the last few decades include electron beams and 'High Linear Energy Transfer' (LET) beams. Electron beams have the advantage that their depth of penetration can be easily adjusted – the electron beam has the characteristic that no energy is deposited in tissues beyond a chosen point (unlike X-ray therapy). High LET releases highly focussed beams of neutrons and charged particles (pi-mesons, protons).

The advantages of modern radiotherapeutic techniques over orthovoltage equipment such as the traditional 250kV machine are shown in Fig. 3.9.

So far, High Linear Energy Transfer radiation remains an experimental tool, trials having failed to show any conclusive advantage over megavoltage therapy. Long-term adverse side effects may be a major problem. The development of better radiotherapy equipment is not simply an academic exercise; much of the improvement in radiotherapy results in the past few decades is due to improved technical ability to deliver high energy radiation directly to the tumour with a minimum of damage to normal tissues. Good examples of the improvement in results reported by major centres are those seen in Hodgkin's disease and cervical cancer.

Biological and Clinical Effects

The biological effectiveness of irradiation is influenced by a number of factors. These include the following:

Cell-cycle position. Cells at or near mitosis are especially sensitive to irradiation, as are those in G_2. The S phase is resistant, as is G_1 to a lesser extent. Resting cells (G_0) are radioresistant – this has major implications for the radiosensitivity of malignant tissues, as in some the proportion of cells in G_0 is very high.

Oxygen effect. The radiation sensitivity of tissues increased rapidly as the oxygen concentration increases. Since tumours often have areas of poor

Fig. 3.9 Advantages of modern radiotherapeutic techniques.

ADVANTAGES OF MODERN RADIOTHERAPEUTIC TECHNIQUES
Megavoltage
Skin sparing dramatically reduces skin reactions Greatly improved depth dose to tumours Less side scatter and sharper beam
Electron Beam
Variation in electron energy controls depth of penetration Ideal for treating superficial cancers Avoids radiation of underlying normal tissues, especially useful over bone
High Energy Linear Transfer
Theoretically, a highly focussed beam releases energy as a burst at a predetermined depth (Bragg effect) Biologically more destructive (but to normal tissues too!)

vasculature and low oxygen concentration, this effect may explain failure to eradicate all tumour cells in some cancers.

When a radiation dose is delivered as two equal fractions with a delay in between, the cell kill of the combined dose is less than that of a single dose at that strength. The overall decrease in cellular sensitivity is a result of there being sufficient time for cellular repair of sublethal damage. Nonetheless, empirical observations of methods of delivering irradiation have shown that multiple small doses (fractions) given over a period of time are generally more effective than a single dose or a short course. This is due to several factors:

- Sublethal repair occurs more rapidly in normal tissue than it does in malignant tissue (Fig. 3.10);
- Protracted fractionation allows redistribution of cells throughout the cell cycle. Thus cells in resistant parts of the cell cycle (G_0) enter sensitive parts of the cycle before further treatment;
- Prolonged treatment plans may gradually reduce anoxic areas in the tumour as it shrinks, increasing sensitivity of cells in these areas.

Radiation Effects on Normal Tissues

The clinical effectiveness of radiation depends on the balance between sensitivity of the malignant tissue and the surrounding normal tissues.

The dose to which a tumour can be treated is, therefore, limited by the tolerance of surrounding normal tissues, and a knowledge of the effects on such tissues is of paramount importance. These effects can be acute or chronic.

Bone marrow: *Acute* – Temporary pancytopenia is common when radiation includes a significant proportion of bone marrow. Whole-body irradiation (up to 1000 cGy) may be used to eradicate bone marrow prior to marrow transplantation. *Chronic* –

Leukaemia is a long-term risk, not as great at therapeutic doses but augmented by alkylating agents.

The gonads. *Chronic* – The testes, are extremely sensitive to irradiation. Hormonal changes in men are, however, uncommon at therapeutic doses. Radiation to the ovaries (100–1500 cGy) may be used to induce an artificial menopause in women. Teratogenicity and mutagenesis are risks of irradiation.

The skin: *Acute* – When external-beam irradiation is used the skin is always exposed and in the past the skin reaction was used as a guide to dose. Modern high-energy equipment gives much less severe reactions. *Chronic* – Many of the long-term effects of irradiation are due to acute necrosis of skin and subcutaneous tissues, leading to fibrosis and change in blood vessels. Skin appendages such as hair follicles and sweat glands will also be damaged. Re-irradiation should generally be avoided.

The eye: *Chronic* – The lens is sensitive to irradiation and should be shielded wherever possible. Radiation-induced cataracts can be excised if they do develop, but perhaps more important is the risk of keratoconjunctivitis sicca caused by lack of tear formation, a consequence of irradiating the lacrymal gland.

Nervous tissue: *Acute* – Radiation to the brain can cause oedema which may be enough to cause a rise in intracranial pressure. Since the patient with a brain tumour has often presented with pressure symptoms these may be temporarily worsened by radiation. Dexamethasone should be used prophylactically. *Chronic* – Vascular damage and demyelination are common and frank necrosis may occur at high doses. The brain stem, hypothalmus and cervical spine are the most sensitive areas.

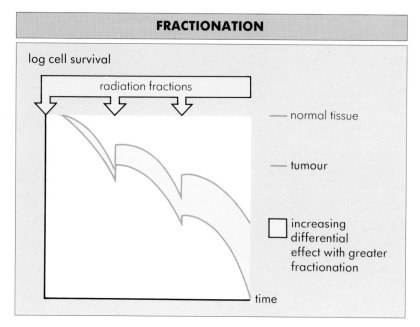

FRACTIONATION

log cell survival

radiation fractions

— normal tissue

— tumour

increasing differential effect with greater fractionation

time

Fig. 3.10 Fractionation. Administering repeated doses of radiation increases the differential cytotoxic effect on normal and malignant tissue.

The bowel: *Acute* – Diarrhoea, colicky pains and tenesmus may occur. Nausea and vomiting are common. Radiation-induced fibrosis and necrosis may result in diarrhoea, proctitis, bleeding, stricture and fistula formation.

Kidney: *Acute* – Renal blood flow and glomerular filtration rate are reduced by irradiation and are slow to recover. Acute radiation nephritis (hypertension, uraemia and proteinuria) may occasionally occur at relatively low doses. *Chronic* – Proteinuria and renal failure may persist.

Liver: Acute and chronic hepatitis may ensue if doses in excess of 2500 cGy are used.

Lung: Acute and chronic pneumonitis occur at relatively low doses. Long term fibrosis may develop.

The dose at which these short- and long-term effects occur varies from tissue to tissue. Therapeutic doses are usually based on the selection of a dose which gives a less than 5% risk of major toxicity.

▬ Chemotherapy

Development of drugs to treat cancer has been a long sought after goal of medicine. However, it was not until the empirical discovery of the effects of nitrogen mustard, at the end of the Second World War, that effective anticancer drugs were developed. Following the bombing of Brindisi harbour by the Germans, a large amount of nitrogen mustard gas was released from an armaments ship. Astute medical officers caring for the injured noticed that myelosuppression was common in those exposed to the nitrogen mustard – subsequently the cytotoxic properties of the drug were shown.

During the First World War cases of lymphopenia following exposure to sulphur mustard had been reported but not followed up. In 1943, however, a patient with Hodgkin's disease had a dramatic response to nitrogen mustard and the era of cytotoxic therapy began.

Since then many thousands of compounds have been screened for anticancer effects and an increasing number of useful new drugs have been developed. One disappointing aspect of new drug development, however, has been an inability to design drugs whose mode of action and effectiveness can be predicted. Indeed, nearly all the currently used compounds were found in empirical screening programmes or are analogues of such compounds.

Although there have been real advances in our understanding of chemotherapy we are far from developing an ideal drug – one which is cytotoxic only to cancer cells. Current drugs lack this specificity, though their effect on normal tissues varies widely.

The Cell Cycle

Anticancer drugs can be classified according to whether they mainly effect cells actively in cycle (cycle specific) or cells not actively in cycle (cycle non-specific); and, if cycle specific, whether activity is confined to one or more phases (phase specific). The sensitivity of tumour cells to anticancer drugs is increased if a large proportion of the cells are proceeding through the cell cycle at the time of exposure to the drug. This is because the mechanism of action of most of these drugs involves processes concerned with cells preparing to divide (DNA synthesis), resting before division or undergoing division.

Cell Kinetics

Cancers are heterogenous collections of cells whose behaviour varies widely. They may be described as belonging to one of three compartments (Fig. 3.11). The proportion of cells in each compartment varies

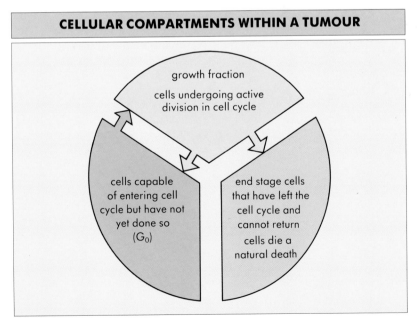

CELLULAR COMPARTMENTS WITHIN A TUMOUR

Fig. 3.11 Cellular compartments within a tumour.

from tumour to tumour, with time and by the type of cancer. The proportion of cells in cell cycle is referred to as the 'growth fraction'. This fraction is the main mechanism for increase in cellular numbers. Though a tumour may grow more quickly by shortening the cell cycle time or by decreasing cell death, a change in the proportion of cells in cycle will be much more significant.

Many tumours, however, are relatively slow growing with low growth fraction; a large proportion of the cells are destined to die naturally. Some haematological malignancies are an exception to this, but even in these tumours cell doubling times are longer than for some normal cells – clearly the potential effectiveness of current chemotherapy does not depend on a kinetic advantage consequent on the rapid growth of cancerous tissues.

Tumour Burden

The interval between malignant transformation of a single cell and the detection of a clinically apparent tumour may be months or years depending on the growth rate of the tumour. Most cancers are a minimum of one gram in weight at the time of diagnosis (1cm diameter mass). As can be seen from Fig. 3.12, the tumour by this time will have existed for three quarters of its life span (expressed as the number of doublings). When it is remembered that a 1cm tumour mass contains one thousand million (10^9) cells, it is not surprising that metastatic spread may have occurred before diagnosis. The doubling time of a cancer is the length of time it takes to double its cell numbers – this is only the same as the cell cycle time if the growth fraction is 100%. Some normal tissues (bone marrow and gastrointestinal tract

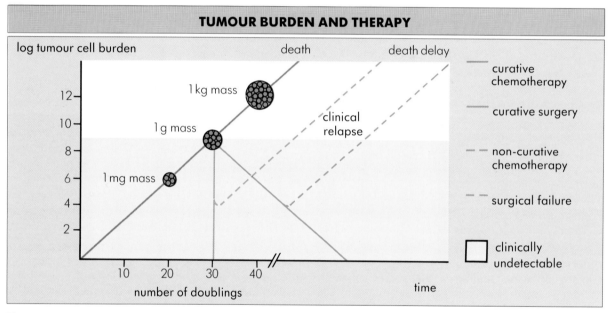

Fig. 3.12 Tumour burden and its relationship to therapy. Tumour burdens of less than 1 gram are generally undetectable. Surgery and chemotherapy will reduce the tumour burden to below this level but cure depends on complete eradication of the cancer. If undetectable residual tumour is left, the cancer will recur.

RELATIONSHIP BETWEEN DOUBLING TIME AND CURE

Cancer	Doubling time (days)	Curability
Burkitt's lymphoma	1.0	Single agent/ combination
Choriocarcinoma	1.5	Single agent/ combination
Acute lymphoblastic lymphoma	3–4	Combination
Hodgkin's disease	3–4	Combination
Testicular teratoma	5–6	Combination
Breast cancer	60	None
Colon cancer	80	None
Adenocarcinoma lung	150	None

Fig. 3.13 Relationship between doubling time and cure in various metastatic cancers. If tumour dissemination is present, cure or long-term remission is possible only with tumours of short doubling time.

mucosa) have a large growth fraction and short cell cycle times and consequently a short doubling time. These tissues are particularly sensitive to cycle and phase specific cytotoxic drugs. Tumours show a wide range in their doubling times though there is a direct relationship between curability and short doubling times (Fig. 3.13).

As has been suggested, most anticancer drugs have an action which directly or indirectly affects cells that are actively dividing. The sites of action of the major anticancer drugs are shown in Fig. 3.14. A detailed discussion of this topic is, however, beyond the scope of this book.

Choice of Drugs

Empirical observation has led to the use of combinations of drugs rather than single agents even when tumours are particularly chemosensitive. Presumably the use of two or more drugs overcomes the development or emergence of a clone of cells resistant to one of the drugs. Combinations are chosen according to the following rules:

- Only use drugs that are active as a single agent;
- Select drugs with a different mode of action;
- Select drugs whose principal toxicities differ;
- Select drugs where there is evidence of synergism.

Since they have a major effect on rapidly growing normal tissues, most combinations of drugs are given intermittently to allow normal tissues to recover between cycles. If the chemotherapy is to be successful, the malignant tissues must either be more sensitive than the normal tissues, or recover from the effects more slowly. The theoretical effects of cyclical chemotherapy are shown in Fig. 3.15 overleaf.

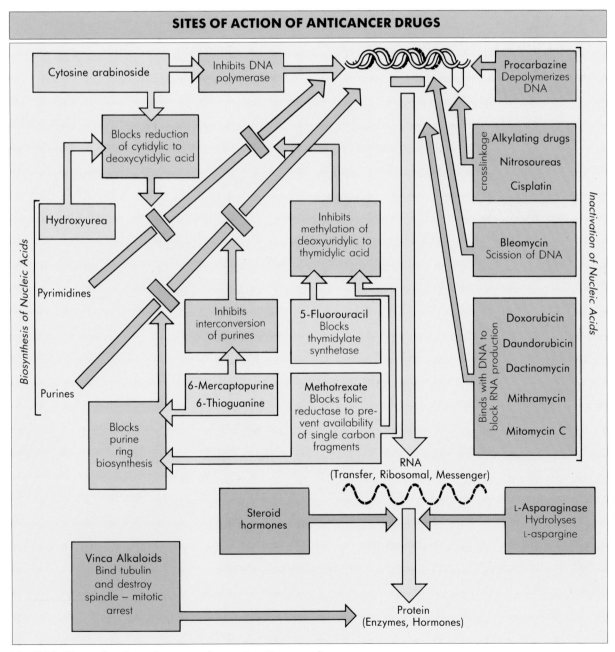

SITES OF ACTION OF ANTICANCER DRUGS

Fig. 3.14 Sites of action of commonly used anticancer drugs.

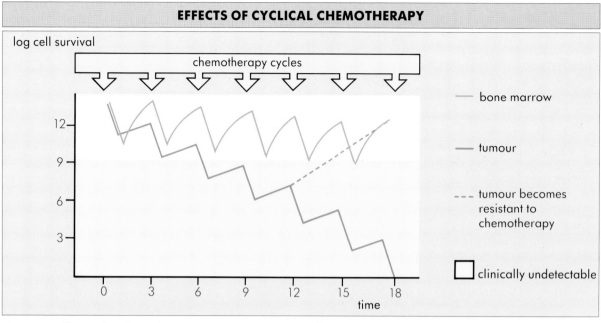

EFFECTS OF CYCLICAL CHEMOTHERAPY

log cell survival

chemotherapy cycles

— bone marrow

— tumour

--- tumour becomes resistant to chemotherapy

☐ clinically undetectable

time

Fig. 3.15 Effects of cyclical chemotherapy on bone marrow and tumour. In this theoretical example the marrow is more sensitive to the effects of chemotherapy than the tumour tissue, but recovers rapidly to almost pretreatment levels before the next cycle. The tumour cells are less sensitive than the marrow, but recover much less quickly so that with repeated cycles their numbers continue to fall rapidly. Unless resistance develops, continual cycles of chemotherapy will eradicate the tumour.

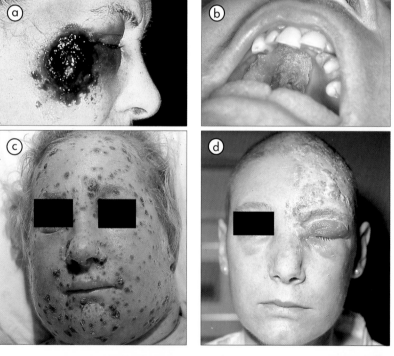

Fig. 3.16 Infection in neutropenic and immunosuppressed patients. (a) Pseudomonas infection in patient with multiple myeloma. (b) Fungal plaque eroding into the hard palate in a patient with leukaemia. (c) Disseminated herpes zoster with encephalitis, pneumonitis and hepatitis. (d) The consequences of trigeminal herpes zoster infection. In this example the infection affected the ophthalmic division of the left trigeminal nerve.

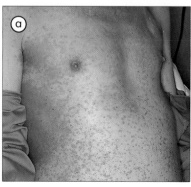
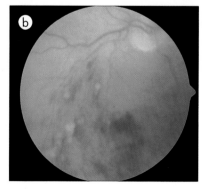

Fig. 3.17 Bleeding complications in thrombocytopenia. (a) Purpuric drug reaction in a thrombocytopenic man undergoing induction chemotherapy for leukaemia. (b) Retinal haemorrhage in a thrombocytopenic patient with leukaemia showing Roth's spots.

Drug Resistance

Sensitivity to chemotherapeutic agents varies enormously. Some tumours (e.g. renal cell carcinoma) appear to be absolutely resistant to all current cytotoxic agents, whilst others are sensitive at the beginning of treatment with resistance emerging later (e.g. breast cancer). In yet others, sensitivity is maintained and the tumour may be eradicated (e.g. teratoma).

The emergence of resistance during treatment is a major problem and may be due to outgrowth of pre-existing clones of malignant cells or to acquired resistance. The mechanisms for resistance that have been described include:

- Decreased cell membrane permeability to the drug;
- Decreased drug-activating enzymes;
- Increased drug-inactivating enzymes;
- Increased levels of inhibiting target enzyme – possibly through gene reduplication;
- Altered affinity of target enzyme for drug;
- Increased DNA repair;
- Increase in an alternative salvage pathway.

Adjuvant Chemotherapy

The realization that many patients with apparently localized and curable solid tumours actually have microscopic metastases has led to the introduction of adjuvant therapy – the use of chemotherapy together with surgery in patients with early stage disease. The advantages of this approach are:

- Chemotherapy is most effective when tumours are small and growing rapidly;
- There will be no avascular areas which may interfere with drug entry;
- Fewer cycles of chemotherapy will be needed to eradicate the tumour, thus reducing the risk of the emergence of resistance.

So far, adjuvant chemotherapy has been rather disappointing. However, the use of chemotherapy or hormone therapy after surgery in selected women with breast cancer has improved long-term survival rates by 10–15%, though advanced breast cancer is incurable with either of these modalities.

Toxicity of Chemotherapy

Since there are no chemotherapeutic agents which are tumour cell selective in their action, they are bound to cause potentially serious toxicities. The major common toxicities of anticancer drugs are described below. Some are acute though others may pose long term problems.

Bone marrow suppression

This is minimized by cyclical administration of cytotoxic drugs. At any one time most marrow stem cells are resting (G_0) – administration of anticancer drugs for a short period results in a temporary fall in white cell and platelet counts, as resting cells are recruited into the proliferating pool. Most cytotoxic drugs have a brief effect with rapid recovery of the counts, although the nitrosourea group often cause prolonged marrow suppression. The risk of infection is related to the level of absolute neutrophil count and the duration of the period of suppression. Once the count falls below 500×10^9 neutrophils per litre there is risk of infection, which increases with time – after 10 days of such low counts infection is almost certain.

Any patient with a lower neutrophil count than this and a fever or other signs of an infection should be started on intravenous empirical antibiotic therapy as soon as cultures have been taken. The treatment of choice is usually a third generation penicillin or modern cephalosporin together with an aminoglycoside. In many cases the organism is not identified and it is clear that the infection may be caused by viruses or fungi as well as bacteria (Fig. 3.16).

Better care of infections has improved the outlook for patients with leukaemia and those undergoing severely myelosuppressive therapy. The recent introduction of haemotopoietic growth factors may help to reduce the period of cytopenia.

Thrombocytopenia rarely causes bleeding when the platelet count is above 20×10^9 per litre. The additional stress of infection may cause bleeding with higher counts. Platelet transfusions are indicated for any frank signs of bleeding, abnormal bruising, retinal haemorrhage (Fig. 3.17), or prophylactically when the count is less than 20×10^9 per litre.

Alopecia

Hair loss is common with cyclophosphamide, vincristine, bleomycin and almost universal with anthracyclines. Patients should be warned before treatment so that they can obtain a wig to match their own hair or to their specifications. Scalp cooling and other devices to temporarily reduce blood flow at the time of chemotherapy have had mixed success at best. Nail changes (Fig. 3.18) are common and can dramatically demonstrate the fact that cytotoxic drugs are indiscriminate cellular poisons.

Nausea and vomiting

Many anticancer drugs cause nausea and vomiting which may be severe in some cases. It is important

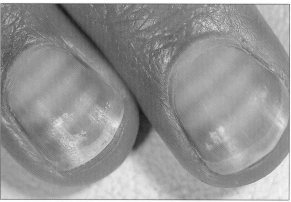

Fig. 3.18 The effects of chemotherapy on nail growth.

to achieve optimum antiemetic therapy right from the beginning since some patients quickly become conditioned. This may become such a problem that they even vomit before treatment, as they associate their surrounding with vomiting. This is often the most distressing adverse effect for patients.

Mucositis

The mucosal cells of the gastrointestinal tract are particularly sensitive to the effects of certain cytotoxic drugs. The mucosa of the mouth is especially affected (Fig. 3.19) and stomatitis may become so severe that the patient cannot swallow. More commonly erythema and pain, with or without *Candida albicans*, presents a week or so after treatment and improves when the neutrophil count rises.

Extravasation

Most anticancer drugs are given intravenously and some may cause local tissue necrosis if allowed to leak from the vein. Great care in administration is required. Because multiple chemotherapy and other drug treatments as well as transfusions may be damaging to veins, patients receiving prolonged intensive chemotherapy often benefit from a long-line placed in the atrium and tunnelled under the skin (Fig. 3.20), or from an indwelling Portacath.

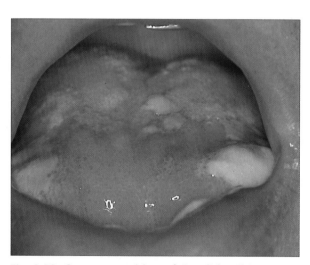

Fig. 3.19 Gross mucositis and *Candida albicans* infection.

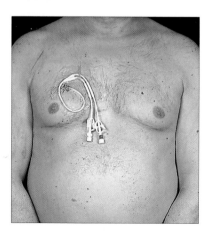

Fig. 3.20 Administration of anticancer drugs. Double lumen long-line catheter ('Hickman line') tunnelled under the skin after placement in the right atrium.

Specific organ toxicities

These may be caused by specific drugs and can affect a variety of systems. They include:
- nephrotoxicity – cisplatin and methotrexate;
- cardiotoxicity – anthracyclines;
- pneumonitis – bleomycin;
- skin – bleomycin (Fig. 3.21);
- neurotoxicity – vinca alkaloids and cisplatin;
- hepatotoxicity – L-asparaginase and methotrexate;
- cystitis – ifosfamide and cyclophosphamide;
- sterility – especially alkylating agents;
- second malignancy, especially leukaemia – alkylating agents and procarbazine are the main risk.

Hormones

Hormones were the first successful systemic therapy for cancer. Beatson showed that oophorectomy was a useful treatment for breast cancer as long ago as 1896, and in recent years a whole new series of hormone preparations has become available. These have replaced oophorectomy, adrenalectomy and hypophysectomy in breast cancer, although orchidectomy is still a standard therapy for prostatic cancer.

Many tumour cells appear to possess receptors for hormones and this finding can be exploited therapeutically. For instance tamoxifen will bind to the oestrogen receptor, blocking the actions of oestrogen (see chapter 8).

Commonly used hormones include tamoxifen (anti-oestrogen), progesterones, oestrogens, androgens, aminoglutethimide and corticosteroids. Although less toxic than cytotoxic drugs they all have adverse effects, though tamoxifen and progesterones are usually well tolerated.

Summary

The management of cancer is complex. The clinician requires detailed knowledge of a wide variety of topics to ensure optimal care. Whilst a thorough knowledge of the mechanics of caring for cancer is paramount, good communication and counselling skills are often equally important for the successful care of cancer patients.

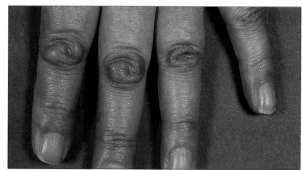

Fig. 3.21 Bleomycin skin toxicity. There is gross thickening of the soft tissues with pigmentation, especially over the joints.

Investigations

Introduction

A number of investigative techniques are used both to confirm the diagnosis and to assess the characteristics and degree of spread of a tumour. This latter function is referred to as staging.

For almost all malignant tumours, treatment decisions are based on a comprehensive evaluation of the tumour stage. In addition to this primary role, staging has an extremely important function in allowing tumours to be accurately described – therapies at different institutions can only be properly compared if there is a widely accepted agreement on how to describe the stage the disease has reached.

The concept of such a common language was recognized as long ago as the 1920s, when the League of Nations supported the development of staging systems in gynaecological cancer. However, it was not until the *Union Internationale Contre le Cancer* (UICC) and the American Joint Committee for Cancer Staging and End-Results Reporting (AJCCS) were formed in the 1950s that the idea came to fruition. In 1978 a common approach was agreed, resulting in a system known as the TNM classification. This can be applied to most solid tumours, but is not used for haematological malignancies. The International Federation for Gynaecological Oncology (FIGO) has continued to produce staging systems for gynaecological cancers which are very widely used.

Staging

Staging is designed to aid the following activities:
- the logical planning of cancer treatment;
- the evaluation of treatment results;
- the exchange of information.

The TNM system was developed primarily to guide locoregional therapy rather than systemic treatment. Because of this there is a considerable emphasis on the extent of primary disease (Fig. 4.1). The system uses a series of subscripts to indicate increasing degrees of tumour extent. In the TNM system used for lung cancer (Figs 4.2 and 4.3) the T stage increases with size of the tumour, its position and the degree of invasion of surrounding structures. N stage increases as more central node areas are

involved. M status is simply recorded as '0' or '1', since the main intent of the system is to record operability.

As can be seen from Figure 4.2 the full TNM classification is too complicated and unwieldy to be useful for comparison of results. For this reason the information is simplified. Patients with groups of TNM stages which are treated similarly and which have a similar prognosis are given a single classification; this process is known as stage grouping. The complex TNM system for lung cancer is thus reduced to just four stages (Fig. 4.4).

Most staging systems are based on an initial clinical assessment supported by appropriate imaging techniques. However, in some tumours (such as breast cancer) surgical information may also be used to define pathological stage. Further information on tumour grade may also be incorporated into staging if it influences choice of therapy, as for example in bladder cancer.

THE TNM STAGING SYSTEM	
T –	extent of the primary tumour
N –	state of regional lymph nodes
M –	presence or absence of distant metastases

Fig. 4.1 The TNM staging system.

STAGING OF NON-SMALL CELL LUNG CANCER	
Stage	Criteria
T1	<3cm diameter
T2	>3cm diameter Involves main bronchus 2cm distal to carina, visceral pleura invaded with associated atelectasis and pneumonitis
T3	Tumour involves chest wall, diaphragm, mediastinal pleura, parietal pericardium Tumour of main bronchus within 2cm of carina atelectasis of entire lung Pneumonitis of entire lung
T4	Tumour invades mediastinum great vessels of the heart, trachea, oesophagus, vertebra, carina Tumour produces malignant pleural effusion
N1	Ipsilateral, peribronchial or hilar nodes
N2	Ipsilateral, mediastinal or subcarinal nodes
N3	Metastasis in contralateral mediastinal or hilar nodes or ipsilateral or contralateral scalene or supraclavicular nodes
M0	No distant metastases
M1	Distant metastases

Fig. 4.2 TNM staging in non-small cell lung cancer.

Staging Investigations

The process of staging begins as soon as the patient is seen – for example, jaundice in the presence of a bowel cancer is highly suggestive of metastatic disease. A thorough history and physical examination gives immediate information and may make more complicated and unpleasant procedures unnecessary. Investigation should ideally be systematic, so that invasive and costly investigations are only undertaken if simple inexpensive tests, such as routine haematology and biochemistry, are negative. Thus, if a chest X-ray shows obvious tumour masses, an expensive CT scan may not be necessary; similarly, grossly abnormal liver function tests may obviate the need for liver imaging or biopsy (Fig. 4.5), though such tests may provide a valuable baseline in assessing response to treatment. With this in mind, the rest of this chapter briefly discusses the optimal use of some common specialist staging techniques.

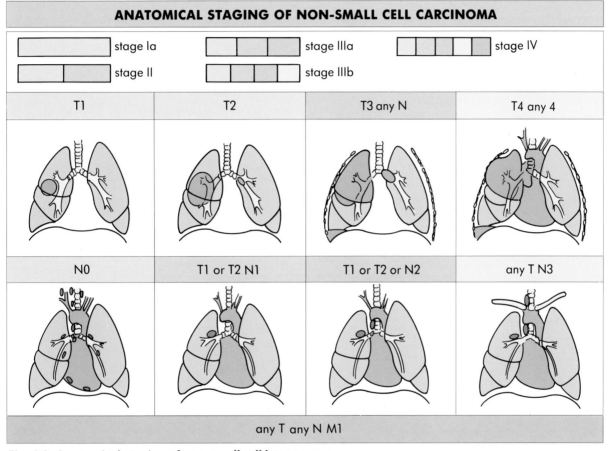

ANATOMICAL STAGING OF NON-SMALL CELL CARCINOMA

stage Ia   stage IIIa   stage IV

stage II   stage IIIb

| T1 | T2 | T3 any N | T4 any 4 |

| N0 | T1 or T2 N1 | T1 or T2 or N2 | any T N3 |

any T any N M1

Fig. 4.3 Anatomical staging of non-small cell lung cancer.

STAGE GROUPING FOR LUNG CANCER

Stage			
I	T1	N0	M0
	T2	N0	M0
II	T1	N1	M0
	T2	N1	M0
IIIa	T1	N2	M0
	T2	N2	M0
	T3	N0, N1, N2	M0
IIIb	Any T	N3	M0
	T4	Any N	M0
IV	Any T	Any N	M1

Fig. 4.4 Stage grouping for lung cancer. [Modified from the AJC Manual for Staging Cancer (3rd edn), 1988.]

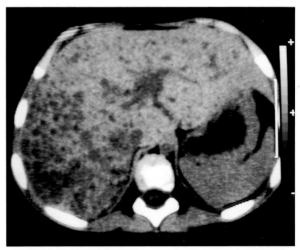

Fig. 4.5 CT imaging showing gross involvement of liver with neuroblastoma. Courtesy of Dr R. Blaquire.

Computed Tomography (CT) Scanning

The introduction of this technique a decade ago allowed a giant leap forwards in the quality of X-ray definition achievable (Fig. 4.6). For example, the sensitivity of CT scanning allows a confident diagnosis of secondary lung metastases, where the chest X-ray might still be normal.

However, this increased information should not allow us to be misled into thinking that the test is infallible. Like any other imaging technique, CT scanning results in both false positive and false negative results, although these can be reduced by the expertise of those conducting and interpreting the test. Disadvantages of the test are its high cost and

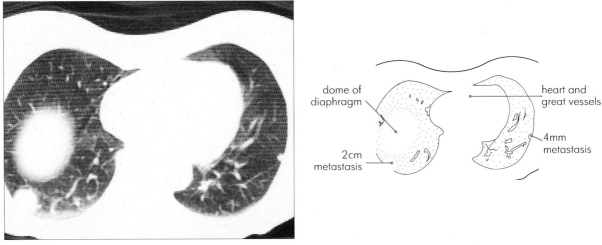

Fig. 4.6 CT image of the thorax of a patient with carcinoma of the rectum. The investigation shows a 2cm metastasis posteriorly at the right base and a 4mm metastasis at the periphery of the left lung. Routine chest X-ray was normal. Courtesy of Dr R. Blaquire.

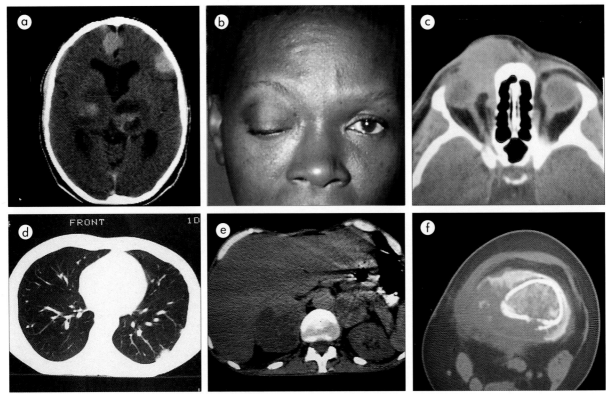

Fig. 4.7 Appropriate use of CT imaging. (a) The CNS: CT image showing enhancement of multiple gliomas. (b) & (c) The head and neck: Patient with an orbital lymphoma, clearly shown on CT image. (d) The thorax: CT image showing small metastasis in the periphery of the left lung of a man treated for a testicular teratoma. Different windows are used to examine the lungs and solid structures. (e) The abdomen and pelvis: CT image showing left adrenal mass in patient with small cell lung cancer. (f) Bone: CT image showing femoral destruction and soft tissue mass in a case of Ewing's sarcoma. Courtesy of Dr R. Blaquire.

the large amount of time and preparation that it requires. It is clearly at its best in the chest and brain, and less reliable in the abdomen and pelvis.

The primary reasons for CT scanning in a patient known to have cancer are:
- to define the extent of the primary tumour in order to help plan surgery or radiotherapy;
- to exclude nodal involvement or visceral dissemination (particularly in the liver and lungs);
- as a baseline from which to monitor response to treatment.

CT scanning is all too often done as a matter of routine without any of the above justifications, which may not only be wasteful, but also result in unnecessary discomfort. Examples of appropriate use of CT scanning are shown in Figs 4.7 and 4.8.

Ultrasound

Ultrasound imaging was developed 30 years ago and has been substantially refined in the last ten years. It uses the echoes created by the different elasticities at tissue interfaces to build up an image of internal body structures (Fig. 4.9).

The main advantages of the technique are that it is quick, non-invasive, inexpensive and easily repeatable. It generally gives a reliable indication as to whether a space-occupying lesion is cystic or solid. The operator can select the direction (or plane) from

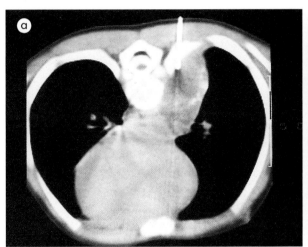
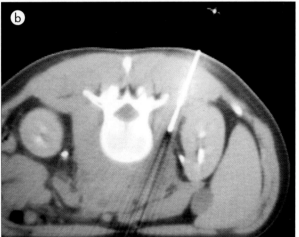

Fig. 4.8 Needle biopsy of masses guided by CT imaging. (a) Biopsy of a mass adjacent to the vertebra in thorax: the needle can be seen posteriorly – a ganglioma. (b) Biopsy of a para-aortic mass: the needle can be seen posteriorly – a seminoma. Courtesy of Dr R. Blaquire.

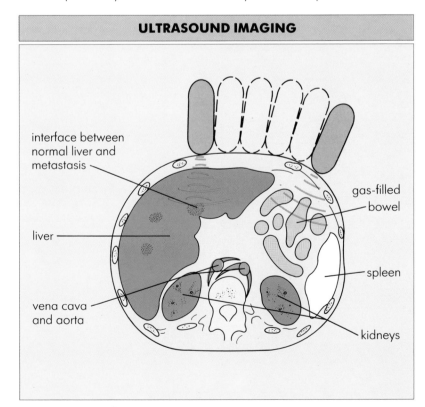

ULTRASOUND IMAGING

interface between normal liver and metastasis

liver

vena cava and aorta

gas-filled bowel

spleen

kidneys

Fig. 4.9 The technique of ultrasound imaging. The high-frequency sound waves produced are reflected at interfaces of different tissue densities, such as that between normal liver and metastases, allowing the computer to construct an image. Gas in the bowel appears as a black shadow obscuring the view.

which he examines the area to be scanned, in order to obtain the maximum information.

Disadvantages include the requirement for an expert operator and an inability to examine behind bone or gas-filled bowel. Its resolving power is not as good as CT imaging, although it is often the investigation of choice because it is so easily repeatable. It is also preferred at a number of sites such as the testis, prostate and thyroid. Cases illustrating the advantages of ultrasound imaging are shown in Figure 4.10.

Magnetic Resonance Imaging (MRI)

Atomic nuclei which have an uneven number of particles (protons or neutrons) normally spin at random. When placed in an electromagnetic field, some of the nuclei align with that field – when the electromagnetic field is removed they revert to their original state and release energy. This signal can be used to construct a computer-generated image of the location of the particles chosen for study. Hydrogen nuclei (protons) are usually used for MRI, since they are ubiquitous within the body.

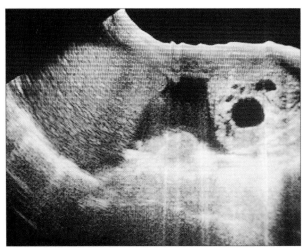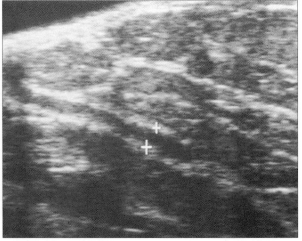

Fig. 4.10 Ultrasound imaging. A technique useful for examining the abdomen and pelvis, being particularly good at detecting cystic areas. (a) Sagittal section showing liver (left) and large complex ovarian cystadenocarcinoma (right). (b) Ultrasonography is also useful at specific sites such as thyroid, testis and breast. This image shows a benign, dilated duct in a breast which was equivocal on mammography. Courtesy of Dr K. Dewbury.

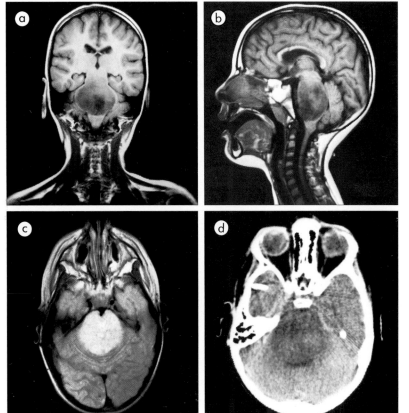

Fig. 4.11 MRI showing a brain stem tumour. (a) (b) & (c) MRI provides excellent images of the head and neck, and the CNS. Comparison with the CT scan of the brain (d) shows the extra information provided by MRI. As well as offering excellent resolving power, particularly for CNS tumours, MRI scanning may be employed as a means of avoiding unpleasant invasive procedures. Spinal lesions, for example, may be adequately imaged by MRI without the need for myelography.

MRI has only recently come into clinical practice (Fig. 4.11). Its advantages are:

- it carries no biological hazard (no radiation exposure);
- several parameters can be varied to enhance the image;
- blood vessels can be seen without contrast;
- anatomical detail is excellent, although in some sites resolution is less than with CT;
- imaging can easily be performed in several different planes.

The main disadvantage at present is the high cost of acquiring and maintaining the equipment (the magnet is supercooled so that large quantities of liquid nitrogen are needed). MRI is still in its infancy and a number of ways of enhancing the image, for example by injection of contrast material such as gadolinium, are being explored. Currently it is developing a role in the investigation of tumour at a number of sites (Fig. 4.11) particularly the brainstem, spine and pelvis.

Isotope Imaging

By judicious choice of isotope and an appropriate vehicle, tumours can be localized in a variety of sites. Localization may be non-specific, depending on the abnormal tumour vasculature; the use of techniques such as technetium-labelled phosphate compounds, which are preferentially taken up by bone, or radiolabelled sulphur colloids, which are preferentially taken up by Kupffer cells in the liver, may add an additional degree of specificity.

As these techniques simply reflect the activity of the organ against which they are targetted, an abnormal finding is relatively non-specific. For example, healing fractures produce changes similar to bone cancer, since both show increased uptake caused by osteoblastic activity (Fig. 4.12). Similarly, both cysts and tumour masses in the liver will produce cold areas. Because of this, experience in interpreting isotope images is important.

The possibility of improving specificity by directing monoclonal antibodies at tumour-associated

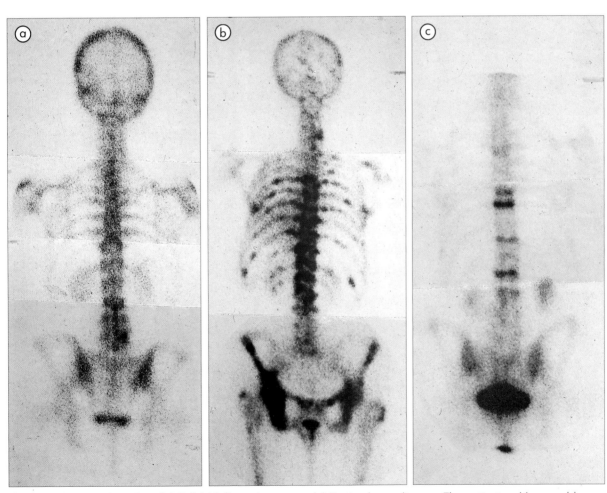

Fig. 4.12 Isotope imaging. (a) & (b) Malignant infiltraton of bone. The patient, a 63-year old woman with T2 N0 M0 breast cancer, was treated by mastectomy. She had no further therapy and remained well until four years later when she developed back pain. The original bone scan (a) was normal whilst a scan 4 years later (b) shows extensive uptake in the spine, ribs and pelvis, typical of metastatic cancer.

(c) Benign bone disease. The patient, a 66-year old woman, presented with back pain but had no prior medical history of note. Her bone image shows markedly increased uptake in multiple vertebrae. These, however, are symmetrical and very different in nature and distribution to those in (b). These images are typical of osteoporotic collapse. Courtesy of Dr D. Ackery.

epitopes has recently excited much interest. Initial studies have produced promising images (Fig. 4.13), but the lack of genuine tumour-specific antibodies, together with many other technical problems, have meant that the hopes for this technique have not yet been fulfilled. If specific monoclonal antibodies could be labelled, they might then be used therapeutically.

Other Radiological Techniques

Contrast studies of the gastrointestinal tract retain an important role in diagnosis (Fig. 4.14), and angiography may be helpful in delineating tumour circulation (Fig. 4.15) before planning surgery.

Bipedal lymphangiography may show spread of tumour to retroperitoneal lymph nodes (Fig. 4.16). This test is cumbersome but it is useful in some cancers, especially lymphomas, as it may reveal involved lymph nodes of normal size. The patient can be easily re-examined at any time so long as the dye persists (often the case for up to two years).

Other special X-ray techniques, such as mammography, are particularly important. Nearly all require specialist interpretation – mammography is a particularly good example of this since the changes are often so subtle. The skill of the radiologist screening for breast cancer is in identifying as many cancers as possible whilst at the same time avoiding unnecessary further investigation of benign lesions that may mimic malignant change (see Fig. 8.10).

Tumour Markers

The development of blood tests which could aid cancer management has long been a goal for oncologists. Such tests might have value not only when making a diagnosis but also when monitoring the response to therapy.

Ideally a marker for cancer would be:
- specific for the tumour;
- produced by all tumours of that type;
- a good indicator of tumour bulk;

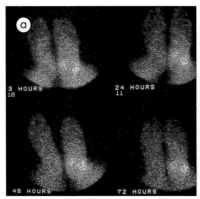
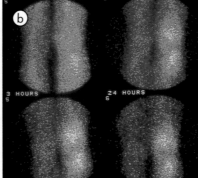
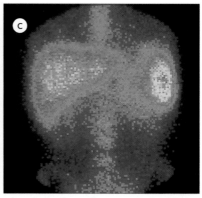

Fig. 4.13 Monoclonal antibodies for tumour imaging. The patient presented with a mass on the sole of his left foot. Biopsy revealed a deeply penetrating malignant melanoma and he underwent a radical excision. However, the tumour recurred rapidly and he was considered for therapy in a phase II study of a radiolabelled anti-melanoma antibody. Prior to this, imaging using the antibody was performed. Images of the feet (a) clearly show uptake in the recurrent tumour. Images of the legs (b) show previously unrecognized tumour around the knee. These images indicate that the monoclonal antibody could be used therapeutically to deliver a high dose of irradiation. However, images of the abdomen (c) revealed extensive non-specific uptake in the liver and spleen, thus precluding therapy. Courtesy of Dr D. Ackery.

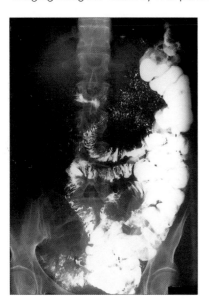

Fig. 4.14 Polyposis coli. Small bowel contrast study showing numerous filling defects. (See Fig. 12.19 for morphological specimen of small bowel.)

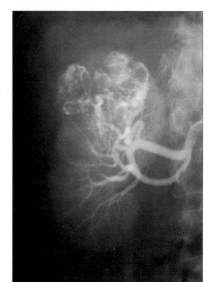

Fig. 4.15 Vascular imaging. Angiography showing an area of abnormal vasculature in the upper pole of the right kidney – a hypernephroma.

- produced equally by metastases;
- easy to quantify;
- detectable at very low levels;
- simple;
- inexpensive.

No current marker fulfils all these criteria, but a variety of very useful markers are available for teratoma and choriocarcinoma. These come closer to the ideal than markers for other tumours and are an invaluable aid to treatment (Fig. 4.17). Other tumour

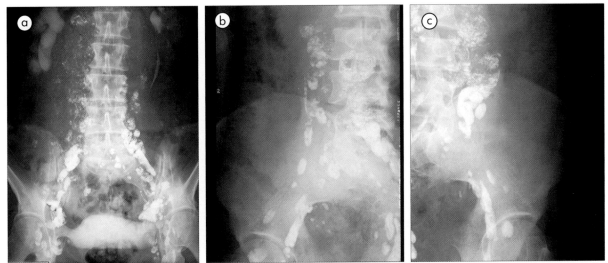

Fig. 4.16 Techniques to display lymph nodes.
(a) Lymphangiogram and intravenous urography showing extensive enlargement of para-aortic lymph nodes. There is hydronephrosis on the left and both ureters are bowed outwards. Urography is a useful adjuvant to lymphangiography since displacement of ureters may be seen in the absence of enlarged nodes – in this case the lymph nodes are so grossly abnormal

that they do not take up the contrast material. This patient has a stage III Hodgkin's disease.
(b) & (c) Oblique left- and right-hand views of a lymphangiogram showing extensive enlargement and disruption of the para-aortic lymph nodes. The changes are due to seminoma though they are similar to those seen in lymphoma. Courtesy of Dr P. Guyer.

TUMOUR MARKERS IN TESTICULAR TERATOMA

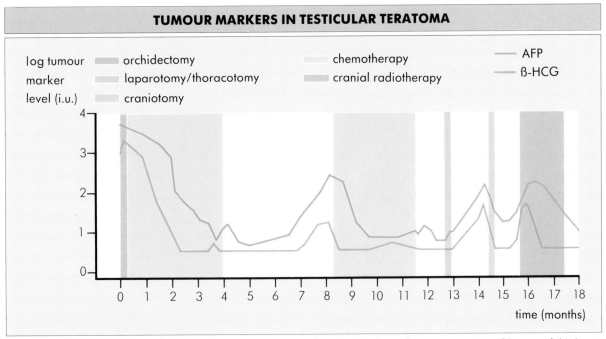

Fig. 4.17 Use of ß-HCG and AFP in the management of testicular teratoma. This patient had markedly raised levels of AFP and HCG at presentation which fell after orchidectomy, but extensive retroperitoneal disease was found. After chemotherapy the levels fell to normal but rose, necessitating further chemotherapy. The levels fell once more. Residual para-aortic masses were removed surgically, but the

levels of both markers rose again – CT scan of the brain revealed a mass, which was removed by craniotomy. However, both marker levels subsequently rose and CT revealed an unresectable lesion in the brain. After cranial radiotherapy the marker levels resolved. At all times during this patient's course the markers accurately reflected disease activity and helped guide treatment choice. Courtesy of Dr G. Mead.

markers can be helpful (CEA in colon cancer, Ca–125 in ovarian cancer) but are rarely of major importance. This is partly because they cannot influence outcome if there is advanced or recurrent disease, since no curative treatment is available at present. Markers are clearly only of real use therapeutically if they can be used to direct highly active therapies.

Another use of tumour markers is to help establish the tissue of origin. Differentiation between anaplastic carcinoma, lymphoma, and germ cell or other tumours is sometimes difficult. Immunocytochemistry (Fig. 4.18) may give clear guidance as to the histogenesis of the tumour; this ensures that treatable tumours are not missed and that unnecessary toxic treatment is avoided in lesions unlikely to respond to intensive chemotherapy.

Surgery

Biopsy of potential metastatic sites, for example lymph nodes, bone marrow and liver, may be used to stage cancer. Laparotomy may very occasionally be used to search for occult intra-abdominal disease, and is most often undertaken in selected patients with Hodgkin's disease, where the decision between radiotherapy or chemotherapy (or a combination of both) can sometimes be difficult.

Biopsy of internal organs (see Fig. 4.8), either by endoscope or percutaneously, can very often give the diagnosis or help identify the extent of tumour spread without the need for a formal operation.

Conclusions

A wide variety of investigations are used to make a diagnosis and stage the extent of cancer spread. The art of the competent physician is to use these in a responsible fashion so that the diagnosis and stage is reached quickly, with as few unnecessary tests as possible. It is always easy to order a battery of tests without thought – a thoughtful selection can save time, money and discomfort for the patient.

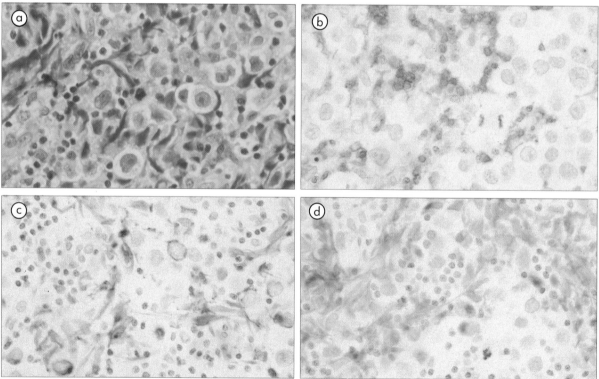

Fig. 4.18 Use of monoclonal antibodies in histopathology. The patient presented with a painless lump in his left supraclavicular fossa. On examination no other evidence of tumour was found and he underwent excision biopsy. Routine histology (H&E), shown in (a), was interpreted as a possible lymphoma. However, immunohistochemistry revealed further information which changed the diagnosis. When stained with CD45 (a panleukocyte marker), the larger tumour cells were unstained (b) whilst the smaller lymphoid cells were stained brown. CK (a cytokeratin marker) produced staining of the large cells (c) consistent with a carcinoma or some other non-haematogenous tumour. Use of placental alkaline phosphatase (PLAP) showed clear staining of the tumour cells (d), strongly suggesting that this tumour was a seminoma. Re-examination of the patient revealed an enlarged left testicle which was excised – histology confirmed a seminoma. Such use of a panel of tissue markers may be helpful in confirming or refuting the putative tissue of origin of a tumour and this may have a major impact on management. Courtesy of Prof D. Wright.

Brain Tumours

Introduction

As a group, brain tumours represent one of the most devastating forms of cancer. They affect both adults and children, and form the largest single group of malignant diseases of childhood after leukaemias. Management problems result not only from the terrible physical effects but also from the profound emotional strain they engender, especially of course where a child is concerned. Almost nothing is known of their aetiology, though childhood cases are occasionally encountered in congenital diseases such as tuberous sclerosis and Fanconi anaemia, or in patients with von Recklinghausen's syndrome (see Fig. 14.8), in which brain tumours may occur at any stage in childhood or early adult life. In addition the brain is an important and common site of secondary deposits in a variety of carcinomas, typically breast cancer (see Fig. 8.9), lung cancer (especially small cell lung cancer) and malignant melanoma, though almost any primary malignancy can produce cerebral metastases. Benign intracranial neoplasms also occur, including neuromas (most characteristically acoustic neuroma, presenting as a space occupying lesion of the cerebello-pontine angle), neurofibromas, meningiomas and of course an important group of pituitary tumours.

A simple classification of malignant brain tumours is shown in Fig. 5.1; pathological features of the most important of these are discussed below.

Clinical Features and Diagnostic Investigations

Three important groups of syndromes may occur. First, the patient may present with a 'focal neurological deficit' relating to the specific site. A tumour of the dominant hemisphere, for example, situated in the cortex close to the motor strip, may produce neurological damage resulting in a hemiplegia. In

PATHOLOGICAL CLASSIFICATION
Primary tumours

Glioma (low to high grade)
    astrocytoma, glioblastoma multiforme,
    ependymoma, oligodendroglioma,
    medulloblastoma
Pituitary tumour (includes functional tumours)
    pituitary adenoma, craniopharyngioma
Meningioma
    benign, malignant (meningiosarcoma)
Pineal tumours (includes germ cell types)
    pinealoblastoma, pinealocytoma,
    germinoma, teratoma
Intracranial lymphoma (usually B cell)
    'histiocytic' lymphoma, microglioma
Acoustic neuroma
Chordoma
Neuronal tumours
    ganglioneuroma, ganglioglioma, colloid cyst

Secondary tumours

Common sites of origin
    lung, breast, melanoma
Less common sites of origin
    ovary, testis, gut, bladder, kidney, pancreas,
    liver, leukaemia and lymphoma
Miscellaneous
    histocytosis X

Fig. 5.1 Pathological classification of benign and malignant brain tumours.

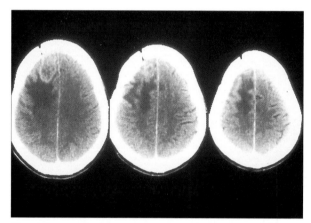

Fig. 5.2 Grade III astrocytoma. This tumour of the frontal lobe produced extensive oedema posterior to the tumour itself. The tumour was partly excised by frontal lobectomy.

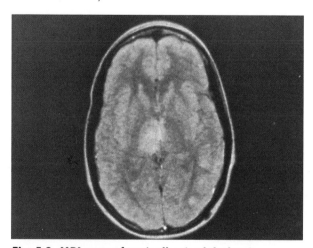

Fig. 5.3 MRI scan of typically sited thalamic glioma. These are invariably inoperable and generally treated by radiotherapy.

addition, there may be expressive dysphasia, either from direct involvement of Broca's area or because of local oedema, often a marked feature with brain tumours (Fig. 5.2). More posteriorly placed lesions, for example in the brain stem or in the occipital cortex, may result in other specific defects such as cranial nerve lesions. More deeply situated lesions (typically thalamic gliomas – Fig. 5.3), which often interrupt the visual pathways, frequently result in a characteristic loss of visual field. Midbrain or third ventricle tumours may cause loss of upward gaze (Parinaud's syndrome). Relatively silent areas of the brain such as the frontal and parietal lobes are less eloquent from the point of view of early neurological damage, and the tumour is often correspondingly larger when first detected (Fig. 5.4). Tumours situated in the non-dominant (usually right) hemisphere are not accompanied by a speech disorder.

Second, the patient may develop 'late onset epilepsy', presenting with a variety of epileptiform seizure patterns. Myoclonic epilepsy, often affecting

the limbs or face, is generally of a consistent pattern and gives important clues to the site of the primary tumour. For example, typical features of temporal lobe epilepsy may occur (Fig. 5.5). In addition to site, an important clinical point is the length of the history. High-grade brain tumours with their characteristically rapid clinical evolution typically produce a short history of only a few weeks or months before clear-cut evidence of clinical deterioration results in the need for further investigation, usually CT scanning, which then gives the diagnosis. By contrast, patients with low-grade brain tumours characteristically present with a lengthy history, often going back several years, and typically with a specific pattern of epileptiform seizures with no permanent neurological damage until much later in the clinical evolution (see Fig. 5.4).

A history of increasingly frequent focal seizures may then result in referral and diagnosis. Typically these lesions are less likely to cause cerebral oedema and midline shift on the CT or MRI scan than are high-grade tumours (see Fig. 5.4). Because they grow more slowly, low-grade brain tumours may attain a large size (particularly in relatively silent areas of the brain) or may show obvious calcification.

The third group of symptoms results from 'raised intracranial pressure' (ICP), the clinical features often occurring together with epilepsy or focal neurological loss. Chief amongst these are headache, nausea, visual disturbance (particularly diplopia) and drowsiness. The headache is often worse in the morning and on straining. The tumours most likely to cause raised ICP are chiefly situated close to the midline near the third and fourth ventricles, and are often not very large, whereas more peripherally placed cortical tumours often do not cause raised ICP symptoms at all. Papilloedema is the most

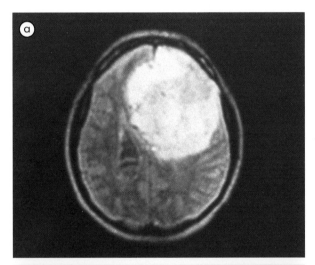
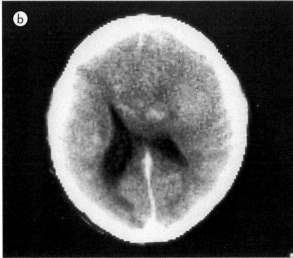

Fig. 5.4 Large frontal lobe low-grade astrocytoma. This tumour is well shown on MRI scanning (a) but less distinctly with CT scanning (b). The patient presented with a grand mal seizure with surprisingly little evidence of frontal lobe symptoms.

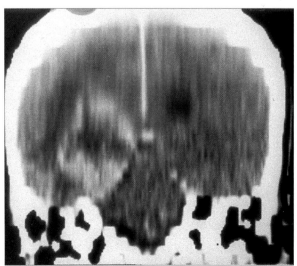

Fig. 5.5 High-grade astrocytoma. Coronal reconstruction of a temporal lobe high-grade astrocytoma which presented with typical temporal lobe features.

common and reliable physical sign (Fig. 5.6). Varying degrees of hydrocephalus are seen on the CT scan (see for example Fig. 5.4).

In addition to these major symptom clusters, pituitary tumours (usually adenomas which are almost never malignant) may cause a variety of endocrine effects as well as local structural damage from direct local extension (Fig. 5.7). Disturbance of the visual pathways is common because of the proximity of the optic chiasm anteriorly. The commonest disturbance is of a bitemporal hemianopia which may present with the patient persistently

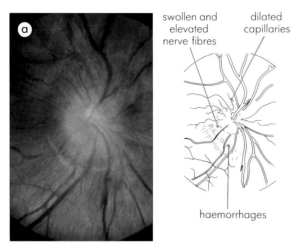

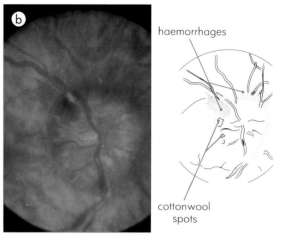

Fig. 5.6 Papilloedema from cerebral tumours.
(a) Early papilloedema. Dilatation of nerve bundle fibres is clearly seen, together with superficial haemorrhages and hyperaemia of the disc margins.
(b) Gross papilloedema. The disc is grossly swollen with dilated nerve fibres masking the blood vessels at the disc borders. There are haemorrhages into the nerve fibre layer around the disc, and cottonwool spots on the disc surface. Courtesy of Mr D.J. Spalton.

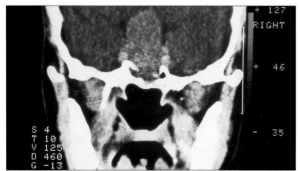

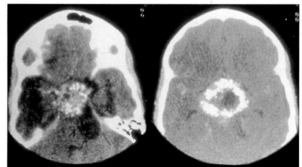

Fig. 5.7 Pituitary adenoma. Coronal CT scan showing large pituitary adenoma with massive suprasellar extension. The lesion, a non-functioning pituitary adenoma, presented with classic bitemporal hemianopia.

Fig. 5.8 Craniopharyngioma. Transaxial CT scan showing characteristic massive local calcification. For this reason, craniopharyngiomas are often not fully resectable. Courtesy of Dr H. Okazaki.

ANTERIOR PITUITARY HORMONES			
Hormones	Molecular weight	Number of Amino Acids	Note
Growth hormone Prolactin	21,800 22,500	219 198	Both hormones are single-chain polypeptides with two disulphide bridges and may have evolved from single ancestral molecules
ACTH ß-Lipotrophin ß-Endorphin	4,500 11,200 4,000	39 91 31	Hormones in this group are single-chain polypeptides, derived from a large precursor molecule, pro-opiomelanocortin
FSH LH TSH	29,000 29,000 29,000	ß,115 ß,115 ß,112	These glycoproteins are composed of a- and ß-subunits, the latter defining biologic specificities of individual hormones. Subunits have 89 amino acids

Fig. 5.9 Anterior pituitary hormones.

bumping into unseen objects, or more worryingly, reporting a series of similar driving accidents. Hypopituitarism is common though generally not profound, and the patient may develop a variety of endocrine abnormalities, including hypocorticism from impairment of ACTH secretion, hypothyroidism from reduction in TSH, and hypogonadism with loss of libido, infertility and amenorrhoea. In children, growth failure is an important clinical feature of a pituitary tumour, which in this age group almost invariably proves to be a craniopharyngioma (Fig. 5.8).

In the adult, pituitary tumours account for 10% of all primary brain tumours and approximately a quarter are functional, that is they secrete excess ACTH, prolactin (PRL), growth hormone (GH) or posterior pituitary hormones (Figs 5.9, 5.10 and 5.11). Of the clinical syndromes produced, acromegaly is among the most common (Fig. 5.12) and can be a life threatening illness. These tumours are not necessarily large, but cause particular problems since they may be difficult to resect entirely, and are less responsive to radiotherapy than non-functional pituitary tumours (see below). Pituitary Cushing's syndrome may be troublesome for similar reasons.

Pathological Spectrum of Brain Tumours

In adults, it is often said that one third of brain tumours are primary malignancies, a further third are secondary deposits and the remainder are benign tumours. Of the primary malignant brain tumours,

PITUITARY ADENOMAS (3073 CASES)		
Type	Number	%
PRL cell adenomas	1095	35.6
GH cell adenomas	584	19.0
ACTH cell adenomas	394	12.8
TSH cell adenomas	11	0.4
Gonadotrophin cell adenomas	52	1.7
Plurihormonal adenomas	169	5.5
Non-secretory adenomas	768	25.0
Non-oncocytic		18.1
Oncocytic		6.9

Fig. 5.10 Comparative frequency of functional and non-functional pituitary adenomas. An analysis of over 3000 cases.

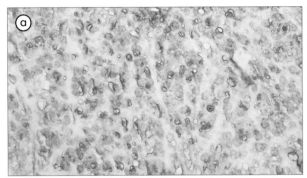

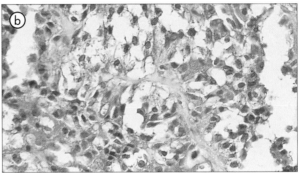

Fig. 5.11 Functional pituitary tumours.
(a) Prolactinoma (medium power photomicrograph). Immunostaining with anti-PRL is limited to the juxtanuclear region. (b) ACTH cell adenoma showing a typical sinusoidal arrangement of cells. Courtesy of Dr Jung H. Kim.

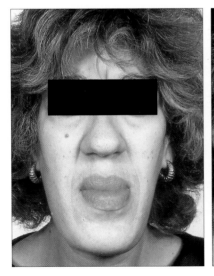

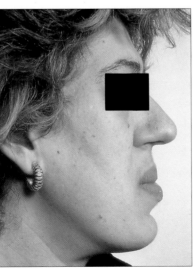

Fig. 5.12 Acromegaly. Typical facial features include enlargement and thickening of the bridge of the nose, lips and chin. Untreated, these patients face life-threatening hypertension and cardiovascular complications.

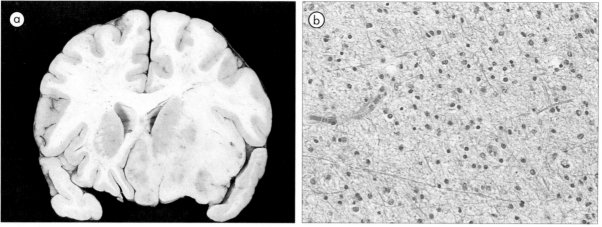

Fig. 5.13 Well differentiated diffuse astrocytoma. (a) This tumour involved chiefly the basal aspect of the right frontal lobe. The demarcation between grey and white matter is obscured. (b) Photomicrograph of the tumour shows slightly increased cellularity but with little deviation from the normal appearance. The formation of cell processes is not conspicuous, a common feature, though pink-staining myelinated nerve fibres show minor irregularities in their contour. Courtesy of Dr H. Okazaki.

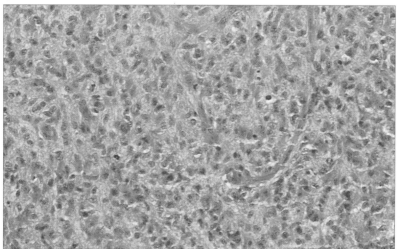

Fig. 5.14 Less well differentiated astrocytoma (Kernohan grade II-III). These lesions show more nuclear atypia, mitotic activity, cellular pleomorphism and hypercellularity. Neither endothelial proliferation nor necrosis is evident in these tumours. Courtesy of Dr H. Okazaki.

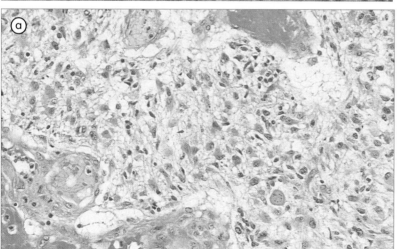

Fig. 5.15 High-grade astrocytoma (glioblastoma multiforme).
(a) Histologically, these tumours are characterized by increased cellularity, pleomorphism, vascular hypertrophy and endothelial proliferation together with areas of necrosis and haemorrhage. (b) This glioblastoma of the left insula shows a low density central area, with visible heterogeneity and a substantial mass effect, displacing the anterior part of the lateral ventricle. Courtesy of Dr H. Okazaki.

the most common are gliomas, resulting from malignant glial transformation. The commonest variety of these is the astrocytoma, varying from low to high grade, with distinct pathological features for each (Figs 5.13, 5.14 and 5.15). Grading is extremely important since this predicts the clinical outcome with a high degree of reliability — there are few human tumours in which the pathological grade carries more prognostic weight (Fig. 5.16). Low-grade (grade 1) tumours are often completely resectable, whereas high-grade lesions (grade 4, often designated 'glioblastoma multiforme') can only rarely be removed. Pathological features of a high grade of malignancy include increased cellularity and abnormality in nuclear characteristics and nuclear/cytoplasmic ratio. The other main types of glioma include oligodendroglioma (Fig. 5.17), often rather diffuse tumours with slow clinical evolution and calcification visible in the CT scan. These tumours are thought to develop from supporting cells within the brain and, typically, have a 'boxed in' cellular appearance. Ependymomas (Fig. 5.18), which occur both in childhood and in adult life, are derived from the cells which line the intracerebral ventricles or

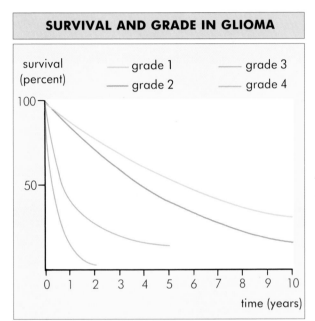

SURVIVAL AND GRADE IN GLIOMA

Fig. 5.16 Survival related to grade in malignant glioma. Note the small proportion of 10 year survivors even with low-grade tumours.

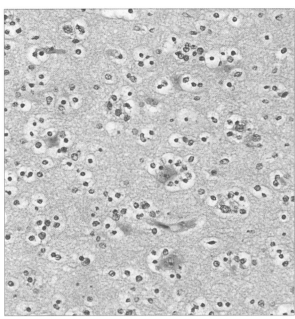

Fig. 5.17 Oligodendroglioma diffusely infiltrating the cerebral cortex. This photomicrograph shows typical 'satellitosis' of neoplastic cells about the neurons. Courtesy of Dr H. Okazaki.

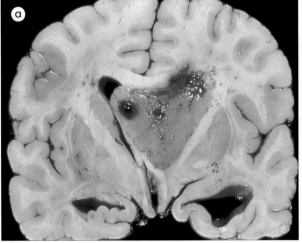

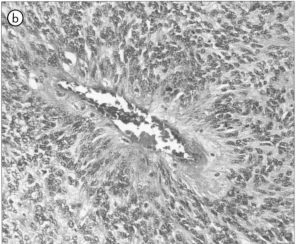

Fig. 5.18 Ependymoma. (a) Coronal section showing an ependymoma filling the right frontal horn of the lateral ventricle. The tumour is well demarcated and homogeneous in texture (haemorrhage from a previous biopsy is visible). (b) Histologically, the tumour is characterized by a tendency to perivascular pseudorosette formation, which may sometimes even result in a papillary appearance. Courtesy of Dr H. Okazaki.

spinal canal, and can therefore arise either as a primary brain or spinal cord tumour (Fig. 5.19). Pathological grade is again important as a predictor of clinical behaviour, and the tumour is able to spread throughout the CNS unlike most other varieties of adult brain tumour. This of course has important implications for clinical management (see below). Medulloblastoma (Fig. 5.20), predominantly a child-hood tumour, can also occur in adults. Although rare, primary intracerebral lymphoma (see chapter 12) is becoming increasingly important as some cases are clearly AIDS related.

In childhood the variety of brain tumours is considerably greater (Fig. 5.21). Although any of the adult brain tumours can occur in children, there are a number of important differences. Gliomas are almost always of low grade – a true glioblastoma

multiforme is a rarity in childhood. Unlike the common primary glioma sites in adult (chiefly cortical tumours, mostly in the parietal, temporal or frontal lobes), the commonest sites for childhood gliomas are the cerebellum and other deep midline structures notably the brain stem, pons and thalamus (see Fig. 4.11). The optic nerves and chiasm are an important site (Fig. 5.22), virtually never seen in adults. In children, pituitary adenomas are never encountered, the commonest pituitary lesion being the craniopharyngioma — which in turn is very un-usual in adult life (see Fig. 5.8).

The commonest of all childhood brain tumours is the medulloblastoma (see Figs 5.20 and 5.21), a tumour arising from the cerebellum, generally in the midline close to the floor of the fourth ventricle. Characteristically it causes cerebellar ataxia, with

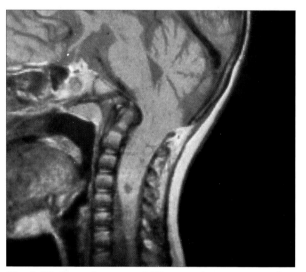

Fig. 5.19 Ependymoma. MRI scan of primary spinal ependymoma showing cord expansion with a small cystic component in the cervical region.

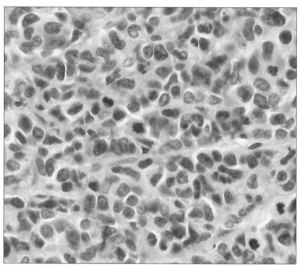

Fig. 5.20 Medulloblastoma. Medium power photomicrograph showing typical features with small, darkly staining, closely packed cells (×200 magnification).

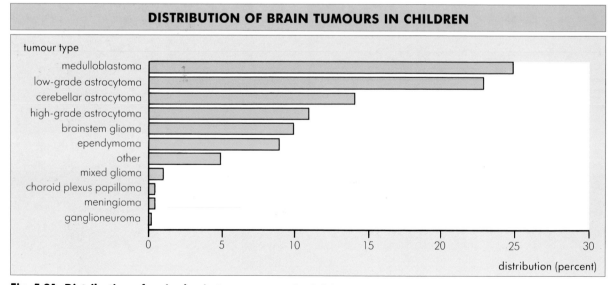

Fig. 5.21 Distribution of major brain tumour types in children.

physical signs including impaired heel to toe walking, poor coordination of the finger–nose test and often marked nystagmus. Symptoms of raised ICP are often marked. The peak age of incidence is four to ten years, and boys are affected more frequently than girls. The tumour has striking histological features often with cell rosettes, and again with a marked propensity for spread within the CNS. This occurs via CSF pathways, and tumour nodules may be present either in the brain itself or thoughout the spinal cord. Medulloblastomas comprise over one-third of all childhood brain tumours, and are often curable (see below).

Another important group includes those arising from the posterior end of the third ventricle which because of their anatomical site tend to cause early symptoms of raised pressure, though they may reach

a substantial size before presentation. They generally originate from the pineal gland (Figs 5.23 and 2.7), and are often germ cell tumours of one type or another, akin to those arising from the testis. These tumours are thought to be due embryologically to cell rests, which can occur almost anywhere in the midline. Although very rare, these tumours are important since they are often curable.

Treatment of Brain Tumours

Surgery
Wherever possible, a brain tumour should be biopsied as its precise nature can hardly ever be determined accurately from the clinical or radiological evidence (Fig. 5.24). Although this point may seem obvious, it lies at the heart of a controversy in neuro-oncology

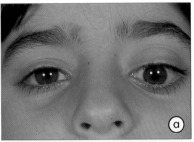

Fig. 5.22 Optic nerve glioma.
(a) Unilateral proptosis of the left eye, the commonest presenting feature. (b) There was a large optic nerve glioma involving the whole of the left optic nerve.

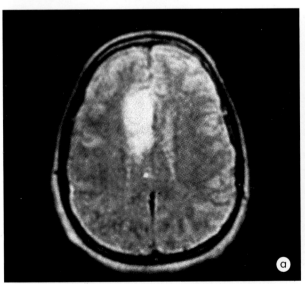

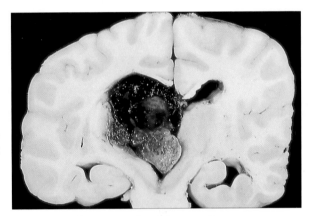

Fig. 5.23 Primary cerebral germ cell tumour. Histology in these cases is widely variable. This was an immature teratoma occurring in a 12-year-old boy, probably originating from the pineal gland. CSF seeding is characteristic of these germ cell tumours (see Fig. 2.7). All types of teratoma, mixed tumours and pure seminoma may be encountered. Courtesy of Dr H. Okazaki.

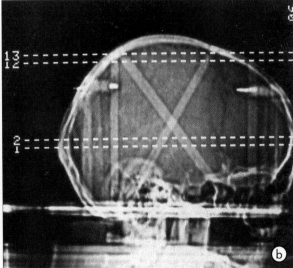

Fig. 5.24 Stereotactic biopsy. (a) MRI showing deeply situated tumour of uncertain histology in the corpus callosum. (b) CT scan of patient taken in the stereotactic frame. The lesion proved to be a low-grade astrocytoma.

since some neurologists feel the treatment of adult glioma to be so unsatisfactory as to be hardly worthwhile. Even with what radiologically appears to be a low-grade glioma, a conservative approach is sometimes taken, the justification being that the tumour has a long natural history anyway. Though many patients have benefitted from this approach, there are certainly those in whom a more aggressive approach would have been productive – for example patients who unexpectedly prove to be suffering from a benign, operable lesion such as a meningioma, or those in whom the glioma has been completely resected with a possible chance of cure. With children expert advice needs to be sought in every case.

Whether or not tumour removal should be attempted is a matter requiring considerable judgement. The neurosurgeon's decision may depend to a great extent on the patient's circumstances and previous personality since there is always a risk of neurological damage, even when the surgery is limited to biopsy. Most surgeons would attempt removal of a frontal lesion thought to be a glioma, or of a parietal tumour which was not too large, potentially completely resectable, and situated in the nondominant hemisphere. Resection of very large or recurrent tumours may even require removal of part of the skull. Tumours close to the motor cortex on the dominant side, or those involving the speech area, are generally regarded as inoperable (see Fig. 5.4). More deeply situated lesions, for example in the thalamus, are unresectable (see Fig. 5.3) though sometimes amenable to stereotactic biopsy using a rigid frame applied to the patient's head, and allowing for fine needle CT-guided biopsy to a very high degree of precision (see Fig. 5.24). Cerebellar tumours are often resectable, and in the case of children with medulloblastoma or cerebellar astrocytoma, an attempt at surgical resection is an essential part of the management in virtually every case. Even where the tumour cannot be delivered in its entirety, partial or subtotal resection is well worth attempting, particularly with low-grade tumours or medulloblastomas, and it is sometimes possible for the surgeon to remove a large portion by suction methods. Postoperatively, some patients recover remarkably quickly, while others, particularly children with medulloblastoma, may remain obtunded, rather silent and withdrawn for many weeks. Increasingly, deep seated tumours of the pineal are also being biopsied or removed, because of the importance of histological clarification at this site.

Complications of surgery include direct damage to local structures (obviously important in tumours near the motor cortex), haemorrhage and infection. The advantages and disadvantages of attempting resection must always be weighed; if partial or subtotal removal seems a vain hope, then the surgeon must consider whether there is anything to be gained by even attempting a biopsy.

Radiotherapy

In many patients with brain tumours, radiotherapy is a critical part of management. Indications for radiotherapy are listed in Fig. 5.25.

INDICATIONS FOR RADIOTHERAPY
Low-grade glioma
Partial resection Inoperable recurrence
High-grade glioma
Postoperatively in virtually every case since complete resection is rarely achieved Palliation of symptoms in recurrent disease (re-irradiation is sometimes possible provided the interval from previous treatment is long enough)
Others
Definitive treatment e.g. medulloblastoma of childhood (often postoperative, pineal germinoma, intracerebral lymphoma) Definitive treatment in large pituitary tumours (often postoperative) Brain metastases Inoperable benign conditions, e.g. meningioma, sometimes in conjunction with surgery

Fig. 5.25 Indications for radiotherapy in brain tumour patients.

RADIATION EFFECTS ON THE BRAIN
Acute
Nausea, vomiting, ataxia, dysarthria, somnolence
Early delayed
At about 2 months, recovery after 6–8 weeks; usually transient—30% improve spontaneously but can progress and prove fatal; probably analogous to l'Hermitte syndrome; somnolence and lethargy common, CT changes may occur; important to recognize and not to assume tumour progression
Late
Occurs 6 months to 5 years after treatment; white matter more sensitive than grey; necrosis relates to dose, fraction size, size of radiation volume; diagnostically difficult as recurrence of brain tumour may occur at the same time; necrosis, demyelination, gliosis, fibrin extravasation, endothelial proliferation

Fig. 5.26 Radiation effects on the brain.

In adults, radiotherapy is not necessary for patients with completely resected low-grade tumours, though the evidence suggests that it adds to the likelihood of local control (and probably survival) in patients where the resection has been incomplete. In high-grade gliomas, the results of radiotherapy, though not very good, are certainly better than those of surgery alone, suggesting a worthwhile degree of biological activity. In patients with glioblastoma multiforme (grade IV gliomas), cure is virtually never seen, though patients with gliomas of slightly lesser degree (typically grade III tumours) have a small chance of cure (about 10%) with radiotherapy (see Fig. 5.16). None are cured by surgery alone. These are common indications for radiotherapy, and the treatment usually involves very generous treatment fields, often to the whole brain or if not, the whole of the hemisphere containing the high-grade tumour. It is generally possible to achieve this without producing further neurological damage, though late adverse effects can be problematic (Fig. 5.26). Hair loss is an inevitable consequence, and this may be very prolonged or even permanent depending of course on the dose employed. Treatment generally takes from three to six weeks depending on the policy of the radiotherapy department, and the normal brain is surprisingly tolerant, though care has to be taken to avoid damage to the eye and upper cervical cord. In primary intracerebral lymphoma radiotherapy is generally the definitive treatment, though prognosis is extremely guarded.

For pituitary tumours opinions with regard to radiotherapy are again varied. There is no doubt that the local control and cure rates of large pituitary tumours and particularly chromophobe adenomas, the commonest variety of all, are improved by radiotherapy, generally following total or subtotal resection in the majority of cases (see Fig. 5.7).

Although this is particularly true for non-functioning tumours, hormone-producing pituitary adenomas (see Figs 5.9–5.12) with their often devastating effects, may not be fully resectable and despite their slightly lower radiation sensitivity, should still be vigorously treated. With the advent of CT and MRI, small precisely localized radiation fields can now be employed to focus on the pituitary, with almost no risk of damage to local structures. Tailor-made immobilization shells are used for such patients, just as with head and neck tumours. Craniopharyngiomas should be treated in a similar way. There is no longer any doubt that radiotherapy reduces their recurrence rate. They are almost always only partly resectable because of the heavy calcific deposits and the tendency to form tumour cysts which recur after surgery alone (see Fig. 5.8). Adult meningiomas should always be resected where possible, though some sites are particularly difficult. Where the surgical resection is incomplete radiotherapy should be offered.

In children, radiotherapy is often curative (Fig. 5.27). This applies particularly to medulloblastoma, the most common of childhood brain tumours and amongst the most radiosensitive. With adequate treatment, at least half can be cured, though the treatment is particularly strenuous since it involves both total excision of the tumour where possible, as well as postoperative radiotherapy not only to the tumour bed in the cerebellum, but also to the whole of the central nervous system. The whole brain and spine need to be given prophylactic treatment in view of the known pattern of spread through the CSF, a treatment taking approximately eight weeks to complete. Because of the skill involved in setting up and treating these children this treatment should only be undertaken in special centres where children are frequently seen, and it is surprising how co-operative most children are, given time, encouragement and the minimum of sedation. Acute adverse effects of treatment are generally quite acceptable, though a careful watch has to be kept on the blood count, in view of the volume of marrow in the child's spine that is exposed to radiotherapy. Long term adverse effects are of course more important, and surprisingly have been recognized only recently. Chief amongst these is growth failure, which is almost inevitable and results from reduction in growth hormone production due to pituitary irradiation, together with loss of spinal height from the direct irradiation. Now that this has been recognized, regular growth clinics for children treated with

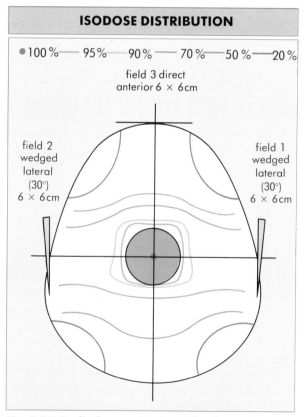

Fig. 5.27 Radiotherapy isodose distribution.
Typical isodose curve with supervoltage equipment using a three field treatment plan for small non-functioning pituitary adenoma.

radiotherapy have been instituted, and once growth failure has been documented, growth hormone is usually given until puberty, often on a daily basis, to ensure that the child's development remains satisfactory. Since this will be a long term requirement, the GP's role is crucial, to say nothing of the emotional support that the child and family will need.

In addition to loss of growth, the child may also suffer some degree of hypothyroidism (generally not severe but recognizable biochemically) due to the exit beam from the direct spinal field, which passes out through the anterior neck. In girls, primary ovarian failure is sometimes seen, presumably as a result of side scatter of the radiation beam at the level of the ovaries. It is therefore essential for any child with a previously treated brain tumour to attend such a clinic on a regular basis until the problem period has passed.

Certain other childhood brain tumours require similar treatment, notably ependymomas and germ cell tumours (usually pineal in origin), which also have a propensity for spread throughout the CSF. In childhood gliomas, radiotherapy is limited to the tumour site itself, though this may be quite extensive, as in the case of the brain stem glioma in which radiotherapy is particularly important because of surgical inaccessibility (see Fig. 4.11).

Chemotherapy

Chemotherapy has not yet established itself as part of the routine management of adult brain tumours, though there is some suggestion that it may be active in certain circumstances. For example, chemotherapy sensitivity testing has documented a degree of drug responsiveness in some cases of high-grade adult glioma, and trials are currently in progress to assess whether or not this treatment could offer clinical benefit. For this reason, some adult patients with glioma may increasingly be recommended to undergo adjuvant chemotherapy. The most commonly used drugs used are cisplatin, procarbazine, vincristine and CCNU (see chapter 3).

In general these drugs are well tolerated and are given only every six weeks or so, on an outpatient basis. Likewise, chemotherapy is sometimes used for recurrent medulloblastoma (or within clinical trials as part of the primary treatment) since there is clearly some degree of responsiveness. It seems that very young patients with local extension of this tumour, where resectability is in doubt, may benefit from chemotherapy, though postoperative radiotherapy clearly remains the more important of the non-surgical modalities.

Pineal germ cell tumours are highly responsive to chemotherapy. Pineal teratomas are probably best treated in this way, though admittedly these tumours are extremely rare, and are therefore best treated only in special centres. The choice of drugs should essentially be the same as those used in testicular teratoma.

Supportive Care

Patients with brain tumours need considerable help though many return to a surprisingly active life after treatment, even where the tumour is of high grade and survival is likely to be limited. Long term treatment with anti-convulsants (usually phenytoin, 300–400mg per day) is often required, particularly if the patient has a history of convulsions. In addition, many patients require dexamethasone during radiotherapy to control cerebral oedema, which results partly from the tumour and is made worse for a period by the radiotherapy. The majority of patients are able to discontinue dexamethasone once the radiotherapy is completed. Indeed, this is one of the major advantages of radiotherapy, since most patients with high-grade glioma accompanied by local oedema would otherwise require long-term steroid therapy, thereby becoming increasingly cushingoid and weakened by the prolonged adverse effects.

Neurological loss associated with brain tumours – particularly hemiplegia and dysphagia – should be managed supportively using the same techniques as for stroke victims, and some cerebrovascular units do accept brain tumour patients for rehabilitation. It is best to encourage patients to return to work and children to resume normal schooling within a month or two of completion of treatment. Patients receiving adjuvant chemotherapy can generally continue working and a good clinical unit will encourage this – for example giving the chemotherapy on a Friday afternoon, so that any residual nausea will have settled by the start of the next working week.

Patients with recurrent disease always present enormous problems of management. In general, the longer the period from the initial treatment, the more possible is a second attempt. In some patients with low-grade gliomas and oligodendrogliomas, this period may be five or ten years, giving at least an opportunity for a second attempt with radiotherapy. The possibility of radiation induced brain damage is much higher second time around, and the radiotherapy is therefore necessarily more limited. Occasionally, a second attempt at surgical resection is possible, though with increased likelihood of surgical damage.

Prognosis

Prognosis in brain tumours varies enormously, from cure of the child with medulloblastoma, with few adverse effects besides growth disturbance and temporary hair loss, to only a few months in the case of most patients with high-grade glioma (see Fig. 5.16). Pituitary tumours and meningiomas are generally cured by surgery and/or radiotherapy. The occasional cure of an adult patient with a grade III glioma is one of the most gratifying experiences for the specialist, and therefore justifies vigorous treatment of these patients, quite apart from the symptomatic benefits that may accrue.

Cancer of the Head and Neck

6

Introduction

Although constituting only 4% of all cancers diagnosed each year in the UK, cancers of the head and neck pose exceptional problems of management and rehabilitation. Not only are they highly visible and sometimes disfiguring, but also the major treatment options of radical radiotherapy and major surgery may themselves lead to serious and long-term secondary problems. Remarkable advances have been made in the past decade, particularly in the field of reconstructive surgery. Patients with locally advanced tumours, though still facing an uncertain prognosis, may now look forward to an improved quality of life with a much reduced probability of irreversible treatment-related damage. From the technical point of view, these tumours often represent the most difficult treatment decisions in cancer therapy, and there is little doubt that a joint clinic, run by a surgeon and radiotherapist but enjoying close links with medical oncologists, pathologists and oral and dental surgeons, offers the best quality of service to the patient.

Aetiology

A good deal is known about the causation of cancers of the head and neck. There is a wide geographical variability with regard to incidence; in Southeast Asia for example, particularly in southern China and Hong Kong, carcinoma of the nasopharynx is the commonest cancer of all. It has been known for many years that the Epstein–Barr virus can often be recovered from tissue samples in patients with this type of tumour. It seems likely, however, that the major causation of nasopharyngeal cancer is a dietary one, with dried smoked fish, often ingested from relatively early childhood, as the culpable agent.

In Western societies a high alcohol (particularly spirit) intake, coupled with excessive cigarette consumption, is a consistent finding in the large majority of patients presenting to head and neck cancer clinics. Males outnumber females by 5:1, and these patients are often socially isolated, from social classes 4 and 5, frequently with a history of poor general nutrition and oral hygiene.

In the past syphilis was an important cause of leukoplakia of the tongue, itself a predisposing feature for carcinoma of the tongue.

In the Indian sub-continent, the practice of chewing betel-nut, particularly where this is placed against the gum and left for long periods, is clearly related to the high incidence of cancer. In some parts of the world, the lighted end of a cigarette is inserted orally, and this is associated with a high incidence of carcinoma of the palate.

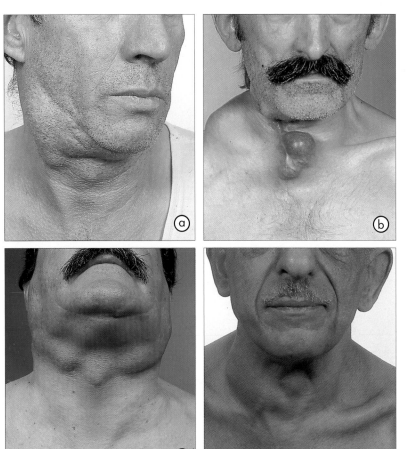

Fig. 6.1 Lymph node metastases in head and neck tumours.
(a) Carcinoma of the tonsil with typical mid-cervical node.
(b) Chordoma with widespread unilateral neck metastases.
(c) Diffuse lymphoma with bilateral bulky lymphadenopathy.
(d) Anaplastic carcinoma of the thyroid with typical mass anteriorly situated in the neck and lower cervical node metastases.

Of the occupational causes of head and neck cancer, the best example is the unusual adenocarcinoma of the nasal fossa, first noticed in and around High Wycombe, England, in hardwood furniture workers, which was clearly related to the inhalation of small particles of wood dust.

In general, it seems likely that alcohol plays a greater part in the causation of cancers of the oral cavity and oropharynx, whilst cigarette smoking is more important as a cause of carcinomas of the larynx.

Pathology

In the UK, the commonest primary sites include larynx, oral cavity, oropharynx and lip, while tumours of the nasal fossa, paranasal sinuses, nasopharynx, hypopharynx and upper oesophagus are less common. Carcinoma of the thyroid gland, though not generally regarded as a typical head and neck tumour, is dealt with separately at the end of this chapter.

Histologically, the majority of these tumours are squamous carcinomas of various degrees of differentiation. Some carcinomas of the oral cavity, particularly those of the tongue and buccal mucosa, may exhibit widespread dysplasia in the surrounding epithelium, and/or areas of carcinoma in situ, presumably as a result of chronic exposure to some carcinogenic insult. This so-called 'field change' is found in a substantial portion of such cases, and it is not unusual to encounter patients with more than one primary site of invasive cancer, sometimes situated within the oral cavity alone, or spread more widely throughout the aerodigestive epithelium as far down as the larynx and hypopharynx. Nasopharyngeal carcinomas are typically undifferentiated and may be difficult to classify, a particular problem for the pathologist and clinician since lymphomas are more common at this site than elsewhere in the head and neck, with the sole exception of the oropharynx (particularly the tonsil).

Patients may of course present not with the symptoms of the primary disease, but with neck node metastases – not an uncommon problem in head and neck cancer, and diagnostically of great importance (Fig. 6.1), since carcinoma of the bronchus, Hodgkin's disease and non-Hodgkin's lymphoma can also present in this way. The precise site of the node metastases in the neck may give important clues to the likely primary tumour; upper cervical neck nodes are more likely to be due to supraglottic laryngeal carcinoma or a tumour of the oropharynx, while those in the submandibular or lower cervical area are more likely to be due to a carcinoma of the tongue or floor of mouth (Fig. 6.2). A node deeply situated in the supraclavicular fossa may be due to a gastric carcinoma, or a carcinoma of the bronchus or thyroid. A tendency to ulcerate makes the diagnosis more likely to be a squamous

Fig. 6.2 The relationship of the neck nodes to the primary site.

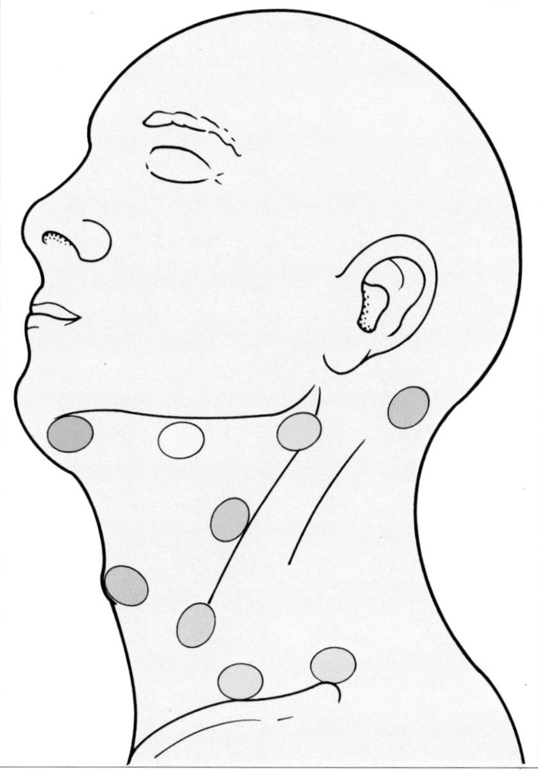

Node(s)	Site
Submandibular triangle	Submandibular gland, oral cavity (especially floor of mouth), lower lip, paranasal sinuses, facial skin
Superior deep jugular (jugulodigastric)	Paranasal sinuses, nasopharynx, oropharynx, oral cavity, hypopharynx, parotid gland, supraglottic larynx, lower pinna
Sub- or post-occipital	Nasopharynx, posterior, scalp, post-auricular skin, exterior ear
Midjugular	Hypopharynx, thyroid, larynx, oropharynx
Prelaryngeal	Thyroid, larynx, lymphoma
Lower jugular	Thyroid, larynx, cervical oesophagus, infraclavicular primaries (including thoracic)
Supraclavicular	Thyroid, cervical oesophagus, infraclavicular primaries (including abdominal)
Submental	Oral cavity, lymphoma, salivary glands

THE RELATIONSHIP OF NECK NODES TO PRIMARY SITES

carcinoma than, for instance, a lymphoma. Bulky bilateral neck disease, particularly in a young person and without any obvious primary site within the head and neck, is more likely to be due to lymphoma than carcinoma. In histologically doubtful cases, the advent of sophisticated immunocytochemical staining has led to much greater confidence in tumour classification.

Rarer tumours include sarcoma, embryonal tumours and melanomas. Salivary gland tumours are discussed below.

◼ Carcinoma of the Larynx

This is the commonest head and neck carcinoma encountered in the UK and almost invariably occurs in smokers, with a male predominance of 5:1. It is commonest in the 50–70 year age group and most frequently effects the true glottis (the vocal cords), although in certain parts of Europe, including Scandinavia, supraglottic tumours are common (Fig. 6.3).

Hoarseness of the voice is much the most common presenting feature; general practitioners should appreciate that any history of hoarseness persisting beyond three weeks should lead to an urgent referral to an ENT surgeon, since early laryngeal carcinoma is easily identified using indirect laryngoscopy, an examination which can be carried out in a matter of minutes in the outpatient department. In difficult cases the newer technique of flexible nasendoscopy which also gives an excellent view of the vocal cords can be used (Fig. 6.4). The hoarseness is of course due to interference of normal phonation due to the irregularity of the cord which results from tumour ulceration or local extension. Other important malignant causes of hoarseness include a paralysed vocal cord from an intrathoracic malignancy such as carcinoma of the bronchus (usually the left cord is paralysed, because of the lengthy and exposed course of the recurrent laryngeal nerve on this side) and direct encroachment of the larynx from other extrinsic malignancies.

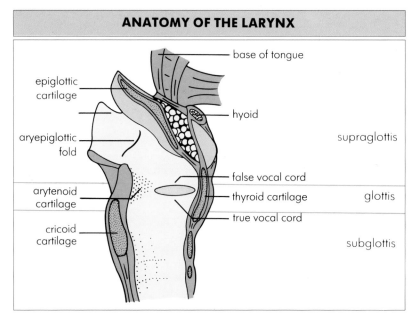

ANATOMY OF THE LARYNX

- base of tongue
- epiglottic cartilage
- hyoid
- aryepiglottic fold
- supraglottis
- arytenoid cartilage
- false vocal cord
- thyroid cartilage
- glottis
- cricoid cartilage
- true vocal cord
- subglottis

Fig. 6.3 Anatomy of the larynx. In most of the Western world, the commonest site of primary laryngeal carcinoma is the vocal cord (glottis), although in parts of Scandinavia supraglottic carcinoma is more often seen. Subglottic carcinomas are very unusual.

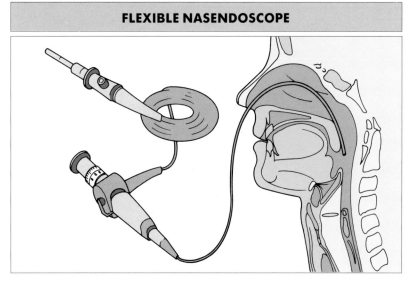

FLEXIBLE NASENDOSCOPE

Fig. 6.4 Flexible nasendoscope. This apparatus, which can be used simply in the outpatient department, gives excellent views of the nasopharynx and the vocal cords. It is particularly useful in patients who cannot tolerate the mirror examination in indirect laryngoscopy.

It is also important to recognize that there are many non-malignant causes of hoarseness, both organic, such as viral laryngitis, and functional, such as dysphonia plicae ventricularis, a disorder in which the patient unwittingly approximates the false vocal cords instead of the true glottis, producing a disordered soft voice which is easily confused with the true hoarseness of malignant origin.

The typical appearance of a carcinoma of the vocal cord is shown in Fig. 6.5, and the most commonly used classification, which is crucial to both management and prognosis, is shown in Fig. 6.6. In fact, this TNM system is widely used for head and neck tumours (and indeed for cancers on other parts of the body) and allows worthwhile inter-departmental comparisons of treatment outcome, as well

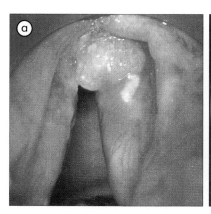
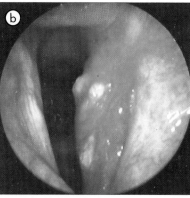

Fig. 6.5 Carcinoma of the vocal cords. (a) Carcinoma of the anterior vocal cords (commissure). (b) Carcinoma of the right vocal cord – direct view.

Fig. 6.6 TNM staging system for laryngeal cancer.

STAGING OF LARYNGEAL CANCER

T–Primary

Tis	Carcinoma *in situ*
T1a	Tumour confined to one vocal cord, with normal mobility
T1b	Tumour involving both cords, with normal mobility
T2	Tumour extending to supraglottic or subglottic region with normal or impaired cord mobility
T3	Tumour limited to the larynx with vocal cord fixation
T4	Tumour destroying cartilage or extending beyond the larynx

N–Regional Lymph Nodes

N0	Cervical nodes not palpable
N1	Homolateral non-fixed palpable lymph nodes
N2	Palpable bilateral, contralateral or midline lymph nodes, non-fixed
N3	Fixed cervical lymph nodes

M–Distant Metastasis

M0	No distant metastasis
M1	Distant metastasis present

Stage Grouping

Stage	Classification
I	T1 N0
II	T2 N0
III	T3 N0 T4 N0 T1 to T4 with N1 T1 to T4 with N2
IV	T1 to T4 with N3 T1 to T4 with N0 to N3 with M1

as providing a consistent method of describing and staging the tumours. Important investigations include a chest X-ray to rule out concomitant carcinoma of the bronchus and careful indirect laryngoscopy by an experienced ENT consultant, who would usually visualize the lesion with confidence and be able to comment on the mobility of the vocal cords. Nasendoscopy, which can be readily performed in the outpatients department using local anaesthetic, will give additional information in difficult cases where, for instance, patients gag with the mirror, or where the anatomy of the primary lesion makes it invisible. Direct laryngoscopy with examination under anaesthetic (EUA) may also be necessary. Radiologically, the early laryngeal carcinoma (T1, T2) is normally best visualized by conventional anteroposterior tomography (Fig. 6.7), though larger lesions may be better demonstrated on CT scanning, which will often give additional information about their local invasiveness. Careful clinical examination must also include palpation of the neck, since nodal involvement is often found, particularly with supraglottic primary tumours. In advanced cases the primary tumour may itself be easily felt, or occasionally even seen externally as a mass at the root of the neck (Fig. 6.8).

Of the three major sites within the larynx, sub-glottic primary carcinomas are the least common in the UK, usually presenting with stridor as well as hoarseness, due to upper tracheal obstruction. Early treatment by tracheostomy (though not necessarily laryngectomy) is often wise, so that the airway is protected during treatment. Many surgeons recommend early laryngectomy if the vocal cord is fixed in such cases, though radical irradiation may be used in an attempt to conserve the larynx, reserving surgery for radiation failure, as with the other varieties of primary laryngeal carcinoma.

For early laryngeal tumours (T1, T2, N0), radical irradiation is the treatment of choice, with the hope that the tumour will prove responsive and a cure will be obtained without recourse to laryngectomy. This is particularly true in glottic lesions (which form the majority of laryngeal tumours) since a total laryngectomy would otherwise be necessary. For T1 tumours radiotherapy alone is undoubtedly the treatment of choice, the cure rate being of the order of 90%. For T2 lesions, that is for those with minimal invasion and no cord fixation, the cure rate by radiotherapy alone falls to about 65%. Some clinics have therefore started to use chemotherapy routinely, in addition to radiotherapy, in the hope that this will yield higher local control rates. Experience in several combined head and neck oncology clinics supports this view. In early glottic cancers, where the incidence of neck node involvement is very low, it is not usually necessary to give prophylactic irradiation to the neck, though for supraglottic primary sites, which have a much higher incidence of node involvement, adjuvant neck irradiation is usually advised. This is particularly so with the higher T stages, which carry a concomitantly higher risk.

For more advanced cancers (T3, T4 and N1–3), there is a wide variety of approaches in current use. It is often worth adopting a non-surgical policy in the first instance, since there is no doubt that some patients in this category are cured without laryngectomy, and return of cord mobility may sometimes occur with recovery of near-normal speech. The possible role of chemotherapy in such cases is discussed at the end of this chapter. Many believe that additional treatment with chemotherapy may give higher response and cure rates – this question is currently the subject of major national trials. Nonetheless, in the majority of cases surgical resection will be required, some clinics preferring to recommend a surgical policy from the outset. Treatment of advanced lesions is rarely straightforward, and the overall strategy will often depend as much on the general fitness of the patient as on the precise details of the tumour anatomy.

A high proportion of deaths are due to causes other than the cancer; such patients are usually in a poor state of health, often with high alcohol and cigarette consumption. As with head and neck carcinomas at other sites, prognosis is critically dependent on the T and N stages and, in particular, on the presence and extent of node involvement.

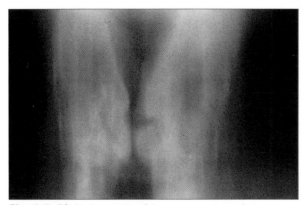

Fig. 6.7 Plain tomographic appearance of a carcinoma of the right vocal cord. Note the obliteration of the laryngeal ventricle and generally bulky appearance of the cord.

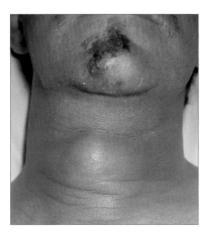

Fig. 6.8 Advanced laryngeal carcinoma. Unusually, the tumour mass is visible in the midline anteriorly, at the root of the neck.

Tumours of the Oral Cavity

The aetiology of these tumours is discussed above. Important sites include the anterior two-thirds of the tongue (the mobile portion), the floor of the mouth, the upper and lower alveolar margins, the buccal mucosa and the hard palate. The lip is considered separately.

Presentation is usually to the patient's GP or dentist, most commonly with an ulcerated and uncomfortable sore area (Figs 6.9 & 6.10). This should be taken seriously if it fails to heal within three to six weeks with no obvious explanation (such as an ill-fitting denture or obvious oral candidiasis). The typical appearance of a carcinoma of the tongue is shown in Fig. 6.11. The tumour is easily visible, although lesions in the floor of the mouth are often missed – a careful inspection with the patient's tongue elevated is critical to diagnosis (Fig. 6.12). Some patients with oral cavity tumours present with a node in the neck, without an obvious primary site visible to the patient.

Apart from careful examination and chest X-ray, an important investigation is the orthopantomogram (OPG), a means of displaying radiologically the whole of the patient's mandible (Fig. 6.13) which gives important information regarding local invasiveness of the tumour. Bone invasion invariably means that the tumour is advanced (T4) and should be treated accordingly. Careful palpation of the neck is mandatory. CT scanning is helpful in selected cases, particularly in tumours of the upper jaw, where local extension to the maxillary air sinuses or nasal fossa can be difficult to determine clinically.

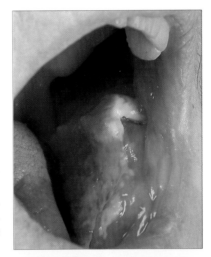

Fig. 6.9 Carcinoma of the oral cavity. This patient presented to her dentist with an oral ulcer which she attributed to ill-fitting dentures. The epithelial lining of the cheek is an uncommon primary site within the oral cavity.

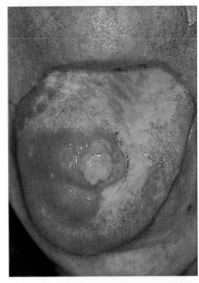

Fig. 6.11 Carcinoma of the tongue. This is a locally advanced tumour which has erupted through the dorsum of the tongue and was also visible on the inferior surface.

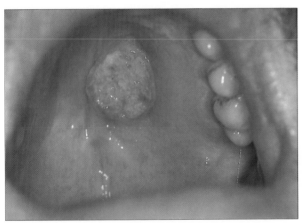

Fig. 6.10 Carcinoma of the palate. This well circumscribed palatal tumour was not noticed by the patient at all and was detected on a routine dental examination.

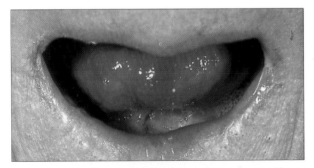

Fig. 6.12 Carcinoma of the floor of the mouth. This oral cavity site is easily missed unless the patient's tongue is carefully elevated. This has the typical appearance of a necrotic, non-healing, clearly demarcated ulcer and is most frequently situated in the midline.

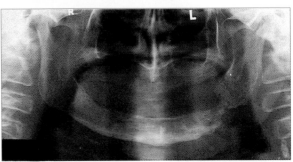

Fig. 6.13 Orthopantomogram (OPG). Note the obvious bone erosion at the angle of the mandible at the left side. The right side is normal in this edentulous patient.

The commonest primary site is the anterior tongue; it is well recognized that even small tumours can be locally very invasive, since the lymphatic and blood supplies to the tongue are so rich and the bulky muscular interior is so closely applied to the relatively thin epithelium.

Small lesions are best treated by surgical excision or a radioactive implant, which should provide excellent local control without unacceptable immobility. One disadvantage of surgery, particularly for tongue cancers, is that a relatively large portion may have to be excised, reducing the quality of speech. With a radiation implant, local control can usually be achieved without loss of tongue bulk, or undue long-term radiation-induced dry mouth. These treatments are best confined to tumours below 2cm in size.

For more advanced lesions, the choice again lies between surgical resection, with or without post-operative radiotherapy, or an attempt at completely non-surgical treatment, possibly employing chemotherapy. The drawback to the surgical approach is that where post-operative radiotherapy is routinely given, the patient necessarily has to face both surgical and radiotherapeutic complications without any clear evidence of benefit, whereas in patients treated by radiotherapy (or chemotherapy) alone there is at least a chance that the surgery can be avoided. Despite this traditionalist view, it is important to bear in mind that impressive advances in surgical technique have been made over the last decade, particularly with the advent of local or free-flap reconstructive grafting (Fig. 6.14) in which wide surgical incision is immediately followed (at the same surgical procedure) by repair of the defect using the patient's own tissues, for example a myocutaneous or vascularized graft using forearm skin. This technique may allow excellent functional results while avoiding the long-term oral discomfort which often occurs with radiotherapy. No formal comparison between these techniques has yet been made.

Where neck nodes are clinically apparent (particularly in N2, N3 cases) the tumour must be regarded

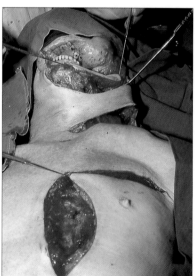
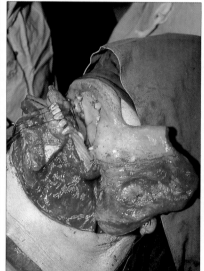
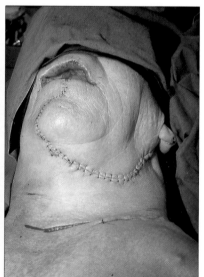

Fig. 6.14 Delto-pectoral flap reconstruction following excision of a recurrent oropharyngeal carcinoma. Although this gives a satisfactory coverage and cosmesis, free-flap myocutaneous grafting is increasingly used.

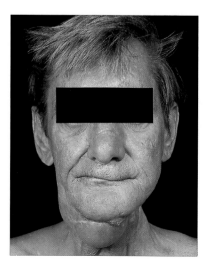

Fig. 6.15 Radical neck dissection. This patient has undergone radical neck dissection on the left and now presents with massive recurrent midline nodes in the submental region. The primary lesion was in the oropharynx and base of tongue.

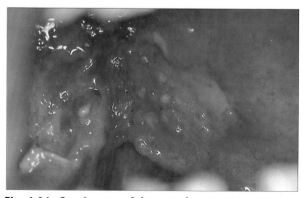

Fig. 6.16 Carcinoma of the oropharynx (retromolar trigone, faucial arch and palate). This was a locally advanced (T3) tumour presenting with dysphagia and marked weight loss.

as likely to be surgically incurable; radical neck dissection followed by local irradiation (Fig. 6.15), or treatment with radiotherapy alone, is generally recommended, in the hope that this will control the nodal disease. 'Salvage' surgical procedures can be safely performed for radiation failure.

Tumours of the minor salivary glands may present as lesions of the oral cavity, and are dealt with towards the end of this chapter, together with tumours of the parotid and other major salivary glands.

Tumours of the Oropharynx

This is a less accessible site than either the larynx or oral cavity and includes the posterior third (base) of the tongue, the soft palate, and the posterior and lateral walls of the pharynx directly behind the oral cavity, including the faucial pillars and tonsil (Fig. 6.16). The primary symptom is dysphagia and the tumours are often more advanced at presentation, perhaps because of their low visibility and symptomatology. They may evade casual inspection and unfortunately spread relatively early, with a marked propensity for early lymph node involvement.

Advances in surgical technique have once again led to primary surgical resection becoming a real competitor to local irradiation. Composite resections of tumours of, for example, the faucial pillar and tonsillar regions can be made using a mandibular splitting operation for access, reconstructed with a free graft at a single procedure (see Fig. 6.14). For small lesions, the alternative of local implantation by radioactive wires or seeds (such as iridium-192 or radioactive gold grains) can yield excellent results. For more advanced tumours (especially those with node involvement), local external beam irradiation, with or without chemotherapy, is the treatment of choice; however, surgical resection is sometimes still feasible, sophisticated grafting procedures, using skin pedicles or jejunal transposition, allowing replacement of substantial portions of the pharyngeal mucosa.

Tumours of the Nasopharynx

These tumours, very common in the Far East, are relatively rare in Western nations; of the cases diagnosed in the UK, a substantial number occur in Chinese immigrants. Because of the inaccessibility of the primary site, presentation is often late, either with a gland in the neck, for which no obvious primary site within the oral cavity or oropharynx can readily be detected, or by nasal obstruction, particularly when the tumour has encroached on the posterior part of the nasal fossa. Otalgia (earache) is also common, particularly where there is obstruction to the eustachian tube. Because of the proximity of the nasopharynx to the base of the skull and inferior surface of the midbrain, focal cranial nerve palsies

are common, especially III, IV, VI and (with more posteriorly placed lesions) IX–XII (Fig. 6.17). Important investigations include chest X-ray and a CT scan of the nasopharynx and nasal sinuses (Fig. 6.18), which will give accurate information on the local extent of the tumour. EUA is always necessary with panendoscopy, particularly in the patient presenting with neck nodes. It is not unusual for the primary site to be undetectable, and blind biopsies of the nasopharynx may give the correct diagnosis.

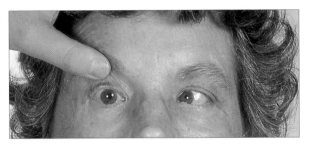

Fig. 6.17 Cranial nerve palsies from local extension to the base of the brain from a large carcinoma of the nasopharynx. This patient has been asked to look towards the right side. The ophthalmoplegia of the right eye is caused by a sixth nerve palsy; she also had a ptosis on the right.

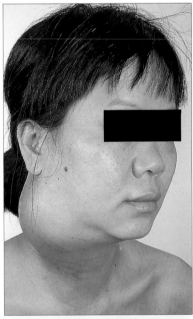
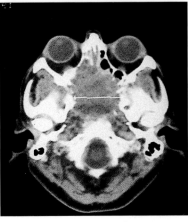

Fig. 6.18 Carcinoma of the nasopharynx. This patient presented with massive nodes in the right side of the neck and CT scan confirmed complete replacement of the nasopharynx and bone destruction by the primary tumour. Following radiotherapy the neck mass resolved entirely.

Treatment is entirely nonsurgical in view of local invasiveness, early nodal spread, and surgical inaccessibility. Radical irradiation is the treatment of choice, including treatment of the neck in every case (whether clinically evident disease is present or not), a difficult technical task because of the large volume irradiated (Fig. 6.19).

Chemotherapy, not usually given as primary treatment, may be valuable in relapsed cases, particularly since many of these patients are young and fit and – unlike other major head and neck sites – surgical salvage is impossible. Although relatively inaccessible, recurrent nasopharyngeal cancer may be treatable by a radiation implant, though considerable skill is required to place the grains accurately behind the palate.

Tumours of the Hypopharynx and Upper Oesophagus

The anatomy of this region is particularly complex (Fig. 6.20), and the sites are difficult to visualize and image accurately. Most patients present with dysphagia or cachexia; in patients with post-cricoid carcinomas (a site, unusually, more common in females) a history of chronic anaemia is often elicited together, in textbook cases, with an oesophageal web (Plummer–Vinson syndrome). Other sites include posterior and lateral pharyngeal walls.

Management of these tumours is extremely unsatisfactory. Early lymph node involvement is common, often to the mediastinum, and the patient may be unable to tolerate any attempt at radical treatment, whether surgical or not, in view of the poor nutrition and weight loss which is so common. Combinations of surgery, radiotherapy and chemotherapy are often used, though surgical resection invariably requires organ transposition, for example using colon or stomach 'pull up', to provide an adequate upper oesophagus. Although occasionally patients do remarkably well, the majority are not curable by any known treatment.

The majority of upper oesophageal lesions are squamous in origin, and are generally thought more suitable for radiotherapy than surgery. The treatment requires a demanding and difficult technique – the common problem of submucosal spread means that the radiation fields must be extended much further down the oesophageal length than seems clinically evident from inspection or barium swallow examination (Fig. 6.21). Many patients are more suitable for palliative than radical treatment, particu-

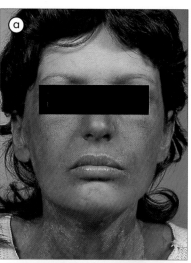
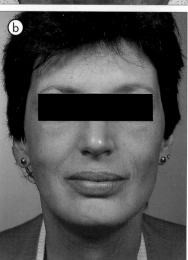

Fig. 6.19 Carcinoma of the nasopharynx. (a) Typical radiation reaction following treatment. (b) The appearance 4 months later, showing complete resolution of the fierce desquamation. The patient is alive and well, five years later.

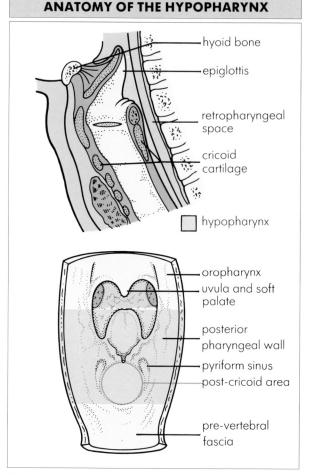

ANATOMY OF THE HYPOPHARYNX

- hyoid bone
- epiglottis
- retropharyngeal space
- cricoid cartilage

☐ hypopharynx

- oropharynx
- uvula and soft palate
- posterior pharyngeal wall
- pyriform sinus
- post-cricoid area
- pre-vertebral fascia

Fig. 6.20 Anatomy of the hypopharynx, showing the major sites.

larly those with local mediastinal node involvement. Tumours of the lower oesophagus are usually adenocarcinomas and are dealt with in chapter 9.

Tumours of the Nasal Fossa and Paranasal Sinuses

These uncommon tumours chiefly present with nasal or facial swelling, skin ulceration or nasal obstruction (Fig. 6.22). With locally invasive tumours, bone erosion may be a prominent feature, leading for example to a sloughing tumour at the roof of the mouth from direct invasion into the oral cavity (Fig. 6.23). CT scanning and OPG are essential investigations (see Figs 6.13 & 6.24). A combination of surgery and radiotherapy has traditionally been recommended and can be achieved with less cosmetic disturbance than one might expect; recently, however, the role of surgery has been questioned and patients are increasingly being treated by radiotherapy alone.

As with nasopharyngeal, hypopharyngeal and upper oesophageal cancers, there is little evidence that chemotherapy plays an important part in the management of tumours of the nasal fossa and paranasal sinuses. Exceptions occur when the tumour

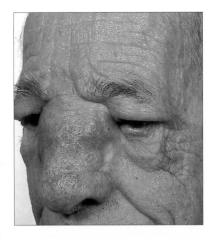

Fig. 6.22 Carcinoma of the ethmoid sinuses and upper nasal fossa. This patient presented with massive swelling and nasal obstruction.

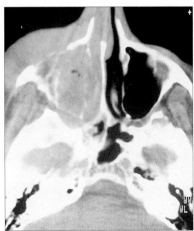

Fig. 6.23 Maxillary lymphoma. This patient presented with a necrotic ulcer in the roof of the mouth, together with erythema and swelling of the cheek.

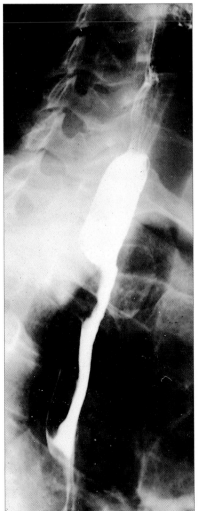

Fig. 6.21 Carcinoma of the upper oesophagus. The obvious constriction in the barium flow is typical of a carcinoma. This patient presented with dysphagia, anorexia and profound weight loss (20kg).

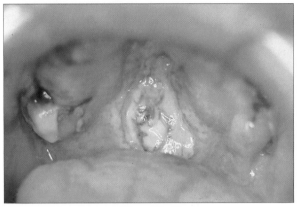

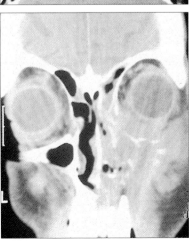

Fig. 6.24 Maxillary lymphoma. CT scanning (previous case) shows both the contour elevation (right cheek) and massive bone destruction of the walls of the maxilla including floor of the orbit, together with the elevation of the right globe.

unexpectedly proves to be a lymphoma or other chemosensitive growth (Fig. 6.25). Maxillary sinus tumours can be surprisingly responsive to radiotherapy, although on the whole the prognosis is guarded (Fig. 6.26). If there is any question of erosion upwards to the orbital floor, the eye will necessarily be included within the radiation field. With careful attention to detail, and with shielding of sensitive structures such as the cornea and lachrymal apparatus, vision may be well preserved, since the remainder of the eye is surprisingly tolerant to well-fractionated irradiation.

Carcinoma of the Lip

These tumours are commoner in males, particularly those who are pipe smokers. They usually present with an obvious non-healing ulcer on the vermilion border of the lip (Fig. 6.27), which may be confused with a benign lesion such as a herpes simplex sore. Nodal involvement is unusual, though the primary lesion itself may reach a substantial size. Typically these are squamous carcinomas. Occasionally two primary carcinomas arise on the upper and lower lips. Such adjacent lesions are known as 'kiss ulcers'.

Treatment is either by local resection or by radiotherapy. For lesions less than 1cm, resection may offer an excellent functional and cosmetic result with a cure in 90% of cases, although larger lesions are probably better treated by radiotherapy because of the surgical defect which an operation will inevitably cause. A popular radiotherapeutic technique is

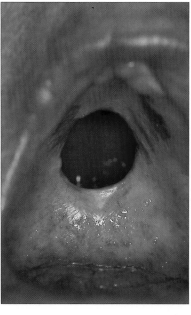

Fig. 6.25 Maxillary lymphoma. The previous case proved highly responsive to chemotherapy and radiotherapy. Four years later the patient is tumour-free, but has a persistent defect in the palate. An obdurator fixed to the upper denture gives excellent rehabilitation of speech, cosmesis and deglutition.

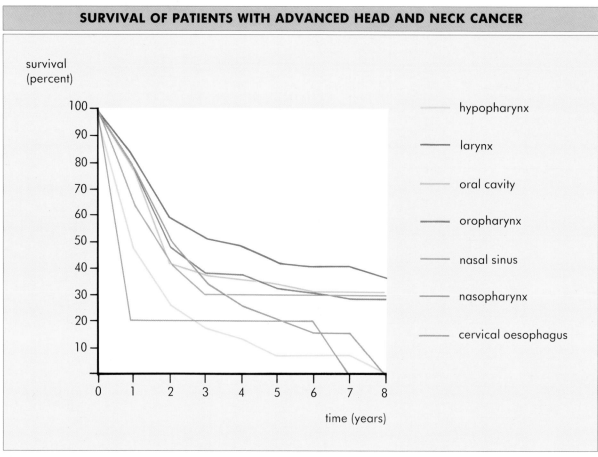

SURVIVAL OF PATIENTS WITH ADVANCED HEAD AND NECK CANCER

— hypopharynx
— larynx
— oral cavity
— oropharynx
— nasal sinus
— nasopharynx
— cervical oesophagus

Fig. 6.26 Survival of patients with advanced head and neck cancer.
This refers to T3 and T4 cases, or any primary tumour with positive neck nodes.

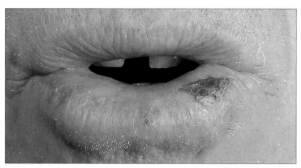

Fig. 6.27 Carcinoma of the lip. In this case the tumour was more extensive than the obvious crust on the left lower lip. In fact the whole of the lower lip is obviously swollen; further biopsies from the right side also confirmed the presence of the tumour.

the use of a radium mould or other implant, although excellent results can also be achieved with external radiation techniques. Chemotherapy is not used for carcinomas of the lip.

Tumours of the Salivary Glands

These tumours are histologically quite different from the other tumours so far described in this chapter. More than 50% of salivary tumours are benign pleomorphic adenomas and are particularly common in the parotid (Fig. 6.28). Other important salivary tumours include mixed malignant tumours, adenocarcinomas, adenoid cystic carcinomas, acinic

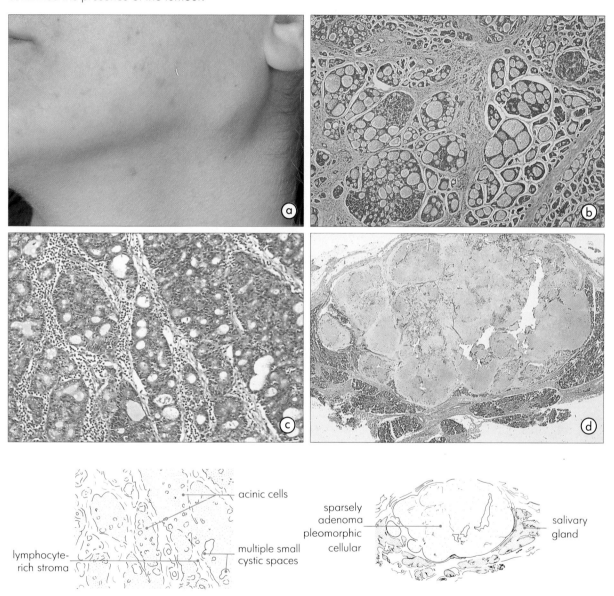

Fig. 6.28 Tumours of the salivary glands. (a) Pleomorphic adenoma: a swelling at the lower pole of the parotid gland is visible. (b) Adenoid cystic carcinoma, showing the characteristic cribriform (cylindromatous) pattern. (c) Acinic cell tumour: sheets of basophilic tumour cells with small intercellular spaces in a lymphocyte-rich stroma. (d) Pleomorphic adenoma: this view (low magnification) shows the tumour to have a poorly defined capsule. Courtesy of Prof R.A. Lawson.

cell tumours, lymphomas (almost invariably non-Hodgkin lymphomas) and, rarely, squamous carcinomas. Some tumours are too poorly differentiated for adequate characterization. Adenoid cystic carcinomas are notable for their local perineural spread, which is thought to account for their unusually painful nature and for a tendency to pulmonary metastasis. Apart from the parotid, salivary tumours may affect other major (sublingual and sub-mandibular) and minor salivary glands. Presentation is usually with a diffuse swelling of the parotid, with elevation of the facial contour just anterior to the ear (Fig. 6.29). Tumours at other sites will of course present differently, and tumours of the minor salivary glands will generally appear as an intraoral or oropharyngeal swelling. Node involvement does not occur with benign tumours but may occur in any of the malignant tumours, particularly lymphoma or squamous carcinoma.

Treatment of all these tumours (apart from lymphoma) is by surgical excision, which should be as complete as possible and preferably without spillage of glandular contents. Ideally this must be achieved without sacrifice of the facial nerve trunk, which is generally possible with a superficial parotidectomy. Some surgeons find it helpful to obtain a sialogram with retrograde cannulation of the parotid salivary duct, to determine whether the precise site of the tumour within the parotid can be demonstrated pre-operatively; CT scanning may also be helpful. With more deeply situated tumours radiotherapy may be preferable, particularly in younger patients for whom sacrifice of the facial nerve would represent a major penalty of treatment.

If the tumour is indeed a pleomorphic adenoma (benign), radiotherapy is not usually recommended unless there is doubt about the completeness of the excision or if there is gland rupture during removal. Under these circumstances local irradiation certainly reduces the risk of local recurrence. If a second excision is required for local recurrence later on, this should always be followed by routine postoperative

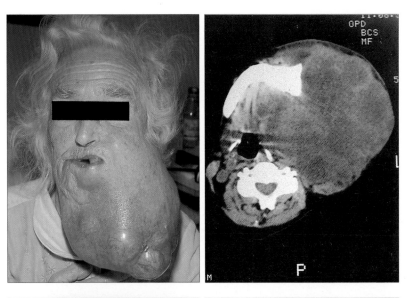

Fig. 6.29 Huge carcinoma of the submandibular salivary gland. This was an adenoid cystic carcinoma producing massive bone erosion, well demonstrated on the CT scan.

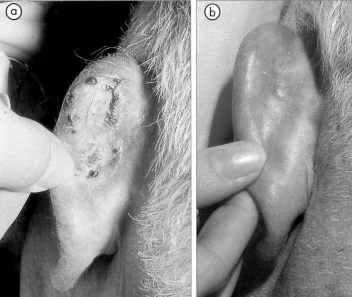

Fig. 6.30 Basal cell carcinoma. (a) Rodent ulcer of the pinna. (b) An excellent result following radiotherapy.

radiotherapy. Excision of malignant tumours should always be made using a generous surgical approach, followed by irradiation of the tumour bed. Adverse effects may include dryness of the mouth, occasional trismus and partial hair loss – with careful planning a field arrangement can usually be achieved which minimizes these effects and prevents damage to the contralateral eye from the exit beam. Adenoid cystic carcinomas are sometimes thought to be resistant, but this is not correct; these tumours should be vigorously treated even though late dissemination, generally to the lungs, is a characteristic feature of such tumours.

Tumours of the Ear

These are, on the whole, unusual cancers, although the pinna is a common site for basal and squamous carcinoma (Fig. 6.30). Although both surgery and radiotherapy are used, radiation has the considerable advantage of producing better cosmetic results, especially in squamous cancers in which large areas of the pinna may have to be resected. Tumours of the ear canal and middle ear are very unusual, the latter most frequently occurring in middle-aged males with a history of chronic otitis media. Local extension may be present, but only detectable by CT scanning. Glomus jugulare tumours, though uncommon, are an important group, arising from neuro-endocrine receptors of the jugular bulb (Fig. 6.31). They produce a cluster of symptoms including tinnitus, unilateral deafness and often severe otalgia, together with lower cranial nerve palsies (Fig. 6.32). Perhaps surprisingly, in view of their slow growth and histologically benign appearance, they can be responsive to radiation therapy, with gratifying relief of symptoms. Surgery is extremely difficult as such tumours tend to be highly vascular.

Tumours of the Orbit and Eye

This is another uncommon site, but a variety of primary and secondary tumours can occur (Fig. 6.33). Proptosis is the commonest physical sign (Fig.

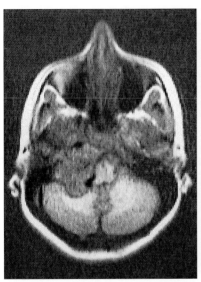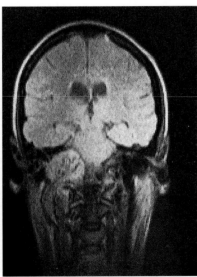

Fig. 6.31 Glomus jugulare and tumours of the middle ear. Axial and coronal MRI scans showing the tumour clearly indenting the cerebellum and brainsteam.

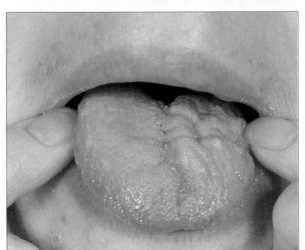

Fig. 6.32 Glomus jugulare and tumours of the middle ear. Obvious left-sided twelfth nerve palsy from tumour destruction from the base of the brain (previous case).

TUMOURS OF THE ORBIT (EXCLUDING GLOBE)	
Benign	Malignant
Haemangioma	Lymphoma
Lachrymal gland tumours	Rhabdomyosarcoma
Meningioma	Optic nerve glioma
Lymphangioma	Metastases
Neurofibroma	Myeloma
Dermoid cysts (Pseudotumour)	Angiosarcoma and other sarcomas

Fig. 6.33 Classification of orbital tumours.

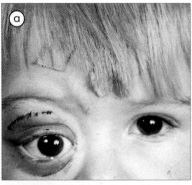

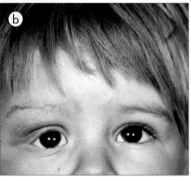

Fig. 6.34 Large orbital rhabdomyo-sarcoma of the right eye.
(a) Proptosis and downward displacement of the globe.
(b) Appearance after treatment with radiotherapy and chemotherapy.

6.34) and is virtually always unilateral, except in the case of optic nerve gliomas (usually a childhood tumour – see chapter 16) involving the optic chiasm, or the orbital 'pseudotumour' or low grade lymphoma (Fig. 6.35). Secondary orbital deposits most frequently arise from cancers of the breast, bronchus or thyroid, although leukaemic deposits may also occur (Fig. 6.36). With large tumours, whether primary or secondary, ophthalmoplegia may develop. Lachrymal gland tumours are very unusual indeed and histologically resemble salivary tumours, usually presenting as a subtle but firm swelling of the outer aspect of the upper eyelid (Fig. 6.37). They are best excised, particularly since radiotherapy is difficult at this site.

Tumours of the eye and conjunctiva are a particularly specialized group. Basal cell carcinomas of the lower eyelid are common and may be locally destructive (Fig. 6.38). In the conjunctiva, both melanoma and squamous carcinoma occur and can sometimes be eradicated by local 'brachytherapy' – locally placed radiation sources using strontium-90

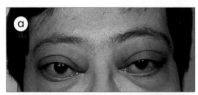

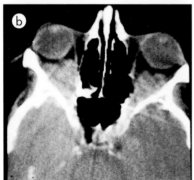

Fig. 6.35 Orbital pseudotumour (low-grade lymphoma).
(a) Chemosis.
(b) CT scan shows bilateral soft tissue swellings in the region of the posterior orbit causing bilateral proptosis and ophthalmoplegia.

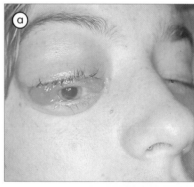

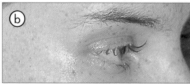

Fig. 6.36 Leukaemic deposits (chloroma).
(a) Severe chloroma.
(b) Taken only one week later, shows dramatic resolution following treatment.

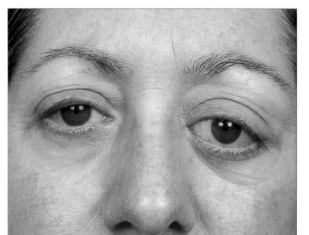

Fig. 6.37 Adenocarcinoma of the left lachrymal gland. Note the fullness of the soft tissues between eyebrow and upper eyelid.

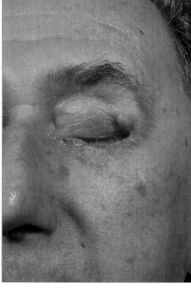

Fig. 6.38 Previously treated basal cell carcinoma of the lower eyelid. In this unusual case, radiotherapy successfully eradicated the primary tumour at the inner canthus but the patient later developed a nodular recurrence at the outer aspect, by direct extension via the upper lid.

plaque applicators. Retinoblastoma, an important hereditary childhood tumour, is discussed in chapter 16. Another childhood malignant tumour, rhabdomyosarcoma, quite frequently presents as an orbital primary and may be locally destructive with wide dissemination. It is usually highly responsive to chemo- and radiotherapy (see chapter 16).

Chemotherapy in Head and Neck Cancer

Despite improvements in surgical and radiotherapeutic techniques over the last thirty years, the long term survival for patients with advanced disease has not appreciably altered. It has become increasingly clear that squamous carcinomas of the head and neck do respond to a variety of chemotherapeutic agents, including anti-folate anti-metabolites such as methotrexate, anti-tumour antibiotics such as bleomycin, and vinca alkaloids such as vincristine. Combinations of these drugs undoubtedly give higher response rates although unfortunately remission duration remains short, and a cure is never seen with chemotherapy alone. The toxicity of multi-drug

regimens is high, so chemotherapy should not be routinely used outside the context of a clinical trial.

Despite these problems, a number of groups have attempted to use chemotherapy in patients with advanced disease and poor prognosis. The head and neck cancer group at Christie Hospital, Manchester, recently published results from a large prospective study (Fig. 6.39), showing that local control rates in some types of head and neck cancer could be improved by adding single agent methotrexate (an outpatient treatment) on two occasions during a standard course of radiotherapy. In patients with advanced oropharyngeal carcinoma there was a striking improvement, with definite increases in survival, as well as local control, from 20% to 45% at a median follow-up of just under three years. This exciting work has been paralleled by others, and a UK multi-centre study has recently been started in order to try and confirm these results. Even if no survival advantage can be demonstrated, it looks as though salvage operations may be less frequently required in patients given chemotherapy, a potential benefit particularly important in the head and neck area where preservation of function is so crucial.

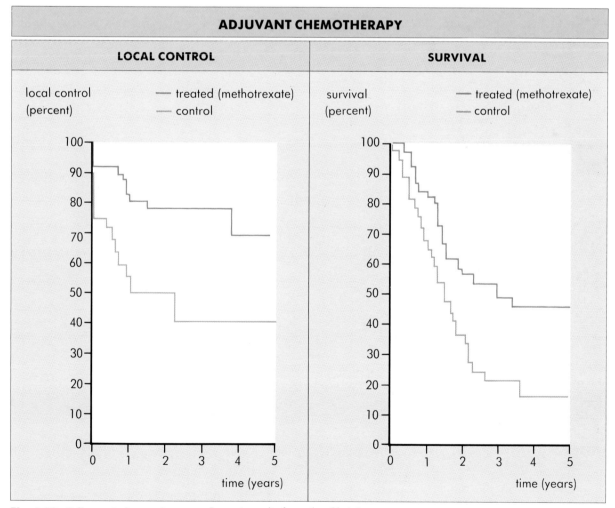

Fig. 6.39 Adjuvant chemotherapy. Recent results from the Christie Hospital, Manchester, confirming the value of adjuvant chemotherapy with methotrexate in oropharyngeal carcinoma.

Rehabilitating Patients with Head and Neck Cancer

A substantial proportion of patients will be cured, including some cases with advanced disease. In some, a cure can be achieved with no long-term adverse effects; a patient with an early glottic carcinoma can be cured with radiotherapy without deterioration of function or, in all probability, any significant long-term damage. On the other hand, some patients are cured only by laryngectomy, maxillectomy, major facial resection, or transposition procedures such as a gastric pull-up. Such patients need to be sensitively treated and offered expert care, for example in prosthesis fitment, speech therapy and stoma care. The remarkable work of skilled speech therapists is often underappreciated, and the teaching of a worthwhile oesophageal voice following total laryngectomy is a critically important part of follow-up care. Some patients cannot ever achieve this, and the development of the Blom–Singer voice prosthesis, which consists of a simple valve placed through a permanent pharyngeal stoma, offers many patients a rather better opportunity for speech and communication. Prosthetic replacement is clearly of particular importance in patients with visible facial defects, such as permanent loss of the nose or facial skin, although recent improvements in plastic surgical techniques, including microvascular anastomosis, mean that such replacements are now required rather less frequently.

Thyroid Cancer

This unusual group of tumours often develops in younger patients, and has a strong female preponderance. The commonest presentation is with a mass either in the thyroid gland itself or in local neck nodes (see Fig. 6.1). In older patients respiratory obstruction is sometimes encountered, particularly with the more aggressive and anaplastic cancers often seen in this age group.

Although the aetiology of thyroid cancer is not fully understood, there are a number of clues. It most commonly develops in young adult women typically at 20–40 years and with a similar age and sex distribution as benign thyroid disorders such as thyrotoxicosis and Hashimoto's thyroiditis. There is evidence that it may be a radiation induced cancer in a minority of cases, and the disease typically runs a lengthy course (particularly in young patients with well differentiated tumours) with long periods of

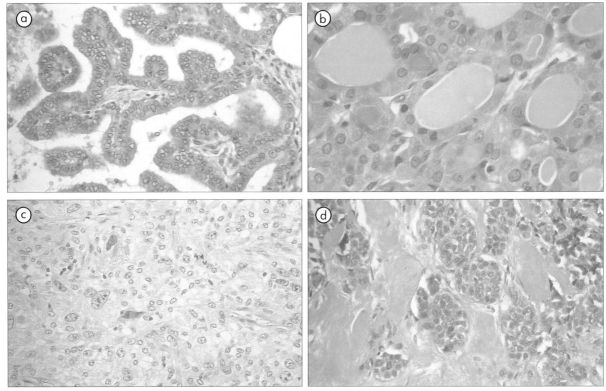

Fig. 6.40 Histological subtypes in thyroid carcinoma. (a) Papillary carcinoma. The papillae are lined by epithelial cells with overlapping, pale, 'ground-glass' nuclei. (b) Follicular carcinoma. This tumour is well differentiated, forming follicles that are indistinguishable from normal thyroid tissue. (c) Undifferentiated (anaplastic) carcinoma. This tumour is too poorly differentiated to be placed in any other category. It is the most aggressive of all thyroid tumours. (d) Medullary carcinoma. The amorphous eosinophilic material between the clumps of tumour cells is amyloid. The tumour cells have the functional and structural characteristics of parafollicular cells.

disease control (often years or even decades), even where cure has not been achieved.

There is considerable variety both in pathology and histological appearance (Fig. 6.40). The commonest type is the papillary carcinoma which accounts for almost two-thirds of thyroid cancer in the USA and Europe and often develops as a multifocal tumour. Lymph node involvement is common in these cases, but unlike most other solid tumours, this may not necessarily herald a more adverse prognosis. Follicular carcinoma, the second commonest type, is also typically a tumour of younger patients, chiefly women, accounting for an additional 15% of cases and with a quite distinct histology and relative lack of lymph node involvement. Unlike papillary carcinomas, these tumours tend more frequently to metastasize via the blood stream, chiefly to lung and bone secondary sites (Fig. 6.41). In older patients, anaplastic carcinomas are much the commonest type, again accounting for 15% of thyroid cancers overall, and often much more rapidly growing and with

a very much worse prognosis than the other well differentiated tumours. Medullary thyroid cancers are far less common, and often form part of the spectrum of disorders of multiple endocrine neoplasia (see chapter 9). Other unusual thyroid tumours are listed in Fig. 6.42.

Management

Patients with suspected thyroid carcinoma should be investigated by means of an iodine uptake scan, which exploits the ability of the normal thyroid gland to take up radioactive iodine. Typically, a 'cold nodule' is seen (Fig. 6.43), and a lesion of this type should always be biopsied or removed. Thyroid ultrasound or CT-scan may be valuable, particularly to delineate whether the lesion is cystic or solid. The diagnosis can generally be confirmed on fine-needle aspiration cytology, though if a carcinoma is discovered, further surgery is invariably required, generally by means of a generous hemithyroidectomy or near total thyroidectomy. These patients will require thyroid supplements for life, particularly in cases where the surgery is followed by postoperative radioiodine therapy to ablate the thyroid and deal adequately with any residual foci of carcinoma. This treatment can be given effectively by mouth.

Radioiodine therapy is valuable not only for residual local disease but also for treatment of secondary deposits elsewhere in the body. These deposits generally retain their ability to take up radioiodine, but only if the normal gland has first been ablated.

Patients with anaplastic tumours cannot be helped by radioiodine treatment since anaplastic carcinoma of the thyroid does not generally respond. Nonetheless, external irradiation of the neck may be very useful for local control in these cases, though this type of thyroid carcinoma undoubtedly has a worse

FREQUENCY OF METASTASES IN THYROID CANCER

	Frequency (percent)	
	Local lymph nodes	Distant
Follicular	28%	14%
Papillary	47%	3%
Medullary	60%	11%
Anaplastic	53%	15%

Fig. 6.41 Metastasis from thyroid cancer.
Frequencies of local and distant metastases for the different histological subtypes vary widely.

UNUSUAL THYROID TUMOURS

Thyroid lymphoma
Hürthle cell tumour
(variant of follicular carcinoma)
Haemangioendothelioma
Primary squamous carcinoma
Plasmacytoma
Thyroid teratoma
Muco-epidermoid carcinoma
Thyroid metastases

Fig. 6.42 Unusual thyroid tumours. Together these tumours constitute approximately 10% of all thyroid neoplasias.

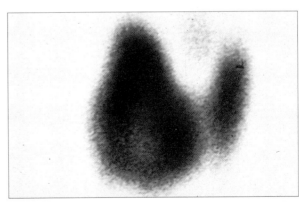

Fig. 6.43 Iodine-123 thyroid scan in a patient with thyroid carcinoma. The 4-hour uptake is above the normal range at 39%. The right lobe is much larger than the left due to previous partial thyroidectomy. The photopenic area in the lower pole of the right lobe corresponds to a palpable nodule. Subsequently, this area proved to be an intrathyroid recurrence of the carcinoma.

prognosis than the follicular and papillary types. In well differentiated tumours, the use of thyroglobulin as a tumour marker is of considerable value for assessing residual or recurrent disease. In medullary carcinomas, both calcitonin and carcino-embryonic antigen (CEA) are useful in the same way.

The results of treatment of well differentiated thyroid cancer are among the best for any solid cancer (Fig. 6.44). In women under the age of forty with papillary carcinomas, a large proportion of the total, the outlook is virtually indistinguishable from the expected survival of a similar age-matched female population. However, with invasive follicular carcinoma, and in particular medullary and anaplastic carcinomas, the results are less satisfactory. In anaplastic carcinoma, even highly aggressive treatment with surgery, external radiation and sometimes chemotherapy have failed to improve the outlook beyond the overall 5-year survival rate of only 5%. In general, chemotherapy has given very poor results in recurrent or metastatic carcinoma of the thyroid, and should not routinely be used.

Non-Hodgkin lymphoma of the thyroid is discussed in chapter 12.

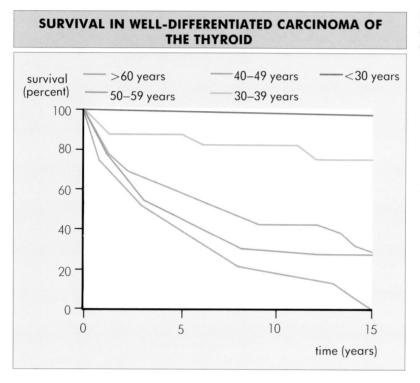

SURVIVAL IN WELL-DIFFERENTIATED CARCINOMA OF THE THYROID

Fig. 6.44 Survival according to age in well differentiated carcinoma of the thyroid.

Lung Cancer

7

Introduction

Lung cancer is now one of the most common fatal illnesses in the industrialized countries. It has steadily risen in incidence since cigarette smoking became popular and widespread, at around the time of the First World War, and is now responsible for almost forty thousand deaths per annum in the UK.

The relationship between lung cancer and cigarette smoking is well established and the important aspects of the epidemiology of this disease as a worldwide problem have been discussed in chapter 1 (see Figs 1.10–1.13). Although men are now smoking less than before, the number of cigarettes smoked by women over the past fifteen years has increased by 50%, so that the ratio of male to female smokers has fallen from 10:1 in the 1950s to 3:1 in the 1980s. In males, there is evidence that the peak incidence of lung cancer may have passed. Other aetiological causes of lung cancer, such as exposure to radiation and carcinogens experienced in certain mining industries (Fig. 7.1) are insignificant when compared to smoking, although the increased mortality from lung cancer in urban areas is thought to be due to the additional air pollution found there. A further significant aetiological factor in thoracic malignancy is the inhalation of asbestos particles, an important cause of diffuse lung damage including the highly malignant mesothelioma, for which current treatments are almost wholly ineffective. Recent data have suggested that high concentrations of radon gas may also play a role in the development of mesothelioma – the gas can accumulate in modern, insulated houses built in areas where radon emission is part of the local geology.

AETIOLOGICAL FACTORS IN LUNG CANCER
Cigarette smoke
Particulate phase Benzypyrene, benzofluoranthenes, dibenzanthracene, nicotine, catechol, nickel and cadmium
Vapour phase Nitrogen oxides, formaldehyde, hydrazine, urethan
Air pollution
Coal and tar fumes, nickel, zinc, benzypyrene
Occupational
Asbestos Radioactivity (uranium mines, radon) Nickel, chromium, iron oxide (metal workers) Arsenicals (sheep-dip workers)

Fig. 7.1 Aetiological factors in lung cancer. Cigarette smoking is much the most important cause (see Figs. 1.10–1.13).

HISTOLOGICAL CLASSIFICATION OF LUNG CANCER
Squamous carcinoma
Small cell carcinoma
Adenocarcinoma Bronchogenic; acinar Bronchiolalveolar
Large cell carcinoma With or without mucin, giant cell and clear cell variants
Mixed squamous and adenocarcinoma
Other tumours Carcinoid, cylindroma, mesothelioma, sarcoma and mixed histological types

Fig. 7.2 Histological classification of lung cancer. (Modified from WHO criteria.)

Pathology of Lung Cancer and Patterns of Spread

Pathology

Most lung cancers arise relatively proximally, from the main or lobar bronchi, whereas tumours arising from the true lung parenchyma are comparatively much less common. The WHO histological classification of lung cancer recognizes four major histological varieties although other, rarer types can also occur as primary tumours (Figs 7.2 & 7.3).

Squamous cell carcinoma

Squamous cell carcinoma is the commonest variety; it accounts for almost half of all lung cancers and is unquestionably related to cigarette smoking. It is similar morphologically to squamous carcinomas at other sites. These tumours are thought to arise by squamous metaplasia, since squamous epithelium is not normally present so low in the respiratory tract.

Small cell carcinoma

Small cell (oat cell) carcinoma is the next commonest type (comprising 25% of all lung cancers) and is also strongly related to cigarette smoking. Its microscopic appearance is quite different from that of squamous cell carcinoma, with tightly packed, darkly staining cells containing neurosecretory granules and very sparse cytoplasm. Small cell carcinomas are the most rapidly evolving form of lung cancer and are most likely to metastasize early, with a particularly wide spectrum of potential secondary sites (Fig. 7.4). Furthermore, small cell carcinoma is the human tumour most likely to produce ectopic hormones such as ADH or ACTH, leading to specific, identifiable syndromes (Fig. 7.5). Bulky lymphadenopathy is also a characteristic feature of these tumours, since major lymphatic invasion is common.

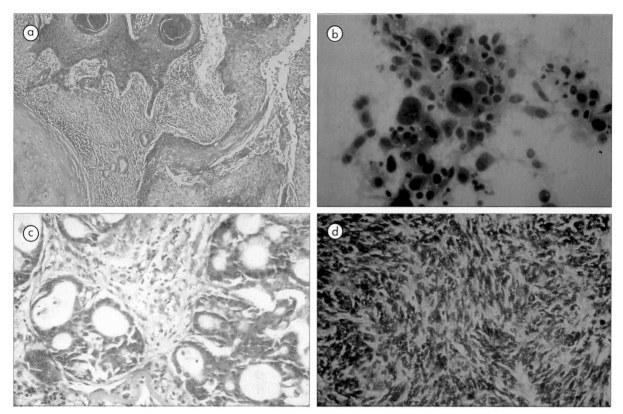

Fig. 7.3 Histological varieties of lung cancer.
(a) Squamous cell carcinoma. Bands of tumour cells show stratification and keratinization with formation of distinctive keratin 'pearls'. (b) Large cell carcinoma (bronchial brushing, cytological preparation). The cells have clear pleomorphic nuclei that lack the denseness seen in small cell carcinoma, and a moderate amount of cytoplasm that lacks evidence of mucus storage and keratinization. (c) Adenocarcinoma, showing prominent glandular differentiation. (d) Small cell carcinoma consisting of spindle or 'oat' shaped shells with dense nuclei, moulded cellular morphology and sparse cytoplasm. Courtesy of Prof B. Corrin.

LOCAL AND METASTATIC SPREAD

brain
supraclavicular nodes
hilar and mediastinal nodes
tumour
bone
adrenal
liver
bone marrow

→ local spread to pleura, ribs, mediastinum, phrenic nerve and oesophagus

Fig. 7.4 Local and distant spread in small cell carcinoma of the lung.

ECTOPIC AND PARANEOPLASTIC SYNDROMES IN LUNG CANCER

Endocrine and Metabolic	
Inappropriate ADH secretion	Low plasma sodium and high urine osmolality with drowsiness and confusion
Cushing's syndrome	Rare, with hyperkalaemia, glucose intolerance, hypertension, weakness, due to excess ACTH production
Gynaecomastia	Increase in glandular and stromal tissue of male breast due to HCG production (?)
Hyperpigmentation	From MSH-like fragments
Neurological	
Peripheral neuropathy	Generally mixed but may be purely sensory or Guillain–Barré type
Cerebellar degeneration	Rapid and progressive with ataxia and diplopia
Eaton–Lambert syndrome	Rare, with weakness, aching of girdle musculature

Fig. 7.5 Ectopic and paraneoplastic syndromes in lung cancer.

Adenocarcinoma

Adenocarcinoma is often regarded as the 'native' form of lung cancer and was in all probability the most prevalent type, often diagnosed in women, before cigarette smoking became popular. Its incidence is rising slightly, particularly in white North American males, a group in which the number of cigarette smokers has actually decreased. These tumours often arise peripherally, sometimes from initially scarred areas, and occasionally involve the pleura.

Large cell carcinoma

Large cell carcinoma has less clear cut histological features. It may, like adenocarcinoma, arise more peripherally than squamous or small cell carcinomas. It is the least common of the four major varieties.

Mesothelioma

Mesothelioma is a particularly aggressive and highly malignant form of pleural tumour which may arise either uni- or bilaterally and is often clearly related to a previous history of asbestos exposure. The histological and radiological appearances are characteristic (Fig. 7.6) with encasement of part or all of the lung by a thickened pleural membrane and, quite frequently, involvement of the medial or pericardial aspect of the visceral pleura as well as the more typical lateral site. Treatment of this tumour is generally unsatisfactory since surgical resection offers the only hope of cure, although this is often impossible due to the widely diffuse nature of the malignancy.

Patterns of Spread

All the main types of lung cancer may spread by local extension, lymphatic metastasis or haematogenous dissemination. In small cell lung cancer, early local and distant dissemination is common. For example, brain metastases are diagnosed in a quarter of all small cell lung cancer patients during their lifetime. At postmortem almost two-thirds of small cell lung cancer patients have evidence of disease within the brain or meninges. Although wide dissemination is less common in other types of lung cancer, it is by no means unusual. Indeed, secondary deposits are so common in lung cancer that a significant proportion of patients may present for the first time as a result of the secondary deposit.

■ Clinical Presentation

General Symptoms

Many smokers suffer from chronic conditions such as emphysema, chronic obstructive airway disease and bronchitis, with regular exacerbations particularly in the winter months. The presenting symptoms of lung cancer and of benign disease are often very similar and therefore difficult to differentiate; they usually include a worsening of symptoms already familiar to the patient, such as exertional dyspnoea, cough, or chest discomfort. Patients are often aware that the symptoms have changed, although this may be less apparent to the doctor. The most significant clue may be the revelation by the patient that the chest problems are now so severe that he/she has

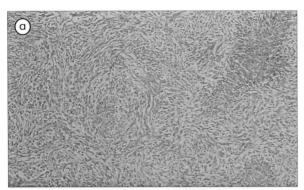
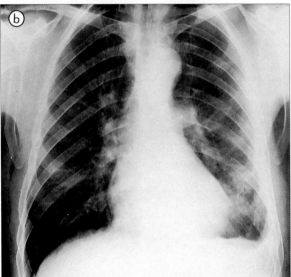
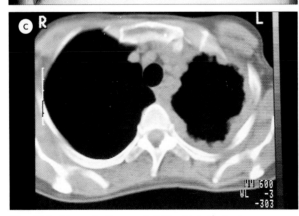

Fig. 7.6 Mesothelioma. (a) The histological appearance is variable but in this specimen the epithelial cell type adenocapillary structures are prominent, and there is an area of necrosis. Courtesy of Prof B. Corrin. (b) Typical x-ray findings, including pleural shadowing with nodulation behind the heart, in the costophrenic angle and along the lateral chest wall, together with partial destruction of ribs. Courtesy of Dr M.E. Hodson. (c) Typical CT scan appearance, with involvement of the whole of the pleura of the left lung with complete sparing on the right.

finally stopped smoking 'for good'. Other features which should be investigated include the following:

- finger clubbing (Fig. 7.7), which is present in about 30% of all cases (although this is far less common in small cell lung cancer, the most rapidly evolving form of this disease);
- haemoptysis, always a worrying symptom, since it is uncommon in bronchitis or uncomplicated emphysema;
- radiating chest pain;
- dysphagia, sometimes caused by direct oesophageal extension but more often by enlarged mediastinal nodes (Fig. 7.8).

Syndromes
Tumours occurring in specific sites often give rise to syndromes whose features depend on local anatomical relationships.

Superior vena cava obstruction (SVCO)
Carcinomas situated in the right main or upper lobe bronchus may cause SVCO, particularly where lymphadenopathy is a prominent feature, as is often the case with small cell lung cancer. Typical findings include bloating and plethora of the face and neck (Fig. 7.9), with fixed high venous pressure sometimes severe enough to cause conjunctival

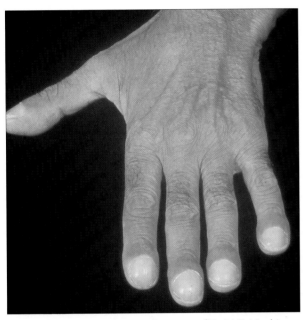

Fig. 7.7 Finger clubbing. Courtesy of Dr M.E. Hodson.

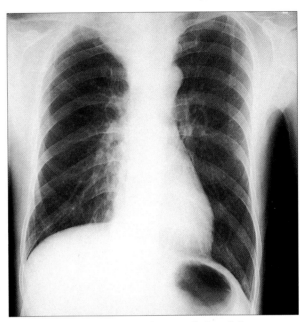

Fig. 7.8 Gross upper mediastinal glandular involvement (right-sided paratracheal lymphadenopathy) causing dysphagia. The small primary lung cancer is not visible in this chest x-ray.

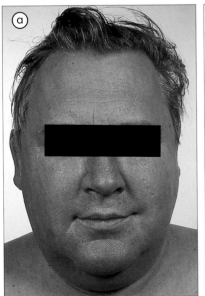
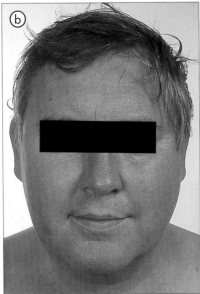
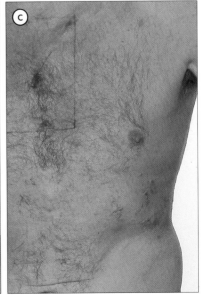

Fig. 7.9 Superior vena cava obstruction. (a) Appearance prior to treatment. (b) Six weeks after palliative radiotherapy. (c) Typical vascular changes over the chest wall, with prominent small purple venules.

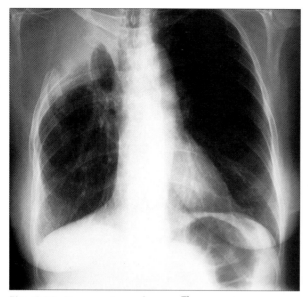

Fig. 7.10 Pancoast syndrome. There is gross destruction of the first four ribs and upper chest wall. The pain was so severe that this patient eventually required a cordotomy.

oedema and retinal changes. The venous pressure may be so high that the level cannot be determined from examination of the neck veins. In such cases one should raise the patient's arms slowly above the level of his/her neck and watch carefully for the point at which the small veins on the dorsum of the hands begin to collapse. This may well be several centimetres above the top of the patient's skull! The commonest physical sign of SVCO, rarely mentioned in large textbooks, consists of a leash of tiny red or purple dilated veins over the precordium – this is much more common than the large collateral vessels coursing over the patient's shoulder, often and wrongly regarded as the most typical physical sign.

The Pancoast syndrome

The Pancoast syndrome, in which the carcinoma arises at the apex of the lungs (Fig. 7.10), also has specific clinical findings, including severe upper chest wall pain, wasting of the small muscles of the hand

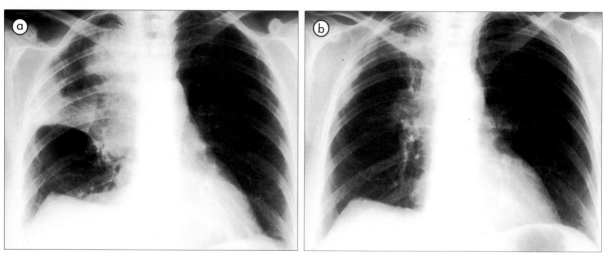

Fig. 7.11 Tenting. (a) Tenting of the right diaphragm due to phrenic nerve erosion from a large right-sided carcinoma. (b) Appearance two months after radiotherapy.

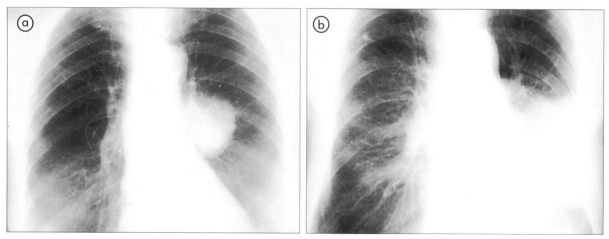

Fig. 7.12 Lung collapse. (a) Massive left-sided hilar lymphadenopathy (small cell lung cancer). (b) Collapse of left, middle and lower lobes (squamous cell carcinoma).

with associated weakness and parasthesia, and Horner's syndrome due to interruption of the sympathetic nerve fibres by tumour erosion. The pain may be extremely severe; typical chest x-ray appearances show rib destruction from direct chest wall invasion.

Other syndromes

Recurrent laryngeal palsy due to carcinomas situated at the left main or upper lobe bronchus produce a characteristic reduction in voice quality and volume, together with a bovine cough.

Where proximal carcinomas erode or compress the phrenic nerve the chest x-ray may also reveal a tented diaphragm on the same side (Fig. 7.11). Apart from the obvious primary tumour, easily visible on the chest x-ray, other radiological features may include pleural effusion, local chest wall erosion, lymphadenopathy in the hila and/or mediastinum and areas of lobar or even total lung collapse (Fig. 7.12).

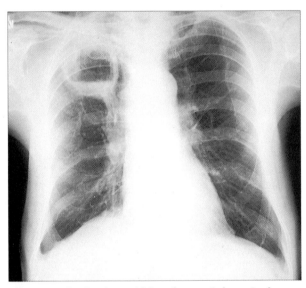

Fig. 7.13 Cavitation within a large right apical squamous carcinoma.

Pulmonary deposits from a primary lung cancer are unusual but by no means unknown.

Squamous carcinomas often cavitate (Fig. 7.13), a rare finding in other types of lung cancer. Such tumours may present as a lung abscess or as a pneumonia which fails to clear on conventional antibiotic treatment.

Investigations

Physical Examination

Physical examination often reveals areas of poor air entry, dullness to percussion, deviation of the trachea and, over the site of the primary tumour, bronchial breathing. Areas of local tenderness may occur, particularly where there is direct invasion of the chest wall. Lymphadenopathy, particularly in the supraclavicular fossa or lower cervical glands, is common; the nodes generally feel firm, rubbery and non-fluctuant. Examination of the hands and wrists may reveal not only clubbing but also, although much more rarely, hypertrophic pulmonary osteoarthropathy (Fig. 7.14). Wasting and neuropathy should be easy to detect. Patients may of course present with features relating to metastatic deposits, particularly bone lesions, although cerebral secondaries and hepatomegaly with or without ascites may also occur. This is especially true in small cell lung cancer which spreads both widely and very rapidly. Indeed, in this particular variety of lung cancer about two-thirds of patients have evidence of disseminated disease at the outset.

Fibreoptic Bronchoscopy

If the chest x-ray suggests a neoplasm, the patient will usually need to undergo fibreoptic bronchoscopy (see Fig. 7.15). This is a procedure generally performed under local anaesthetic using agents such as diazemuls, which may well permit the investigation to be performed as a day case. Typically the primary tumour will be visible, since most lung cancers are

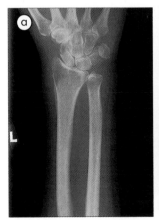 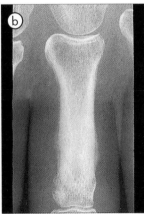 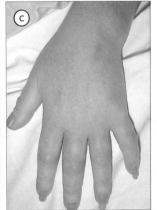 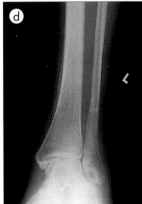

Fig. 7.14 Hypertrophic pulmonary osteoarthropathy. (a) Involvement of the distal ulna and radius, the commonest site. (b) Involvement of middle phalanx of left third finger, an unusual site. (c) Clinical appearance. (d) Involvement of distal tibia and fibula.

FIBREOPTIC BRONCHOSCOPY

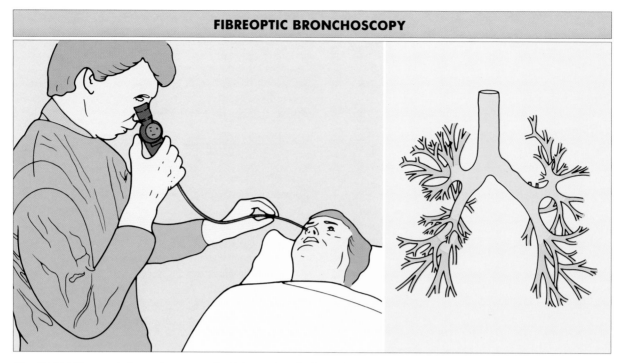

Fig. 7.15 Fibreoptic bronchoscopy. (Left) Insertion of a bronchoscope into the right nostril under direct vision. (Right) This diagram shows the limits of the technique. Courtesy of Prof M. Turner-Warwick.

proximally situated; this enables the chest physician to undertake fibreoptic biopsy with brushings for cytology as well. An important consideration is an estimation of the distance from the carina to the edge of the lesion since this may determine operability. Where fibreoptic bronchoscopy is normal then percutaneous biopsy, often CT-guided, is often used although the patient may have to be admitted into hospital because of the risk of pneumothorax. Once the diagnosis is established a full blood count and simple blood tests are both important, to exclude abnormalities of liver function. The blood count may reveal an unexpected anaemia, usually normochromic. Fibreoptic bronchoscopy will already have given information on the site of bleeding in patients with haemoptysis.

CT Scanning and Mediastinoscopy

Two further important investigations are frequently performed, and are chiefly designed to confirm operability in doubtful cases. First, CT scanning of the chest is now an established technique with excellent reliability in demonstrating mediastinal lymphadenopathy (Fig. 7.16) as well as giving useful information to the surgeon about the anatomy of the tumour. Most radiologists agree that glands above 1.5cm in diameter, easily seen on CT scanning, are likely to contain metastatic tumour, although biopsy may be indicated before surgery since enlarged nodes may be uninvolved in some patients.

Central mediastinal node disease is always an absolute contraindication to surgery. Where the involvement of these nodes is in doubt, mediastino-

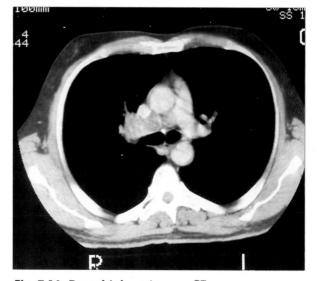

Fig. 7.16 Bronchial carcinoma. CT scan appearance, showing unequivocal mediastinal involvement which was not evident on the chest x-ray.

scopy can be performed. The procedure is simple, requires only one night in hospital, and gives histological confirmation of mediastinal contents (Fig. 7.17).

Other important criteria of operability include the site and local extensiveness of the tumour and the patient's general condition (particularly where pneumonectomy has to be considered). Some surgeons routinely request CT scanning of the abdomen and brain as well, since silent metastases may be present in 5–10% of apparently surgically

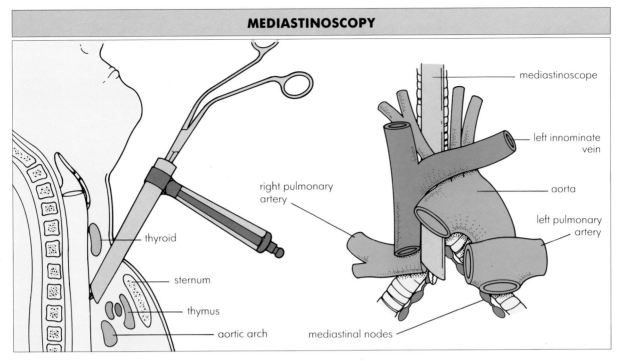

MEDIASTINOSCOPY

mediastinoscope

left innominate vein

right pulmonary artery

aorta

left pulmonary artery

thyroid

sternum

thymus

aortic arch

mediastinal nodes

Fig. 7.17 Mediastinoscopy. (Left) The technique of mediastinoscopy. (Right) Position of the mediastinoscope in relation to the major local structures. Courtesy of Prof M. Turner-Warwick.

CRITERIA FOR OPERABILITY

No obvious distant metastases

Usually only non-small cell varieties considered

General condition of the patient adequate for the planned operation

No clinically evident pleural effusion

Hilar lymphadenopathy may be acceptable, but not central mediastinal disease

Tumour >2cm from carina

Negative abdominal CT scanning

Age *per se* unimportant

Fig. 7.18 Criteria for operability in non-small cell lung cancer.

suitable cases. Clearly any operation in these circumstances should be avoided if at all possible. The aim of staging is to select all patients who are suitable for surgical resection and so avoid unnecessary thoracotomy wherever possible.

▮ Treatment

It is customary to consider small cell lung cancer, which accounts for about 25% of all cancer cases, as a distinct management problem, grouping all other types together (so called 'non-small cell lung cancers'). This latter group includes the squamous carcinomas, which are the commonest tumour type, together with adenocarcinomas and large cell, anaplastic and unclassifiable lesions. With adenocarcinomas, which characteristically arise rather peripherally in scar tissue, it is particularly important to confirm that the lesion is indeed a primary bronchial tumour, since it may well be a secondary deposit from another primary site masquerading as a genuine lung cancer.

The reason for the distinction between small cell and non-small cell lung cancer is that small cell lung cancer, because of its aggressive nature, is almost never regarded as potentially operable except in rare instances of small peripheral lesions. Furthermore, this tumour is undoubtedly more chemosensitive than the other types; indeed, chemotherapy has become the mainstay of treatment for small cell lung cancer.

Surgery

For non-small cell lung cancers, surgery is clearly the treatment of choice, although sadly not possible in the majority of cases (Fig. 7.18). In considering surgical resection for patients with non-small cell lung cancer the thoracic surgeon will need to know the patient's lung function, particularly where a pneumonectomy is contemplated. Age is not critically important, provided that the patient's general condition is adequate. In exceptional cases, patients of 80 years and over may legitimately be considered for resection of a lung cancer.

In the common situation of a surgically unresectable non-small cell lung cancer, the patient's symptoms should govern the choice of therapy – treatment in such cases is essentially palliative. For troublesome complaints such as chest pain, haemoptysis, unremitting cough, and major obstruction of bronchus, radiotherapy can be extremely valuable and is the mainstay of conventional treatment (Fig. 7.19).

Radiotherapy and Laser Treatment

Small cell carcinoma is undoubtedly the most radiosensitive type of lung cancer (Fig. 7.20) but also has the lowest survival rate, due to its rapidly aggressive nature. Radiotherapy is also the treatment of choice for bone metastases (Fig. 7.21), and is essential in patients with cord compression, sometimes with surgical decompression (selected cases) or imminent

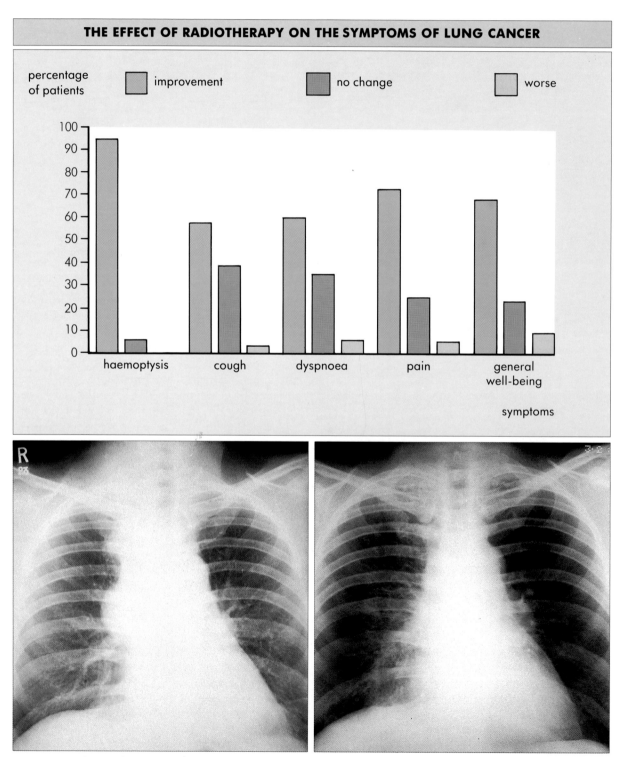

Fig. 7.19 Therapy. (Top) Radiotherapeutic palliation of symptoms in inoperable lung cancer. (Bottom) This patient with gross hilar and mediastinal involvement (left) presented with severe dysphagia, which fully resolved following radiotherapy (right).

fracture of a weight bearing bone. In such cases, a combination of radiotherapy with surgery is generally the best treatment. Radiotherapy is also useful for brain metastases and is generally used in combination with high doses of dexamethasone. In general, radiotherapy is given palliatively over short periods, since lung cancer patients have limited survival and prolonged treatments are unwarranted. When patients have widespread metastases, other aspects of supportive care are also important, for example close attention to metabolic effects of the tumour (such as hypercalcaemia) and nutrition. Corticosteroids, often undervalued, may be given for their effects on appetite, motivation and diet. These points are fully discussed in chapter 3.

Adverse effects of radiation include:
- dysphagia from radiation oesophagitis, occasionally complicated by oesophageal stricture;
- acute skin reaction, although not generally so severe as to warrant discontinuation of treatment;
- radiation cord damage (myelopathy), described more fully in chapter 13.

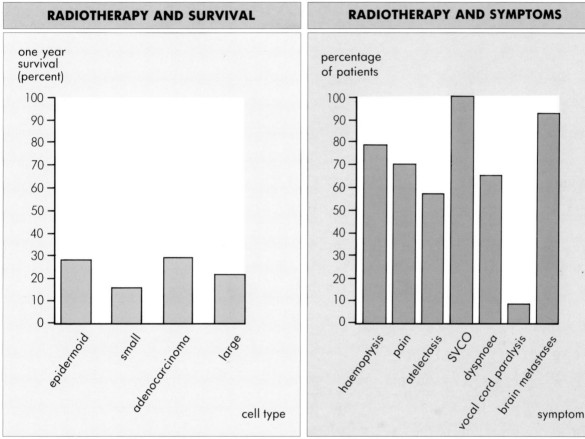

Fig. 7.20 Radiotherapy of lung cancer. (Left) One year survival in inoperable lung cancer. Small cell carcinoma shows the worst survival. (Right) Symptomatic response to radiotherapy in small cell lung cancer.

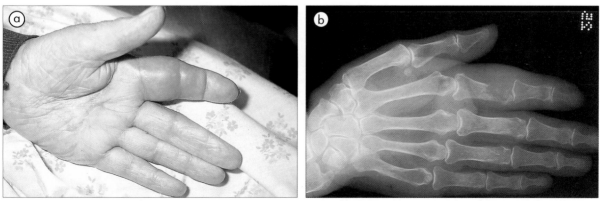

Fig. 7.21 Bone metastasis in carcinoma of the bronchus. (a) Clinical appearance. (b) Typical x-ray change in this unusual site.

In patients with locally recurrent disease and where further radiotherapy is judged to be unwise, laser therapy may be helpful. It can be used to stop bleeding or to re-establish the airway. A patient with a severely obstructive proximal lesion, often gasping and stridulous, can sometimes be transformed overnight by a single laser treatment. Unfortunately, this technique is not widely available.

Chemotherapy

Although chemotherapy has no established role in non-small cell carcinoma of the bronchus, it is increasingly used since newer regimens of cytotoxic drugs have been shown to produce worthwhile responses, particularly in patients with limited disease (that is, limited to a single hemithorax, without evidence of widespread metastases). The

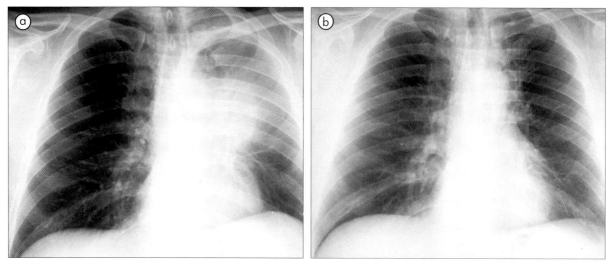

Fig. 7.22 Small cell carcinoma of the bronchus. (a) Appearance before treatment. (b) Dramatic tumour reduction following three months of combination chemotherapy.

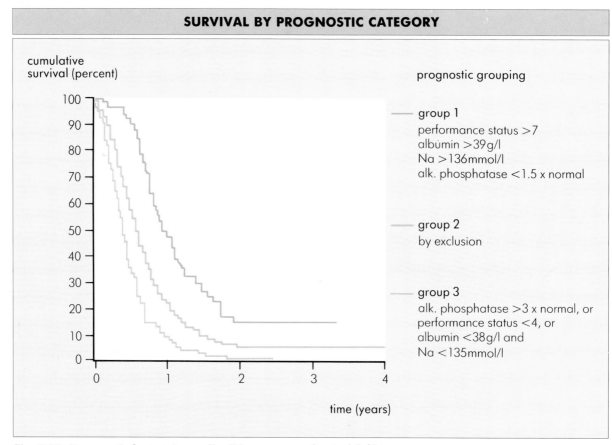

Fig. 7.23 Prognostic factors in small cell lung cancer. Survival (left) in relation to prognostic grouping (right). Courtesy of Prof R.L. Souhami.

combination of mitomycin, ifosfamide and cisplatin has produced response rates of over 50%. Such patients should ideally be treated within clinical trials, and patients receiving these drugs are usually admitted to hospital on a regular basis every three to four weeks. It is common for this treatment to be followed up by local radiotherapy to the primary site, and initial results of such treatment are encouraging.

For small cell lung cancer, chemotherapy is now accepted as the treatment of choice, and may produce remarkable responses (Fig. 7.22). Response to chemotherapy may to some extent be predicted by simple tests (Fig. 7.23), but the most valuable indication is a complete response to the treatment (Fig. 7.24). Overall, less than 10% of patients survive small cell lung cancer, and even in the relatively favourable group with only limited disease (30% of all patients), the results from the very best centres in the world are rarely better than 20% survival at five years. Although these figures have led many to question the role of chemotherapy, there is no doubt that the symptomatic benefits are substantial, quite apart from the slim chance of cure. No one regimen has established itself as clearly superior, but combinations of vincristine, doxorubicin, etoposide and cyclophosphamide are often used (see chapter 3). Common adverse effects include nausea, vomiting,

hair loss and weakness although supportive care with anti-emetics and steroids can greatly limit these disadvantages, and most treatments are now well enough tolerated to be given without hospital admission.

Treatment Combinations

Combinations of chemotherapy and radiotherapy probably produce the best overall results with small cell lung cancer, though this form of lung cancer still carries a very poor prognosis, a grim paradox in view of its extreme short-term responsiveness to both types of treatment. Radiotherapy alone is now not generally used other than in elderly or frail patients, because of the frequency of widespread metastases even when this is not apparent at diagnosis.

With combination treatments, radiotherapy is generally employed after induction with chemotherapy, preferably at the point of 'complete remission' where the chest x-ray has returned to normal. Because of the high rate of brain metastases some patients are offered prophylactic radiotherapy to the brain if they have achieved a complete response to chemotherapy. Radiotherapists are aware that previous chemotherapy administration may increase radiation-related adverse effects, particularly radiation pneumonitis which is characterised clinically

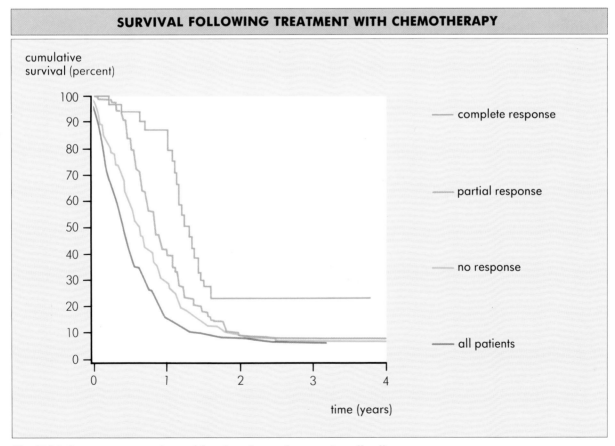

SURVIVAL FOLLOWING TREATMENT WITH CHEMOTHERAPY

cumulative survival (percent)

— complete response

— partial response

— no response

— all patients

time (years)

Fig. 7.24 Response rates to combination chemotherapy (small cell lung cancer). The attainment of a complete response is the most critical prognostic feature of all.

by cough, dyspnoea and tightness of the chest and radiologically by an often striking density within the hilar/mediastinal nodes and lung fields, clearly outlining the previous radiation field (Fig. 7.25). Treatment with oral or inhaled steroids can be extremely beneficial in such cases.

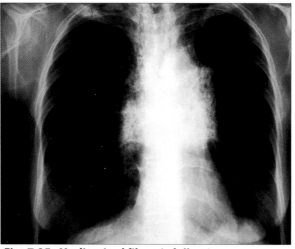

Fig. 7.25 Mediastinal fibrosis following radiotherapy for lung cancer. The radiation portal is clearly outlined, and the patient suffered from recurrent dry cough and dyspnoea, responsive to oral steroid therapy.

Summary

Lung cancer still has a gloomy prognosis, a particularly tragic admission in an almost entirely preventable disease. Careful counselling, stressing both the dangers of cigarette smoking and the large number of smokers who die each year from lung cancer, may be helpful in encouraging patients to cut down or stop smoking. Although opinions are divided, many feel that nicotine chewing gum can be a useful halfway house for patients who do wish to stop.

Lung cancer rates in the Western world will probably fall over the next twenty years, due to better health education measures and a slow decline in the number of male smokers. However, this is not the case in the Third World, where both cigarette consumption (Fig. 7.26) and lung cancer incidence are increasing in line with the emergence of a powerful commercial lobby. We are clearly still a long way from defeating this common and lethal condition.

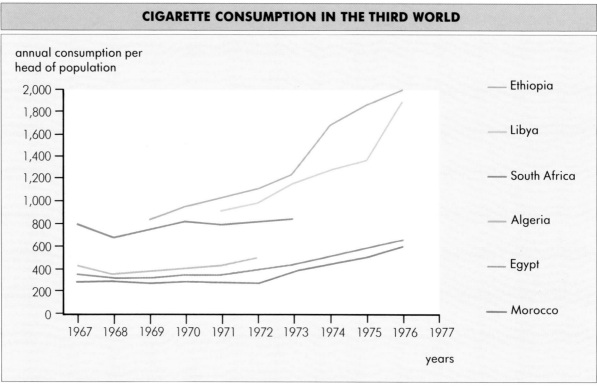

CIGARETTE CONSUMPTION IN THE THIRD WORLD

annual consumption per head of population

— Ethiopia
— Libya
— South Africa
— Algeria
— Egypt
— Morocco

years

Fig. 7.26 There is an increasing trend of cigarette consumption in Third World countries.

Breast lumps are notoriously difficult to evaluate, even in experienced hands, and any mass that feels suspicious should be referred for a surgical opinion, preferably from a specialist working within a breast clinic. Patients who have fibroadenosis, a benign and widespread condition often affecting both breasts, may have such granular breasts that they prove particularly difficult to assess. Other important benign breast conditions include fibroadenoma, breast cysts and breast abscesses. Fibroadenoma typically feels like a firm, spherical, mobile mass and occurs characteristically in relatively young women. Breast cysts can be single or multiple, may feel firm and be very worrying. However, they often transilluminate and are readily detectable by fine needle aspiration, when they typically yield a yellowish or greenish fluid with consequent disappearance of the mass. They are almost always benign. Breast abscesses are usually more obvious clinically, with local inflammation, tenderness and erythema. Abscesses often occur in association with pregnancy. A history of benign breast disease, however, cannot be regarded as an indication that a new lump is benign, since the incidence of breast cancer is actually higher in such patients. Apart from the mass itself, other features of malignancy may include the following:

- inversion of the nipple (Fig. 8.3), often long-standing but particularly important if there has been a recent change;
- distortion of the skin, often best noted with the patient bending forward and the breast hanging away from the body;
- nipple discharge, which may be caused by an intraduct carcinoma although benign disorders are also important here;
- inflammation of all or part of the breast, which may categorize the patient as having inflammatory carcinoma, a particularly serious and rapidly growing form of breast carcinoma (Fig. 8.4);
- fungation of the mass through the skin, which may occur in advanced cases and which is virtually pathognomonic of malignancy (Fig. 8.5);

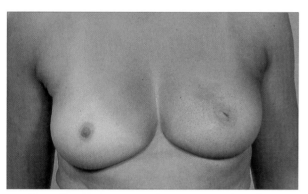

Fig. 8.3 Nipple inversion. An important clinical sign in breast cancer.

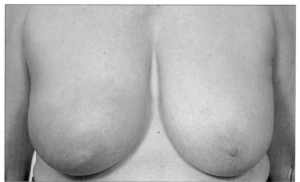

Fig. 8.4 Inflammatory carcinoma. With obvious discolouration of a large portion of the right breast.

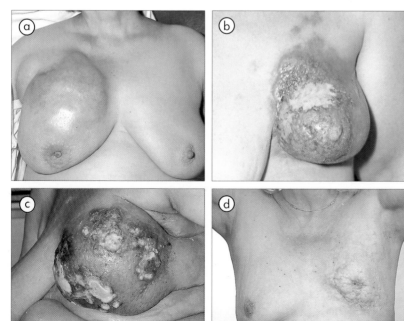

Fig. 8.5 Locally advanced breast cancer. (a) Massive tumour occupying most of the right breast and about to fungate. There is nipple inversion, visible axillary lymphadenopathy and *peau d'orange*. (b) & (c) Fungating tumour occupying whole breast with skin satellite nodules. (d) Automastectomy with almost complete destruction of the left breast.

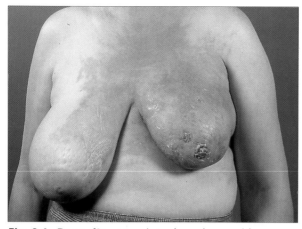

Fig. 8.6 *Peau d'orange.* Intradermal spread from carcinoma of left breast can be seen, with the carcinoma now affecting the opposite side.

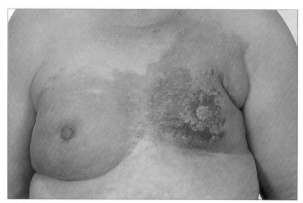

Fig. 8.7 Automastectomy. Contralateral spread can also be seen.

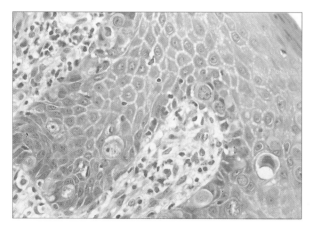

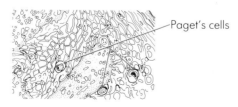

Paget's cells

Fig. 8.8 Paget's disease of the breast. This preparation shows individual atypical cells infiltrating the otherwise unremarkable epidermis of the nipple. H & E stain. Courtesy of Dr L. Bobrow.

- *peau d'orange*, due to local lymphatic permeation and blockage, is a characteristic appearance (Fig. 8.6);
- evidence of intradermal spread may be clinically evident (Fig. 8.7);
- Paget's disease of the nipple has a characteristic appearance (Fig. 8.8) and is generally associated with an underlying carcinoma;
- supraclavicular nodes may be enlarged.

It is of course critically important to examine for nodes in the axilla and to note whether they are fixed or mobile. The breast may be a site for secondary deposits (Fig. 8.9).

Because of the reported improvement in survival in trials testing the value of breast screening, and following the recommendations of the Forrest report published in 1986, the UK has now adopted a policy of breast screening in patients aged 50 to 65 years. The recommendation is that screening mammograms should be performed every three years in patients of this age group, though clearly it will be several years before the policy is fully implemented throughout the country. Workers in Europe have discovered that the detection rate of subclinical breast cancer is sufficiently high to warrant the small radiation exposure and other hazards of screening – the additional risk is more than outweighed by the expected reduction of mortality due to the detection of relatively small cancers. The rapid response of many women to screening programmes has already led to a change in the type of tumour now being detected, with very small tumours and lesions of doubtful invasive behaviour now being recognised more frequently. Ductal carcinoma *in situ* in which no frank invasion has yet developed is now a frequent histological feature of screen-detected early cancers and one which presumably would not have come to light for some years without the screening intervention. We are still learning how best to manage such cases.

Typical mammographic features of a breast carcinoma (Fig. 8.10) include the demonstration of an abnormal mass with microcalcification and spiculation, often with radiating fibrous bands from the

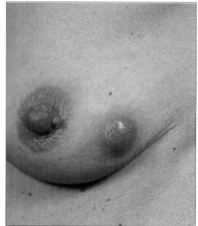

Fig. 8.9 Secondary deposits. This deposit in the left breast originated from a carcinoma of the bronchus.

main lesion. Mammography will not be performed in every suspected case of breast cancer, particularly where the mass is already large, or has the characteristic firmness of a carcinoma. However, surgeons will often request a mammogram in more difficult cases, when the mass is indistinct and the needle biopsy therefore likely to fail, or if he is anxious to have radiological information about both breasts.

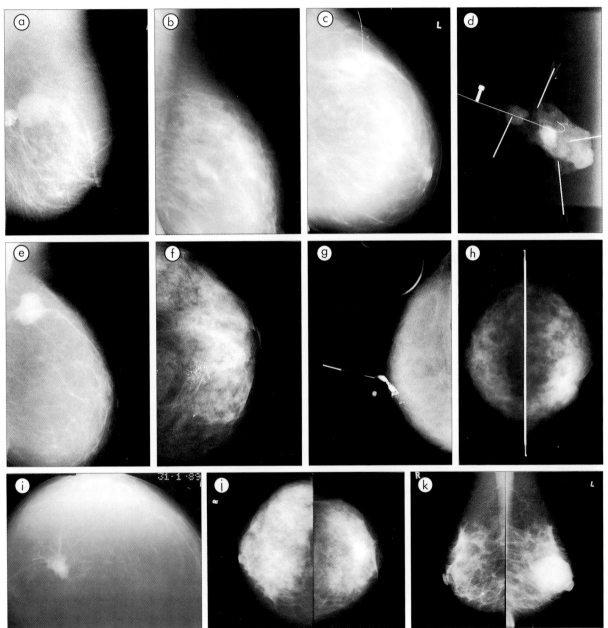

Fig. 8.10 Typical mammographic features in breast carcinoma. (a) Large benign cyst (anterior) and a smaller fibroadenoma (posterior) with characteristic macrocalcification. (b), (c) & (d) This discrete rounded mass looked benign, but there was a slight suspicion about the anterior inferior margin. It was therefore localized and removed with wire; it turned out to be fibroadenoma. (e) Carcinoma. Malignant lesion with fibrous strands and overlying skin thickening. (f) Intraductal carcinoma with extensive microcalcification (defined as fine pieces of calcification of branching irregular pattern) which is characteristic of malignancy and should be investigated further. (g) Investigation of bloody discharge from nipple by galactography showed a blocked duct with an intraluminal rounded filling defect, indicative of an intraductal papilloma.

(h) This large dense area had few of the normal features of malignancy. On biopsy it was adenosis. (i) Carcinoma. Elderly patient with fatty breast. It is easy to identify the malignant lesion, which is intraductal with vascular and neural invasion. Branching microcalcification, a characteristic feature, can be seen following the duct. Strands emanating from the lesion indicate a fibrous reaction generated by the tumour along the stroma and suspensory ligaments. (j) Infiltrating ductal carcinoma. In the younger breast small lesions are more difficult to detect, although this one is big enough to see. (k) Cystosarcoma phyllodes tumour (a benign condition). Relatively well circumscribed with a very large and suspicious posterior margin which is slightly hazy, possibly due to infiltrates. Courtesy of Dr P. Woodhead.

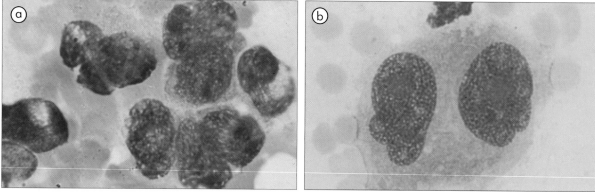

Fig. 8.11 Fine needle aspiration cytology of the breast. (a) Cluster of pleomorphic cells showing coarse chromatin pattern indicative of a duct-type breast carcinoma. MGG stain, ×40. (b) A single cell, with bizarre nuclear features and prominent nucleoli, from the stroma of cystosarcoma phyllodes tumour. MGG stain, ×100. Courtesy of Dr G. Kocjan.

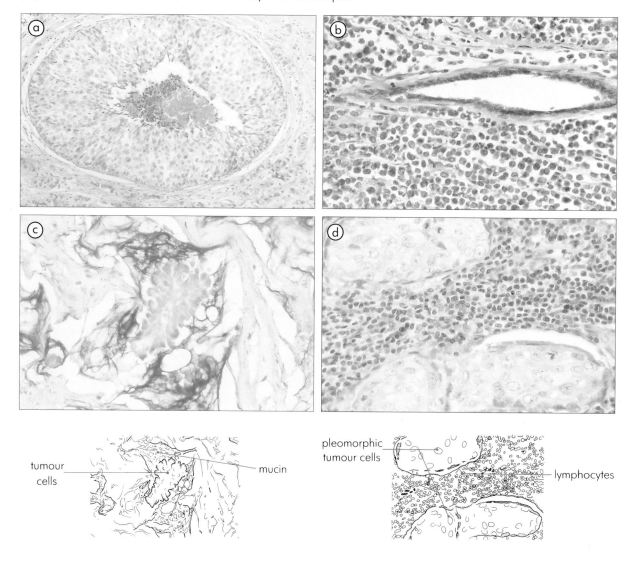

Fig. 8.12 Pathology of the breast. (a) Intraduct carcinoma of the comedo type. The duct is expanded by malignant cells and central necrosis can be seen. H & E stain. (b) Infiltrating lobular carcinoma surrounding a non-malignant duct. H & E stain. (c) Mucinous carcinoma demonstrating extracellular mucin production by tumour cells. Periodic acid–Schiff stain. (d) Medullary carcinoma. Sheets of pleomorphic tumour cells are separated by a heavy infiltrate of lymphocytes. H & E stain. Courtesy of Dr L. Bobrow.

Fine needle aspiration cytology (FNAC) has largely replaced other methods of biopsy since it is quick, can be rapidly performed on an outpatient and gives reliable results in the hands of an experienced cytologist (Fig. 8.11). Some surgeons prefer the Trucut biopsy, which has the advantage of providing histological material, but it is clearly more traumatic for the patient. Breast pathology is extremely varied (Fig. 8.12); in malignant cases tumour grade is a critically important prognostic determinant.

Where there is a clinical suspicion of cancer but the FNAC or Trucut have failed to show a positive result, the patient may need to be admitted for excision biopsy of the mass. Although some surgeons still proceed at the same anaesthetic to a mastectomy if the frozen section of the lump is positive, most agree that this practice is to be discouraged (unless the patient specifically requests it), since it gives no time for the woman to consider the alternative approaches to treatment. One of the GP's important roles is to act as his patient's advocate, and it is worth exploring this when first referring a patient with an obvious lump in the breast to a surgeon. Patients can now be told with confidence that it is by no means essential to undergo mastectomy in every case, even if the lump is confirmed as a cancer (see below).

Management of Breast Cancer

Surgery

During the early part of this century radical mastectomy was the preferred operation for patients with breast cancer. The operation consisted of removal of the entire breast and underlying supporting structures (pectoralis muscles), together with a formal lymph node clearance (Fig. 8.13). It was undoubtedly a mutilating procedure, leading not only to loss of the breast but also a major change in body contour from the loss of muscle bulk. Although there are still a few adherents to this policy, most surgeons now accept that more conservative forms of mastectomy or even lesser operations are adequate; several well controlled studies have shown that simple mastectomy – removal of the breast without any attempt at further resection of supporting structures or nodes – gives equivalent results when combined with postoperative radiotherapy. Although the local recurrence rate following a radical mastectomy is low, typically under 7%, this figure can be achieved by simple mastectomy and routine postoperative radiotherapy (Fig. 8.14). Some surgeons combine this with a total or partial axillary clearance, chiefly for the information that this gives rather than for its therapeutic value in reducing local or regional recurrence. The presence of axillary node metastases is probably the most important prognostic feature in patients with breast cancer (Fig. 8.15), and many surgeons feel such information to be essential. However, unless it alters the approach to management,

RADICAL MASTECTOMY

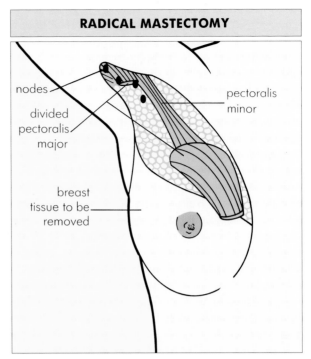

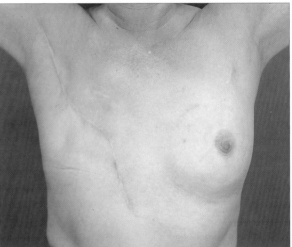

Fig. 8.13 Radical mastectomy. (Top) The pectoralis major is divided and often removed with the axillary contents and all the breast tissue. (Bottom) Postoperative appearance showing loss of chest wall contour.

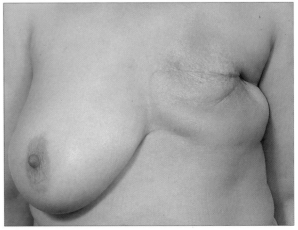

Fig. 8.14 Simple mastectomy and radiotherapy. It is now generally accepted that this procedure is just as effective as radical mastectomy.

such information might be clinically valueless in the individual case.

More recently, large randomized studies have shown that results equivalent to mastectomy can be achieved by a breast-conserving operation followed by local irradiation (Fig. 8.16). After many years of opposition to the concept of breast conservation, many surgeons have now adopted this approach in suitable patients – this is discussed in the next section. Attempts at surgical reconstruction of the breast after mastectomy have met with variable success (Fig. 8.17). Simple silicone implants, though providing valuable contour, are rarely completely acceptable.

Radiotherapy

The real surgical issue over the past decade or so has been the question of whether or not *any* form of mastectomy is necessary. Series from Europe and the USA, in which large numbers of patients have been treated by local excision ('lumpectomy') together with postoperative radiotherapy, have shown

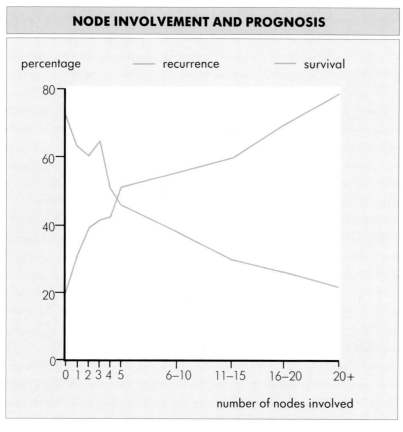

Fig. 8.15 Lymph node involvement and progression in breast cancer. In patients with early carcinoma, confined to the breast itself, the degree of nodal involvement is still the best guide to the final outcome. Other important prognostic features include tumour size, histological grade and oestrogen receptor status. The presence of distant metastatic disease at the outset naturally confers a very poor prognosis.

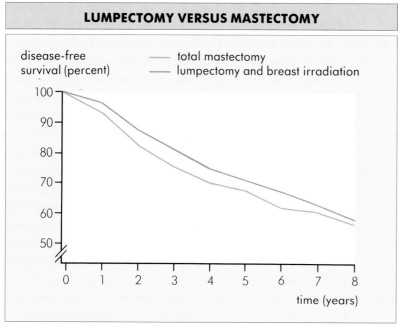

Fig. 8.16 Lumpectomy and breast irradiation compared with total mastectomy. This large, randomized study (over 1,200 subjects) showed that these very different procedures can give quite similar survival rates. [Modified from Fisher *et al.* (1989) *N Engl J Med*, 320, 822–8.]

excellent local control and survival rates, with remarkably good cosmetic appearance in the majority of cases (Fig. 8.18). It seems important to remove the cancerous lump with a narrow rim of normal tissue, in order to avoid local recurrence. However, in some series larger tumours have been treated with radiotherapy alone, to avoid deformity. Even in these cases many patients have had excellent local control and survival. The largest single series to date, from the *Fondation Curie* in Paris, compared ten year survival and local control data with results from the Memorial Sloan–Kettering Cancer Center in New York, which predominantly treated patients by radical surgery. The results were identical (Fig. 8.19), although the majority of the French patients were treated without an initial mastectomy. In addition, preservation of the breast occurred in an overwhelming majority of cases.

Since the surgeon is usually able to provide adequate local excision, radiotherapy for the microscopic residual disease can generally be given to a modest dosage with a correspondingly low level

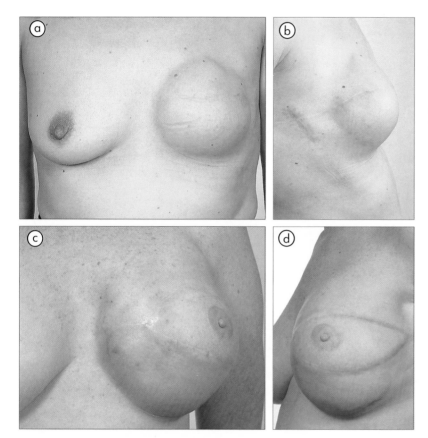

Fig. 8.17 Prosthetic replacement.
(a) & (b) Simple silicone implant giving contour but unsatisfactory aesthetic appearance. (c) & (d) A more sophisticated breast reconstruction with free flap grafting and modelling of nipple, taken from vulval skin.

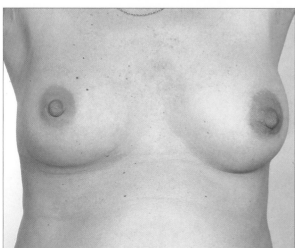

Fig. 8.18 Typical cosmetic appearance following lumpectomy and local irradiation for early carcinoma of the right breast. Taken approximately five years after treatment.

SURGERY VERSUS RADIOTHERAPY

Stage	Disease-free survival at ten years (percent)	
	Memorial Hospital (Radical Surgery)	Fondation Curie (Local excision + Radiotherapy)
T1 N0 N1a	89	90
T2 N0 T1/T2 N1b	52	53
T3 N0 T3 N1b	29	27
total	55	51

Fig. 8.19 Differing philosophies in breast cancer management. The results are identical, even though the French centre avoided mastectomy wherever possible. [Modified from Calle *et al.* (1978) *Cancer,* **42,** 2045.]

of adverse effects. Though rare, these effects can include fibrosis and upward retraction of the breast (Fig. 8.20), telangiectasia of the skin (Fig. 8.21), stiffening of the shoulder (Fig. 8.22) and brachial plexus damage. Acute radiation-induced skin damage subsides rapidly after treatment (Fig. 8.23).

Although the psychological aspects of mastectomy and breast preservation have not been fully assessed,

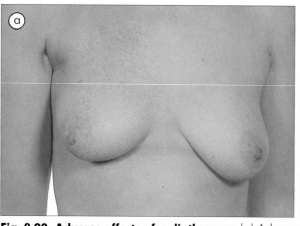
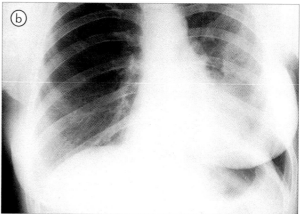

Fig. 8.20 Adverse effects of radiotherapy. (a) Adverse effects of radiotherapy to the right breast with fibrosis and upward retraction although the skin quality is good. (b) Radiation pneumonitis and upward breast retraction, following high-dose radiotherapy for very large carcinoma of the left breast.

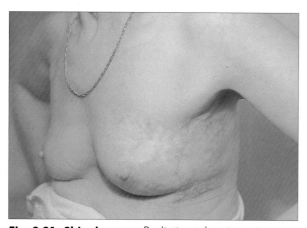
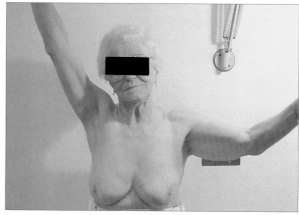

Fig. 8.21 Skin damage. Radiation telangiectasia, evidently a result of excessive radiation.

Fig. 8.22 Shoulder capsule stiffening. Same patient as Fig. 8.21.

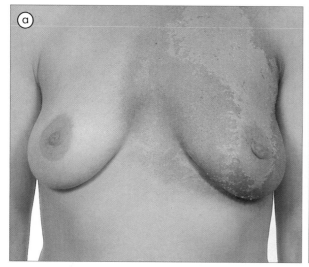
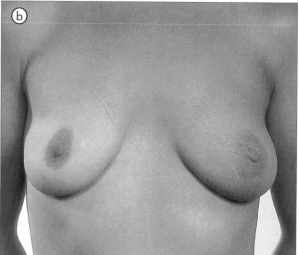

Fig. 8.23 Resolution of radiation-induced skin damage. (a) Acute skin damage (dry desquamation) following radiotherapy. (b) Early resolution after one month.

it seems clear that most patients prefer to have the tumour treated without mastectomy. Careful explanation and support is always necessary from both the surgeon and the GP, to ensure that the patient realises that both are confident in the radiotherapist's approach.

In the USA a few years ago, the issue of breast treatment for early breast cancer became so contentious that the State of Massachusetts passed a law, requiring that all surgeons explain to their patients that an alternative treatment to mastectomy was now widely accepted as safe and effective! Although some surgeons remain sceptical as to the long term local control rate, most large series have confirmed that there is no disadvantage in withholding mastectomy, and that mastectomy can indeed still be performed in the event of local recurrence without serious problems of healing or other major sequelae.

Adjuvant Treatment in Breast Cancer

The other major revolution of the past ten years has been the increasing acceptance that adjuvant treatment – additional systemic approaches for control of unrecognised micrometastatic disease – have now proved themselves, at least in certain circumstances. In postmenopausal patients over the age of fifty there is no longer any serious doubt that treatment with tamoxifen, an oral agent with predominantly anti-oestrogenic but some oestrogen-like properties, is both well-tolerated and beneficial. A large Cancer Research Campaign (CRC) study, in which patients aged over 50 took a single tablet (20mg) of tamoxifen daily for two years, confirmed that this group of patients had a better outcome than the control group, both in terms of the disease-free interval after treatment and also overall survival (Fig. 8.24). This important finding, subsequently confirmed in an even larger Scottish study, is particularly significant because some two-thirds of breast cancer patients fall into this age group; very few had to discontinue tamoxifen because of adverse effects (hot flushes, vaginal discharge or bleeding, occasional thrombocytopenia and hypercalcaemia). A further study is in progress to discover whether five years of treatment offers even greater protection and still other trials are investigating different hormone

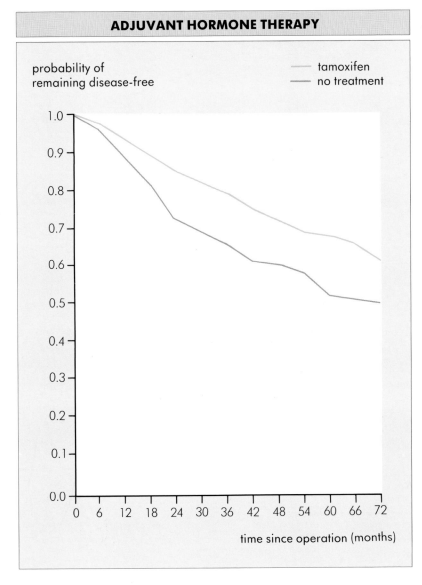

ADJUVANT HORMONE THERAPY

probability of remaining disease-free

— tamoxifen
— no treatment

time since operation (months)

Fig. 8.24 Adjuvant hormone therapy. Data from the original NATO ('Nolvadex' Adjuvant Treatment Organisation) study of adjuvant tamoxifen for early breast cancer. Relapse-free survival was clearly improved by the treatment, which was given as two years continuous oral medication (20mg/day). [Modified from 'Nolvadex' Adjuvant Treatment Organisation (1988) *Br J Cancer*, 57, 608–611.]

approaches, such as the use of radiation-induced menopause (ovarian irradiation), to see whether this gives similar results. Interestingly, tamoxifen appears to work even in patients who apparently have oestrogen-receptor negative tumours. In younger (premenopausal) women, the role of tamoxifen has still to be defined; the CRC group is currently mounting a study to look at this.

More contentious is the use of adjuvant chemotherapy, which has been increasingly used since the report by a major Italian group (published over ten years ago) which suggested a real advantage in both disease-free and overall survival for premenopausal women with a limited number of positive axillary nodes when treated with six courses of adjuvant chemotherapy (Fig. 8.25). The point has been hotly

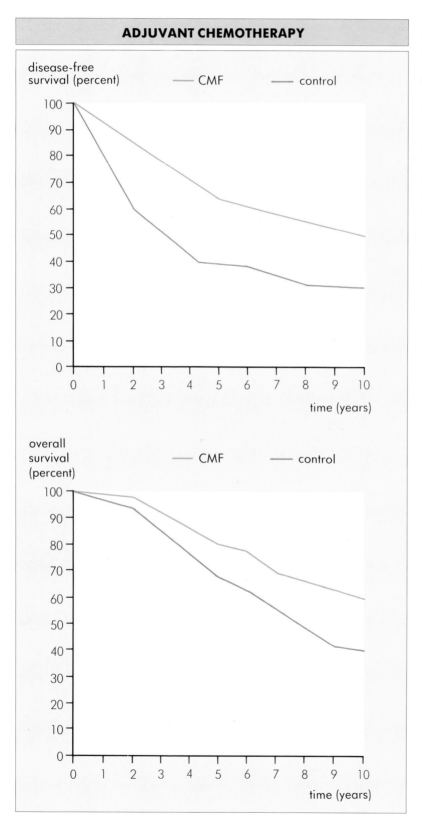

Fig. 8.25 Adjuvant chemotherapy. Data from Milan study showing the benefit of six courses of adjuvant chemotherapy in premenopausal node-positive patients. Treatments consisted of monthly cycles of CMF (cyclophosphamide, methotrexate and 5-fluorouracil). [Modified from Bonadonna and Valagussa (1987) *Seminars in Oncology*, 14, 8–22.] Other studies from the same institution (Istituto Tumori Nazionali, Milano) had previously confirmed that 12 courses of adjuvant CMF chemotherapy were no more effective than 6 courses. These data are included in the world overview shown opposite.

debated and British cancer surgeons have on the whole taken a more conservative line than their colleagues in the USA and mainland Europe. The argument has been that such treatment is hazardous, extremely unpleasant, of dubious benefit and in any event might perhaps only work by providing a chemotherapy-induced menopause, which is no more than ovarian irradiation would offer. Nonetheless, a recent worldwide overview of prospective randomized studies surprisingly showed that the use of adjuvant chemotherapy in node-positive premenopausal patients was genuinely effective, both for prolongation of disease-free survival and also in improvement of overall survival rate (Fig. 8.26). Apart from demonstrating the value of looking at very large numbers of properly randomized patients, this overview analysis demonstrated that the small but definite improvement in survival in such patients could benefit thousands of patients worldwide. In our view, patients with node-positive breast cancer who are fit, premenopausal and willing to undergo chemotherapy should be treated in this way. The potential additional value of hormone manipulation in these premenopausal patients is currently the

subject of further studies. Very recently, randomized trials testing the value of adjuvant chemotherapy and hormone therapy in node-negative breast cancer have reported improved disease-free survival. However, until these and subsequent studies are mature such therapy cannot be recommended.

All such studies, though crucially important, present real difficulties both for hospital doctors and GPs. Many patients like to have a full explanation of what the trial is all about (though some prefer to take a more passive role) and, increasingly, local ethical committees are demanding that each patient give fully informed consent – admirable in principle but often difficult in practice, especially in busy outpatient clinics! GPs can help enormously, particularly if they appreciate the value of the study and also the fact that many patients are happy to know that they are making a useful contribution to medical understanding. The important point to get across is that the potential treatments on trial all represent the very best of current knowledge and that patients on clinical trials are always particularly well looked after, by experts in the field who have access to the most up-to-date information.

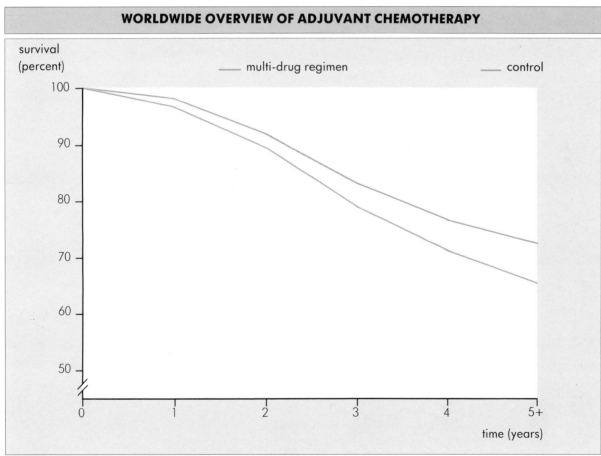

Fig. 8.26 Overview of world data on adjuvant chemotherapy in premenopausal patients with operable breast cancer. This analysis showed conclusively that there is a small benefit from treatment. The power of the study was greatly enhanced by the large sample size. [Modified from Early Breast Cancer Trialists' Collaborative Group (1988) *N Engl J Med*, 319, 1681–1692.]

Breast cancer is a prime example of a disease in which a standard treatment (radical mastectomy), performed for many years on the bland assumption that it was necessarily superior to all other approaches, has rapidly fallen from favour since clinical trials clearly demonstrated that it is, after all, no better than much more conservative approaches.

Treatment of Metastatic Disease

Sadly, many patients with breast cancer develop distant metastases, generally within a few years of the initial treatment, but sometimes with a delay of 20 years or more. It was this capricious behaviour that forced us to the realization that most patients with breast cancer had undetectable micrometastases throughout the body at the time of the initial mastectomy. If one looks at survival curves following breast cancer treatment (Fig. 8.27) it becomes clear that excess mortality over at least the first 20 years (probably rather more) is seen even in the group of patients in whom mastectomy was, at the time, thought likely to be curative. Common sites of spread include the skeleton (particularly ribs, pelvis and spine), liver, lung and brain.

The main types of treatment available for disseminated disease include palliative radiotherapy, chemotherapy and/or hormone therapy. For bone metastases, which are common, painful and often extremely troublesome to the patient, there is no doubt that radiotherapy is the treatment of choice. Short, moderately intensive courses of treatment (given over periods of as little as a week, or even by a single fraction of irradiation) produce pain relief in the large majority of patients. In patients with large deposits in long, weight-bearing bones (particularly the femur), it may be combined with internal orthopaedic fixation, generally undertaking surgery first and postoperative irradiation over the following two weeks. Spinal cord compression is a particularly urgent indication for treatment, either by radiotherapy alone or, where patients have relatively few sites of disease and are in good general condition, by surgical treatment (decompression laminectomy). The shorter the history of spinal cord symptoms and the slower the onset, the more likely the patient is to make a full recovery. If a patient has been completely paraplegic or severely weak for more than seven days, full recovery is extremely unlikely.

At the first sign of tumour recurrence after the initial treatment, the traditional approach has been to treat patients with hormone therapy. In the past, postmenopausal patients were given oestrogen supplements and premenopausal patients treated by surgical oophorectomy. About 30% of patients responded (those who were strongly oestrogen-receptor positive), often with a relatively long-lasting remission and a particularly good symptomatic response where the metastases were predominantly

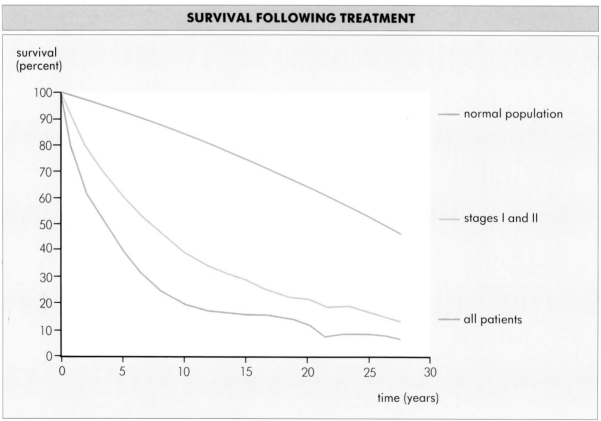

SURVIVAL FOLLOWING TREATMENT

survival (percent)

normal population

stages I and II

all patients

time (years)

Fig. 8.27 Breast cancer survival rates. 25-year survival of patients treated for breast cancer compared with that of an age-matched control population. [Modified from Brinkley and Haybittle (1975) *Lancet* ii, 95–97.]

bony. Nowadays the approach has altered somewhat and surgical oophorectomy has largely been replaced by two competing approaches. The first is the use of radiation-induced menopause, which stops the menstrual periods and does not require a surgical operation or any time in hospital, but simply a week of pelvic irradiation. The second is the use of tamoxifen, which randomized studies have shown to be as active as oophorectomy in premenopausal women. Other approaches include the use of hormones other than tamoxifen (progestational agents for example) and aminoglutethimide (a drug which inhibits steroid synthesis by producing 'medical adrenalectomy' as well as reducing peripheral aromatization). In *postmenopausal* patients tamoxifen has become the drug of first choice in relapsed patients who have not previously received it, although an increasing number of patients now take tamoxifen as part of their primary therapy. Many physicians are disinclined to treat elderly patients with chemotherapy, so a common choice in the event of a relapse is a second–line hormonal preparation, for example progestogen (as medroxyprogestogen acetate), or aminoglutethimide with hydrocortisone – all agents which can be taken orally. Another useful means of hormonal manipulation is to use an androgenic steroid such as nandrolone decanoate (Deca-Durabolin) which is generally given by intramuscular injection every month – because of their virilizing properties, these drugs are less commonly used. All of these agents can produce responses, but it is generally fruitless to persist with hormonal medication if the patient has never shown any benefit from the first- or second-line hormone therapy.

Judicious use of combination chemotherapy may, under these circumstances, be justified; obviously one has to balance the advantages against the possible adverse effects. The UCH breast clinic has frequently used cytotoxic chemotherapy as *primary* treatment for elderly patients with advanced fungating tumours, and we have been impressed at both the tolerance and effectiveness of chemotherapy when used in this setting (Fig. 8.28). If given prior to local irradiation, it may provide good partial healing of the primary lesion by the time that radiotherapy is offered. Chemotherapy, used appropriately, can provide genuine palliation and should not be rejected out of hand. However, it is senseless to persist with it in the face of progressive disease.

Summary

The management of breast cancer has changed rapidly over the past ten years and will doubtless change further. The increased emphasis on conservative surgery with breast conservation, and the demonstration that systemic adjuvant therapy can prolong both disease-free and overall survival, have led to a new sense of optimism in the management of this common and fatal type of cancer.

Breast Cancer in Men

This is a rarity, 100 times less common in men than it is in women (Fig. 8.29). Little is known of the aetiology, but some family clusters have been reported and there may be a connection with Klinefelter's syndrome, in which gonadotrophin levels are raised. Gynaecomastia or hyperoestrogenism following liver damage (cirrhosis, for example) have also been

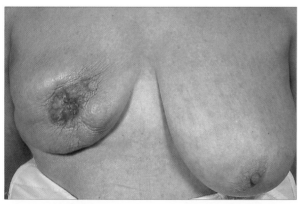

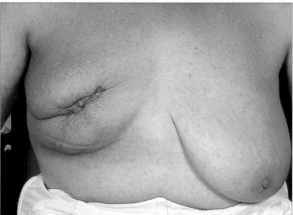

Fig. 8.28 Locally advanced breast cancer treated with cytotoxic chemotherapy. Substantial healing is seen after six cycles of out-patient treatment.

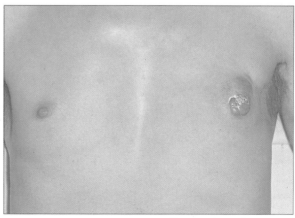

Fig. 8.29 Male breast cancer. The nipple is almost completely destroyed. Courtesy of Mr P.B. Boulos.

implicated. Most patients present with a tender area close to the nipple, sometimes with a discharge or crusting. The chest wall is usually involved early. Local and distant dissemination follows the usual pattern.

The preferred treatment is simple mastectomy. This procedure is chosen by many surgeons because the breast is smaller and the cosmetic result less important. As with women, there is a considerable risk of local recurrence when the axillary nodes are involved. Radiotherapy should be considered in such patients, although there is a high incidence of lymphoedema following this treatment. For distant metastases, orchidectomy is the treatment of choice. Responses have been reported in two-thirds of patients, a reflection of the high incidence of hormone receptor positivity in males. Other hormone treatments include tamoxifen, progestogens, cyproterone and hypophysectomy. Where hormone treatment fails, chemotherapy may give a brief remission.

Whether the prognosis is different from that of female breast cancer remains a matter for debate, but it seems likely that, stage for stage, the outlook in men is no worse.

Gastrointestinal Cancer

9

Introduction

This large group of tumours includes those from the upper oesophagus along the whole of the gastrointestinal tract to the anus, together with carcinomas of the liver, gallbladder and pancreas. The relative incidence of these cancers is shown in Figure 9.1.

Aetiology of Gastrointestinal Cancer

A good deal is known about the aetiology of gastrointestinal tumours, a number of clues coming from their geographical distribution (Fig. 9.2), which is so widely variable that dietary factors are probably important. For example, oesophageal cancer is common in the southern tip of Africa, the shores of the Caspian Sea and in the Far East, with a high incidence belt running across part of the USSR. It is more common in lower socioeconomic groups and in US Blacks (particularly males). There is a clear link to smoking and high alcohol intake. In western Europe, patients with long-standing achalasia have a high incidence of oesophageal cancer, as do those with the Plummer–Vinson syndrome of congenital oesophageal web with a predisposing history of iron deficiency anaemia and recurrent glossitis, recognized mainly in female patients. In northern France, the consumption of calvados (apple brandy) has long been thought to predispose to a high incidence of oesophageal cancer.

Stomach cancer also has a marked social and geographical heterogeneity, again with a preponderance of cases in lower social classes and amongst Blacks. The high risk areas include parts of China and Japan (with the highest incidence in the World at 80 cases per 100,000 male population), other parts of the Far East and South America (Fig. 9.3); Europe has a lower incidence. In the UK and the USA, the prevalence rate of carcinoma of the stomach has fallen markedly since the war (see Fig. 1.5), in direct contrast to the rate for carcinoma of the pancreas, which has risen. Gastric cancer is much more common in patients with pernicious anaemia, chronic gastritis, or those with blood group A. The mechanism appears to involve gastric atrophy and alteration in intragastric pH, resulting in production by the stomach of nitroso compounds which are known to be carcinogenic in animals.

Cancers of the duodenum and small bowel are extremely uncommon, unlike those of the large bowel, in which the incidence of both colonic and rectal tumours remains high. Indeed, in the Western World, cancers of the large bowel comprise up to 15% of all malignant neoplasms. Large-bowel cancers are uncommon in Africa, South America and Asia, again suggesting a possible dietary cause. This may relate to the high fat/carbohydrate, low fibre diet traditionally enjoyed in many western countries (though the position is now changing rapidly) with the inevitable consequence of a slow stool transit time, low frequency of defaecation and thereby a higher exposure to any potential carcinogen passing through the intestine, particularly the large bowel. These ideas, initially postulated by T.L. Gleave and Denis Burkitt, were greeted with ridicule when first proposed, but

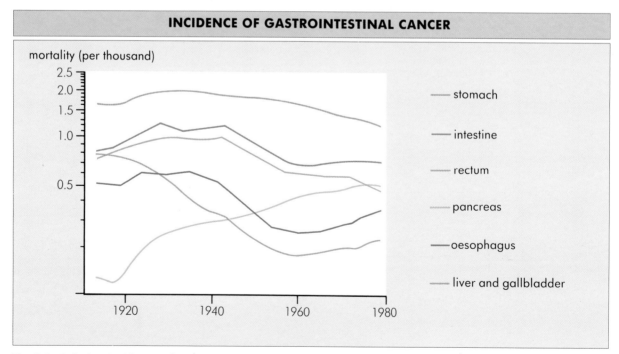

Fig. 9.1 Relative incidence of gastrointestinal cancer, over a sixty year period. The major changes are in the gradual decline of carcinoma of the stomach, together with an increased incidence of carcinoma of the pancreas over the same period.

have been more widely accepted in recent years. As with other tumours, Japanese immigrants to the USA show an increased incidence of colorectal cancer within two or three generations (see Fig. 1.3). In general there appears to be a strong global connection between consumption of meat and incidence of colonic cancer (see Fig. 1.14).

Several genetic or acquired conditions are known to predispose to the development of cancers of the large bowel. These include ulcerative colitis, particularly where the patient has been diagnosed in early life and has extensive involvement, and polyposis coli, a familial condition with autosomal dominant inheritance in which affected family members later

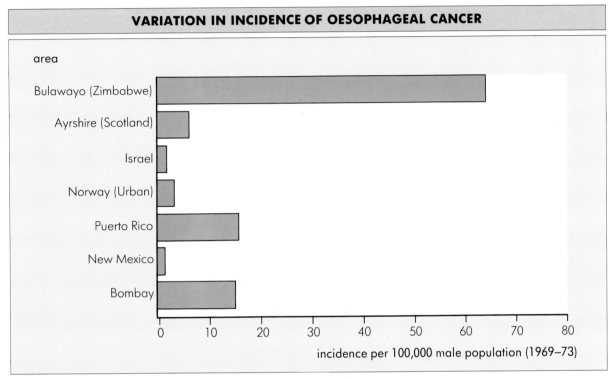

Fig. 9.2 Geographical distribution of oesophageal cancer. These figures show the remarkable variation in incidence throughout the World.

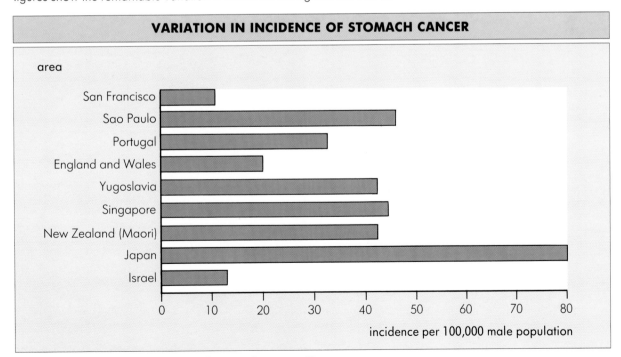

Fig. 9.3 Geographical incidence of stomach cancer. The rates are approximately double for US Blacks compared with Whites. The highest incidence in the World is in Japan, with much lower rates in Europe.

develop colon cancer; prophylactic colectomy is recommended for this reason, though frequent (preferably annual) colonoscopy is considered to be adequate in some centres. Likewise, the rarer Gardner's syndrome of multiple polyps of the bowel together with skull, mandible and skin lesions should also be regarded as a premalignant condition. A much more common condition is the occurrence of sporadic colonic polyps which occasionally undergo malignant change, but with insufficient frequency to warrant colectomy as a prophylactic measure. Such patients should be regularly reviewed, and the advent of colonoscopy has permitted frequent inspection and biopsy without recourse to extensive surgery.

Within the large bowel the frequency of carcinoma varies between specific sites, with a high incidence in the rectum itself and in the sigmoid colon, but a much lower incidence in the transverse and ascending colon (Fig. 9.4). The anus, although an unusual site, is receiving increasing attention because of the probability that anal carcinoma is an HIV related tumour. The incidence of anal cancer appears to be rising, and there seems to be a predisposition to malignancy in patients who harbour anal condylomata or those in whom wart virus can consistently be identified.

Liver, Gallbladder and Pancreas

The aetiology of carcinomas of the liver, gallbladder and pancreas is also well defined. Primary cancers of the liver (Fig. 9.5) are far less common in the West than are secondary deposits, which often arise from gastrointestinal tumours, though the liver is a common site of metastasis from many solid carcinomas. In the West there is a preponderance of primary

hepatic cancer in males, but these tumours are less common than cancer of the pancreas. However, in parts of Africa the incidence is almost a hundredfold greater, presumably as a result of difference in the incidence of viral hepatitis, diet or food preparation. In Europe and the USA, the commonest type of primary hepatic tumour is hepatocellular carcinoma (sometimes termed 'primary hepatoma') most frequently arising in a cirrhotic liver, particularly where it follows a hepatitis B infection or where there is heavy alcohol intake.

There is a strong male preponderance in this condition with a significant incidence (perhaps 20%) in men who have survived with a cirrhotic liver for 20 years or more. A less common type of primary liver cancer, the angiosarcoma, is of importance since it is essentially an occupational condition occurring in workers with long-term exposure to PVC (polyvinyl chloride), a material used in the plastics and clothing industries.

Cancer of the gallbladder is of greater numerical importance in the West, particularly since gallstones, which are so common in the normal population, apparently have a role in their aetiology. This tumour is unusual in patients without a previous history of gallstones or at least the identification of cholelithiasis at the time of diagnosis of the gallbladder cancer. Elsewhere in the world, infestation by the liver fluke is of importance as these parasites produce a sclerosing cholangitis which may be genuinely premalignant.

Pancreatic carcinoma generally affects the head rather than body or tail of the organ, and is more common in patients with diabetes and, possibly, in patients with a past history of chronic pancreatitis. It

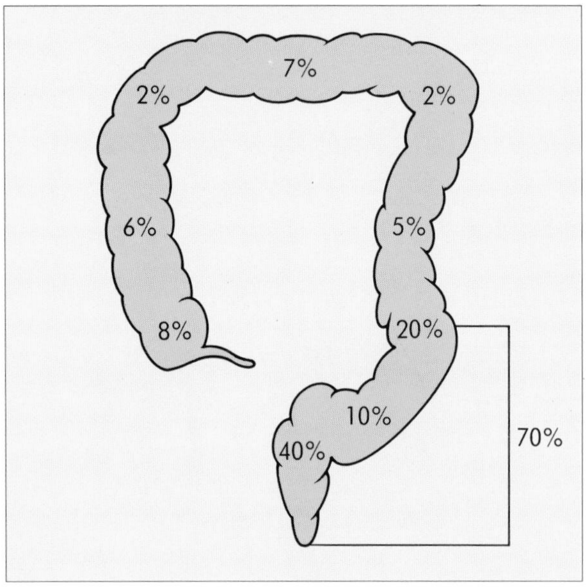

Fig. 9.4 Distribution of colorectal carcinoma, by large bowel site.

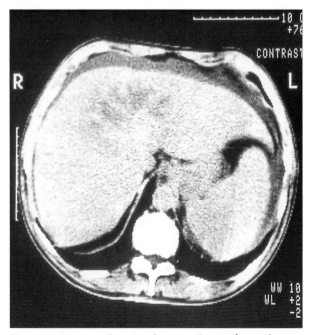

Fig. 9.5 CT scan showing large primary hepatic carcinoma. This was a hepatocellular carcinoma, with a grossly elevated AFP level.

may also be related to high alcohol and cigarette consumption, and is found mainly in the elderly, with a slight preponderance in males. Some years ago it was proposed that increased coffee consumption could be an independent variable, but this has not been confirmed by other studies. In addition, a very rare type of pancreatic sarcoma occurs in childhood.

Tumours of the endocrine pancreas are uncommon but nevertheless important, and may form part of a group of exotic conditions in which clusters of endocrine neoplasms occur with specific genetic patterns (Fig. 9.6). These are the multiple endocrine adenomatosis syndromes (MEAs) of which there are three distinct varieties: Wermer's Syndrome (MEA type I); Sipple Syndrome (MEA type II); and Mucosal Neuroma Syndrome (MEA type III). Other tumours of the pancreatic endocrine system include insulin-producing *insulinoma* (originating in the beta cell islet) resulting in symptomatic hypoglycaemia with dizziness, confusion and loss of consciousness, and *gastrinoma* (the well known Zollinger–Ellison Syndrome) which, in contrast to insulinoma, is generally malignant. The tumour arises from the delta cells of the pancreas and may be single or multiple. It results in recurrent peptic ulceration due to high levels of circulating gastrin constantly stimulating the gastric parietal cells and producing chronic diarrhoea in up to half of all cases. Other rarer tumours of the endocrine pancreas may also occur, all tending to produce recurrent diarrhoea due to secretion of vasoactive mediators and suppression of pancreatic exocrine function. Many of these rare tumours have a higher propensity for malignant transformation.

Cancers of the Oesophagus and Stomach

Symptoms and Diagnosis

Oesophageal cancer is sometimes associated with surprisingly few symptoms. Most patients present with dysphagia and weight loss, often very profound, leading to cachexia. Patients are sometimes able to describe the precise level in the chest where food lodges, and it is common for them to report much greater difficulty with solids than liquids. Dysphagia can progress rapidly, some patients presenting with complete inability to swallow even their own saliva. By this time, weight loss of 10 kg or more is not unusual, but surprisingly there may be few if any physical signs, other than the obvious signs of malnutrition and possibly chronic anaemia. It is important to search for nodal metastases, particularly in the neck of supraclavicular fossa, and of course for hepatic enlargement which may be due to malignant deposits. The oral cavity and oropharynx appear normal on inspection, though the tongue may be coated and furred through dehydration and/or candidiasis.

Although patients with carcinoma of the stomach may present with weight loss and dysphagia, together with nausea and upper abdominal discomfort or bloating, the condition is more difficult to diagnose reliably from the clinical history alone. This problem is often compounded by a history of peptic ulceration. For this reason, carcinoma of the stomach may not be recognized until there is an obvious epigastric mass or a sign of metastatic spread such as lymphadenopathy (classically a node – Virchow's node – in the left anterior triangle), ascites or hepatomegaly.

MULTIPLE ENDOCRINE ADENOMATOSIS TYPES I, II AND III		
Type I Wermer Syndrome	Type II Sipple Syndrome	Type III Mucosal Neuroma Syndrome
Parathyroid adenoma and/or hyperplasia (with hypercalcaemia)	Bilateral medullary carcinoma of the thyroid gland	Bilateral medullary carcinoma of the thyroid gland
Pancreatic islet adenomas (B or non-B cell)	Phaeochromocytoma (bilateral or extra-adrenal)	Phaeochromocytoma(s)
Pituitary adenomas (functioning or non-functioning)	Parathyroid hyperplasia	Parathyroids usually normal
Adrenocortical adenomas	No specific phenotype	Specific phenotype (mucosal neuromas of lip, tongue, mouth, gut)
Thyroid adenomas	Familial inheritance, autosomal dominant	Infrequently familial
Autosomal dominant; presentation 20–60 years	Medullary carcinoma of thyroid relatively 'benign'	Medullary carcinoma of thyroid 'aggressive' Rare survivors aged 30

Fig. 9.6 The multiple endocrine adenomatosis (MEA) syndromes.

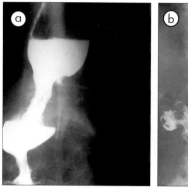
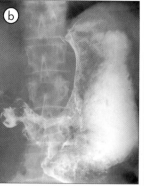
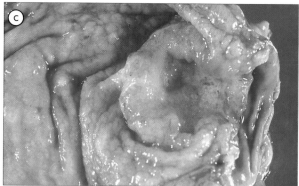

Fig. 9.7 Barium contrast studies in upper gastrointestinal cancer. (a) Barium swallow showing typical features of a malignant stricture of the oesophagus. There is obvious 'shouldering' of the barium column, and the length of the stricture is clearly demonstrated. (b) Large malignant gastric ulcer of the inferior prepyloric portion of the stomach. (c) This large, exophytic gastric adenocarcinoma has a central ulcerated area, which gives it a fungating appearance. Courtesy of Dr F.A. Mitros.

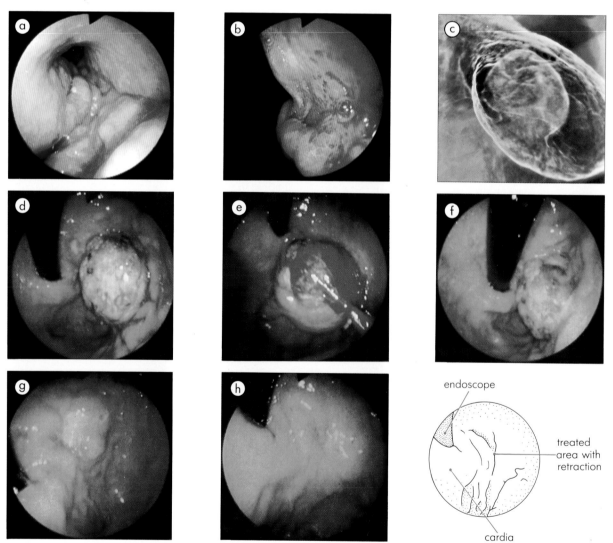

Fig. 9.8 Endoscopy in carcinoma of the stomach.
(a) Type IV adenocarcinoma (linitis plastica). The mucosa covering the diffusely infiltrating tumour appears normal. (b) Extensive linitis plastica of the corpus and fundus with abnormal erythematous mucosa. (c) X-ray of gastric carcinoma in an elderly woman who presented with GI bleeding. (d) Endoscopy revealed a large polypoid cancer in the cardia. The tumour is best seen on retroflexion. (e) The tumour began to bleed while being inspected endoscopically. (f) After partial Nd-YAG laser therapy, the tumour is smaller and there is no evidence of bleeding. (g) Several weeks later after more laser therapy, no cancer is seen. Only a small ulcer is noted in the area of treatment. (h) Finally, the area is completely healed. Biopsy of the area was negative for residual tumour. The only abnormality is a slight retraction in the treated area. Courtesy of Dr F.E. Silverstein.

Patients with suspected carcinoma of the oesophagus or stomach should be investigated with a barium swallow and/or meal, which may reveal typical features of a malignant ulcer (Fig. 9.7). In the oesophagus, the true extent of the tumour is always greater than is apparent from the barium examination. In the linitis plastica variant of carcinoma of the stomach, in which the whole mucosa may be involved, the barium meal may be surprisingly normal. CT scanning is now increasingly used to demonstrate the extent of disease, especially if surgery is contemplated. In such cases, ultrasound or CT of the liver should be performed, to avoid unnecessary surgery.

These tests are generally supplemented by endoscopic examination (Fig. 9.8), allowing direct inspection and biopsy. In the case of oesophageal cancers which prove inoperable because of the patient's age, frailty or extent of disease, a Celestin or other semi-rigid oesophageal tube can be inserted during the examination, giving rapid palliation of symptoms (Fig. 9.9), though patients with total dysphagia often cannot be helped in this way. Immediate laser therapy holds considerable promise in this situation and may lead to rapid reduction of the dysphagia or bleeding.

Pathologically, the commonest cell type is adenocarcinoma, though in high oesophageal lesions (particularly those of the cervical oesophagus) squamous carcinoma is more common. These are similar to other squamous carcinomas of the head and neck, at least in terms of patterns of spread and clinical management. Squamous carcinomas of the oesophagus are not usually identified below the midthoracic portion. Both types of tumour metastasize to local lymph nodes in the neck (particularly the supraclavicular fossa), mediastinum and upper mesentery. Liver metastases are common, though bone, lung and other deposits may occasionally occur.

Management
Radiotherapy or surgery?
These are difficult tumours to treat successfully and there is vigorous debate as to the best approach. In general upper oesophageal (squamous) carcinoma is best treated by radical irradiation, which can sometimes be curative – the best figures (though never confirmed) coming from a Scottish study yielding a 25% survival rate after five years (presumed cures). Radiotherapy has several advantages over surgery. The treatment-related mortality rate is very low, unlike surgical mortality which may be as high as 10–20% even in experienced hands, and moreover radiotherapy is generally more acceptable to frail, elderly patients. The surgical alternative requires not only radical resection, but also sophisticated reconstruction, using colonic interposition or a stomach 'pull up' procedure to provide a satisfactory replacement for the normal oesophagus. Very high oesophageal lesions may also require surgical excision of

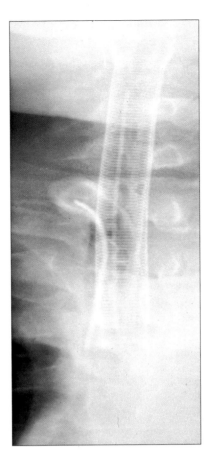

Fig. 9.9 Celestin tube *in situ*. Patient with inoperable carcinoma of the upper oesophagus, which had recurred locally after radiotherapy. The tube allowed adequate nutrition with a semi-solid diet. Note also the tracheostomy tube.

the hypopharynx and larynx in order to achieve control. Such operations are unsuitable where there is extensive nodal or other metastatic spread. There is no evidence that radical oesophageal surgery gives better results than radiotherapy, though there can be little doubt that its morbidity is greater. Where patients are felt to be unsuitable for radical treatment, palliative radiotherapy, to a modest dose, may also be worthwhile. In addition laser treatment, still in its infancy, may be helpful for some patients, with the possibility of repeating the treatment (unlike radiotherapy) if the dysphagia returns and the clinical situation warrants a further attempt. An alternative to these approaches is the use of interstitial radiation therapy, in which the patient literally swallows the irradiating source for a few minutes, an easy out-patient procedure which is gaining in popularity.

For lower oesophageal carcinomas (usually adenocarcinoma), surgery is generally the treatment of choice. Clearly any attempt at a curative operation is contraindicated if the tumour has spread beyond the primary site. In doubtful cases, a careful intra-abdominal exploration should be the first procedure at laparotomy, before a decision on resection is taken. In the case of oesophageal cancer it is generally best to use the mobilized stomach as the method of reconstruction, particularly for mid-oesophageal cancer. Particular problems exist, however, when a substantial portion of the oesophagus has to be resected and some surgeons still prefer colonic transposition. Radiotherapy may also be considered in conjunction with these surgical techniques. If the local extent of tumour has been underestimated pre-operatively, it is best to cut short the operation and rely on radiotherapy. In young, fit patients, however, some surgeons are prepared to proceed to oesophagectomy if there is minimal nodal involvement, with the intention of referring the patient for post-operative radiotherapy. It is occasionally possible to cure node-positive patients in this way, or even, very rarely, by radiotherapy alone.

For carcinoma of the stomach, surgical resection is the only treatment likely to be curative. This is generally confined to young, fit patients who show no evidence of metastatic disease. Clearly with large lesions which are thought to be operable (including linitis plastica), a total gastrectomy may have to be considered. This involves removal of the entire stomach, part of the duodenum and sometimes part of the transverse colon, though fortunately it is sometimes possible to perform a more limited operation (partial gastrectomy). Radiotherapy plays a very minor part in the management of carcinoma of the stomach due to the proximity of radiosensitive organs such as the small bowel and kidneys, the relative insensitivity of adenocarcinoma of the stomach to radiotherapy, and the frequent need for surgery as a palliative procedure.

Complications of surgical treatment include anastomotic leaks, local infection, abscesses and fistulae, quite apart from the considerable mortality, particularly when oesophagectomy is attempted. Complications following radiation treatment of the oesophagus include acute oesophagitis and late radiation stricture from fibrosis. This may be a troublesome and recurrent problem particularly since the length of irradiated oesophagus is generally quite substantial in view of the known submucosal spread of the disease, and the necessarily large treatment volume. It may require intermittent dilatation for satisfactory management. Although successful treatment may provide both symptom relief and considerable weight gain, it is extremely difficult to help patients with total obstruction and absolute dysphagia.

For oesophageal cancer, the results of surgery and radiotherapy are both very poor, but broadly similar in the long term, with a one year survival rate of about 20% and a five year survival rate of under 10%. Approximately one quarter of patients with resectable carcinoma of the stomach will be alive five years after treatment, though only two-thirds of patients undergoing surgery prove to have resectable cancers. If vigorous screening programmes are undertaken, as for example in Japan (where the incidence is the highest in the world), there is no doubt that these cancers are generally identified earlier whilst still operable, and the surgical resectability and long term results are correspondingly better.

Chemotherapy

Chemotherapy has little if any rôle in the management of oesophageal and stomach cancer, though squamous carcinomas of the upper oesophagus may show a similar response rate to squamous carcinomas at other head and neck sites. For carcinoma of the stomach, the situation is slightly different, and these tumours seem to be slightly more responsive to chemotherapy than those at other sites in the gastrointestinal tract. For relatively young, fit patients with extensive disease (for example those with liver metastases) whose general condition is nonetheless reasonably good, the combination of 5-fluorouracil, mitomycin C and doxorubicin have yielded response rates of 30–40% in several reported series, though randomized trials have failed to show survival benefit.

Cancers of the Small Bowel

Symptoms and Diagnosis

Small bowel tumours are rare, accounting for less than 5% of all gastrointestinal malignancy. Consequently they are seldom diagnosed before surgical exploration. The usual clinical presentation is with abdominal pain or obstruction, and an abdominal mass may sometimes be felt. Adenocarcinomas, lymphoma and carcinoid tumours are the most common, and the major sites of spread include the liver and mesenteric lymph nodes. Carcinoids are curious, yellow coloured tumours arising many from neurosecretory cells in the appendix and caecum (Fig. 9.10). In about 25% of carcinoids the tumour is functional (i.e. secretory), particularly where hepatic metastases are present. The carcinoid syndrome (Fig. 9.11) results from secretion of 5HT (5-hydroxytryptamine) and/or bradykinin and prostaglandins. Clinical features incude borborygmi and flushing. This syndrome is readily diagnosable by a 24-hour urine analysis for the 5HT metabolite 5HIAA (5-hydroxyindoleacetic acid). Another curiosity is the appendiceal tumour pseudomyxoma peritonei, a mucinous tumour which can eventually coat the entire peritoneal lining, producing a clinical picture very similar to advanced ovarian cancer (Fig. 9.12).

Management

Small bowel tumours are difficult to treat and often misdiagnosed. Wide surgical resection is generally the best approach. Small bowel lymphomas (see chapter 12) pose a particular problem since these are much more responsive to chemotherapy, but there is a real risk of chemotherapy-induced bowel perforation, presumably due to rapid lysis of a plug of tumour which was maintaining the integrity of the bowel wall. This may prove fatal, and bowel lymphomas should be treated with caution in the initial stages. They may affect a surprising length of bowel (see chapter 12) and multiple skin lesions are common.

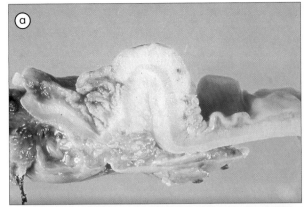

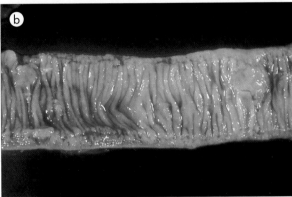

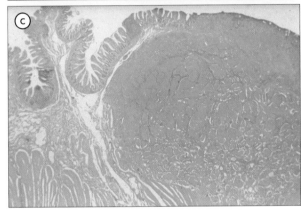

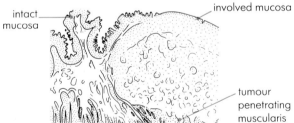

intact mucosa — involved mucosa — tumour penetrating muscularis

Fig. 9.10 Small bowel carcinoid tumour. (a) In this ileal lesion, the tumour has resulted in formation of a knuckle of bowel, with hypertrophy of the involved muscle, which is expanded by tumour, together with direct involvement of the serosa. (b) In this relatively short segment of ileum, there are four grossly identifiable carcinoids. The largest lesion, towards the right, is ulcerated, an unusual feature, and has a typical pale yellow colour. (c) This carcinoid of the terminal ileum is typical of an early lesion. Islands of bland-appearing oval cells expand the submucosa, while the overlying mucosa is intact but involved in its deeper aspects. At the base, tumour clusters penetrate muscularis propria. Courtesy of Dr F.A. Mitros.

FEATURES, TREATMENT AND DISTRIBUTION OF THE CARCINOID SYNDROME

Features
Flushing attacks
Diarrhoea
Bronchospasm
Valvular heart lesions (chiefly tricuspid incompetence from endocardial fibrosis)
Facial telangiectases

Treatment
Pharmacological blocking agents (often used postoperatively)
Cyproheptadine
Aprotonin
Methotrimeprazine
Methysergide

Distribution of gastrointestinal carcinoids	
Stomach	2.5%
Duodenum	4%
Small bowel*	28%
Colon	45%
Appendix	45%
Rectum	16%

*Chiefly terminal ileum

Fig. 9.11 The carcinoid syndrome.

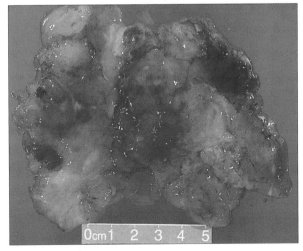

Fig. 9.12 Pseudomyxoma peritonei. The appearance is typical of mucoid material from the peritoneal cavity, here due to an appendiceal primary. Courtesy of Dr F.A. Mitros.

117

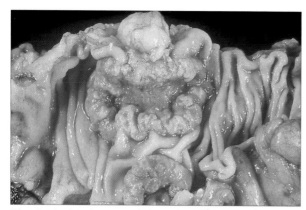

Fig. 9.13 Carcinoma of the colon. The central irregular eroded area and everted rolled edge are typical features. Histologically the lesion was a typical adenocarcinoma. Although the tumour was relatively small, obliteration of the muscle and puckering of the wall both indicate transmural extension. Courtesy of Dr F.A. Mitros.

DUKES STAGING SYSTEM FOR RECTAL CANCER	
Stage	Description
A	Confined to mucosa and submucosa (80%)*
B	Invasion through the musculature with no lymph node involvement (50%)
C	Metastases to regional lymph nodes
C1	Lymph nodes not involved up to the point of vascular ligation (40%)
C2	Nodes involved up to the level of vascular ligation (12%)
*5 year survival	

Fig. 9.14 The Dukes staging system for rectal cancer. Extensive regional nodal involvement has a particularly adverse prognosis. Tumour grade and depth of penetration are also important.

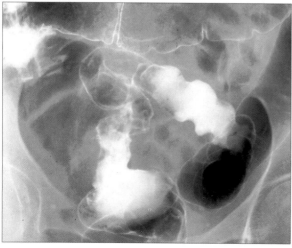

Fig. 9.15 Rectal carcinoma. Barium enema appearance in rectal carcinoma showing typical malignant stricture formation.

Cancers of the Large Bowel

Symptoms and Diagnosis

Large bowel cancers are much more common and chiefly affect the distal large bowel, particularly the rectum and sigmoid colon. Characteristically they occur as fleshy, polypoid growths (Fig. 9.13) and tend to spread locally, through the bowel wall to the exterior (serosal) surface, unlike oesophageal tumours which spread up and down. Haematogenous spread is usually via the portal vein to the liver, though other sites such as bone and lung can be involved. The degree of penetration of the bowel wall and involvement of local lymphatics together form the basis of the Dukes staging system (Fig. 9.14) which gives an excellent indication of the likely outcome following surgery.

Clinical presentation includes abdominal pain, change in bowel habit, rectal bleeding, weight loss and obstructive symptoms, though the frequency of these features clearly varies with the site of the tumour in the bowel. For example, with rectal carcinomas, change in bowel habit and rectal bleeding are generally present, though obstructive symptoms are uncommon. There is usually no palpable abdominal mass though a rectal examination generally reveals the correct diagnosis without difficulty. On the other hand, in tumours of the ascending colon, abdominal pain with a palpable mass are fairly consistent features, while overt rectal bleeding, constipation or diarrhoea are less common. Careful abdominal and rectal examination of patients with any of these symptoms is mandatory, and early referral should be considered. Sigmoidoscopy, colonoscopy and barium enema studies usually give a reliable pre-operative diagnosis (Fig. 9.15), though CT scanning may give additional information and may also confirm inoperability without subjecting the patient to an unnecessary laparotomy. Although there is no reliable plasma marker for these tumours, the serum CEA (carcinoembryonic antigen) level is often elevated, and can be useful either at diagnosis or as a means of predicting relapse following treatment, even before any symptoms supervene.

Management

These tumours are the province of the surgeon. Wide excision is undoubtedly the treatment of choice and the operative details of course depend on the site of the lesion. It is generally possible to perform either a left or right hemicolectomy (Fig. 9.16) with end-to-end anastomosis for sphincter preservation. Low rectal tumours may, however, require abdomino-perineal resection with a permanent colostomy. Recent surgical advances have permitted sphincter preservation for an increasing number of patients with rectal tumours. In clearly inoperable tumours, local irradiation should be considered (especially for rectal carcinomas) as they are partly responsive, and treatment can often produce an improvement in symptoms. Bowel diversion by colostomy can be particularly helpful in such cases, allowing a reasonably high dose of radiotherapy to be given, with a correspondingly more durable remission. Though surgical mortality is now low, complications are still quite common, and include anastomotic leak, pelvic abscess, abdominal fistulae and post-operative wound sepsis. Local recurrence remains a major problem, but it now seems clear that this may be reduced by the routine use of post-operative radiotherapy.

Most patients find life with a colostomy tolerable, though care must be taken to teach correct maintenance techniques from the outset. Patients should be reassured that modern colostomy bags are extremely reliable and do not burst or allow escape of offensive gas. It is important to avoid local spillage of bowel contents onto the skin as this causes subsequent excoriation. Most large hospitals have stoma nurses to help with support, and patients should generally be able to take over their own care without undue difficulty.

Apart from its palliative value, there is increasing evidence that radiotherapy could become an important part of routine management of rectal cancers. Two large American multicentre studies comparing surgery alone with surgery plus radiotherapy, have shown survival benefit (Fig. 9.17), particularly in the more advanced tumours. This approach has not yet been widely accepted in the UK, but a large MRC study is in progress which is attempting to

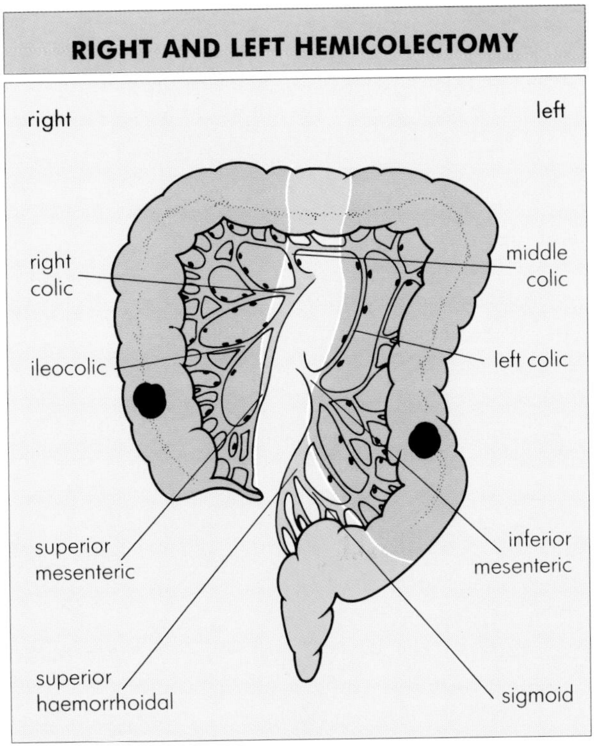

RIGHT AND LEFT HEMICOLECTOMY

Fig. 9.16 Extent of resection in right and left hemicolectomy procedures for carcinomas of the colon. For tumours of the ascending colon, resection should be undertaken well beyond the hepatic flexure. For lesions of the descending colon, this part of the bowel together with the splenic flexure will need to be resected. End-to-end anastomosis can generally be performed at the primary procedure. Major arteries are indicated.

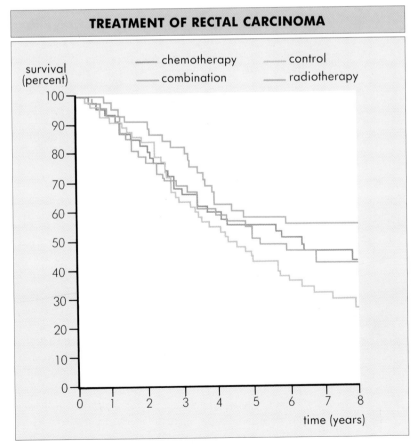

TREATMENT OF RECTAL CARCINOMA

Fig. 9.17 Survival distribution of rectal carcinoma according to treatment. Effect of radiotherapy and chemotherapy in locally advanced carcinoma of the rectum, showing benefit, at 5–8 years, particularly from the combination of both modalities given shortly after initial surgery. [Modified from the Gastrointestinal Tumor Study Group (1986) *N Eng J Med,* **315,** 1294.]

confirm these American findings. In cancers of the anus, radiotherapy has also begun to compete with surgical excision, since surgical removal almost invariably means permanent sphincter loss (Fig. 9.18), while radiotherapy does not usually interfere with normal sphincteric function. This is another site where interstitial radiation therapy techniques have been developed. One further exciting advance, still not fully established, is the use of concomitant radiotherapy with chemotherapy, which may result in remarkable local control even in bulky tumours.

Chemotherapy alone is not very successful in the management of large bowel tumours, though responses are seen with 5-fluorouracil and the nitrosourea group. However, chemotherapy for recurrent disease does not appear to improve survival substantially. Although response rates are only of the order of 25%, the drugs may be more useful given as adjuvant therapy after primary bowel resection, particularly since 5-fluorouracil is so well tolerated. One randomized trial of peri-operative intraportal 5-fluorouracil has shown improved survival compared to control patients undergoing surgery alone. Results from several large studies investigating this technique are awaited.

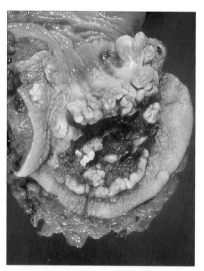

Fig. 9.18 Carcinoma of the anus. This very large squamous carcinoma arose in the perianal skin, and secondarily involved the anal skin and rectum, necessitating extensive resection. Courtesy of Dr F.A. Mitros.

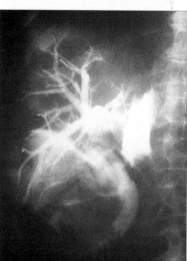

Fig. 9.19 Carcinoma of the biliary tract. Preoperative contrast study showing dilated biliary tree with distal irregularity. This proved to be an obstruction caused by a carcinoma that was largely periampullary. Courtesy of Dr F.A. Mitros.

Overall prognosis depends largely on the stage of the tumour (see Fig. 9.13) and early stage carcinomas confined to the mucosa and submucosa have an excellent five year survival rate. Careful follow-up is essential for all patients since some recurrences are essentially local in nature, and further surgery may still be curative.

Cancers of the Liver, Gallbladder and Pancreas

Liver and Gallbladder

Primary cancers of the liver are uncommon in the West, but the most frequent type is the hepatoma (hepatocellular carcinoma). This tumour occurs either as a diffuse hepatic lesion or as a more defined mass, with residual normal (or cirrhotic) liver even when the primary mass has reached a very late stage (see Fig. 9.5). Since many patients already suffer from cirrhosis or are known to be persistently positive for hepatitis B antigen, vigilance in patients with these disorders can lead to early diagnosis, particularly where rapid deterioration of hepatic function has occurred. Characteristic symptoms include jaundice, hepatic tenderness, abdominal mass and ascites. Liver function tests are always abnormal, and the AFP (alphafetoprotein) is typically raised (out of proportion to benign liver disease) and can often be identified histochemically in the biopsy. Ultrasound or CT imaging is generally conclusive, and careful assessment of the radiology is important since surgical resection can be curative. Wide excision is not, however, performed in many centres, and successful resection is particularly unlikely in cirrhotic patients, thus automatically excluding the majority. Neither radiotherapy nor chemotherapy are very helpful, though these approaches may be worth considering in relatively fit patients for whom surgery is not possible, and particularly where symptoms warrant intervention. Other types of primary liver cancer are much less common, though most carcinoid tumours remain non-secretory (i.e. non-functional) unless they have metastasized to the liver.

Cancers of the gallbladder and biliary tract (Fig. 9.19) also cause right upper quadrant pain, nausea, weight loss and obstructive jaundice, features which make them difficult to distinguish from hepatocellular carcinoma. However, gallbladder and biliary cancers are together more common than hepatoma (in the West) and are generally seen in patients without pre-existing cirrhosis. The distal common bile duct is the most common site and the tumours are typical adenocarcinomas, spreading locally to draining lymph nodes and producing hepatic deposits. It is important to investigate such patients to exclude non-malignant causes of obstructive jaundice and to allow for assessment with a view to surgical resection. This is likely to include sophisticated radiological procedures including CT scanning and/or ERCP (endoscopic retrograde cholangiopancreatography).

Pancreas

Pancreatic cancer presents many difficulties in diagnosis and management. It is increasing in incidence, is found more frequently in males, and has a steep age relationship such that many cases are diagnosed in patients aged 65 years and over. It is a typical adenocarcinoma. Often a firm histological diagnosis is never established since patients may present late and with clinical or radiological evidence of inoperability, making histological diagnosis redundant. Because of the extensive lymphatic drainage of the exocrine pancreas, local nodal spread is extremely common, and these tumours also tend to metastasize early to the liver (Fig. 9.20). Two-thirds are located in the head of pancreas, producing obstructive jaundice and epigastric or back pain as the chief symptoms. In tumours originating in the body or tail, jaundice occurs later so that they are likely to be even more locally advanced by the time of diagnosis, even though back pain is a predominant feature. Other local sites commonly involved by direct extension include the duodenum, bile duct, spleen, transverse colon and retroperitoneal sites. Distant metastases are common.

Pain from pancreatic cancer can become very severe, requiring coeliac plexus block or other sophisticated techniques, and most patients require analgesia for control. Weight loss can be profound, and the clinical course is often extremely short.

Barium meal shows characteristic displacement of the duodenum and stomach, but for definitive diagnosis a CT scan is generally more rewarding (Fig. 9.21). Simple ultrasound of the abdomen may be sufficient if CT facilities are not available. Percutaneous CT guided biopsy is simple and safe, and the number of histologically unverified cases is now

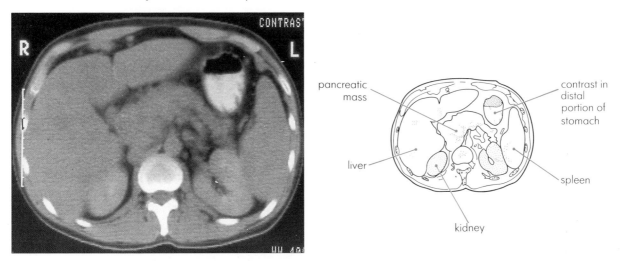

ADENOCARCINOMA OF THE PANCREAS

Spread	Symptoms
Duodenum	Pain, vomiting, obstruction
Bile duct and pancreas	Jaundice, pancreatitis
Retroperitoneum	Back pain
Spleen and colon	Left upper quadrant pain
Portal and splenic veins	Varices, splenomegaly, hepatic disorders
Peritoneal cavity	Ascites
Lymph nodes	Obstructive jaundice
Blood stream	Distant metastases

Fig. 9.20 Sites of spread and production of symptoms in adenocarcinoma of the pancreas. Courtesy of Prof R.L. Souhami.

Fig. 9.21 CT scan showing large carcinoma of the head of the pancreas. CT scanning has largely replaced barium contrast studies, and can be used to guide percutaneous biopsy.

declining. ERCP may also be helpful, but is only justifiable if the patient's condition is reasonably good, and if the investigation is carried out to assess operability.

Cancer of the pancreas is particularly difficult to treat effectively. Although radical surgery offers the only prospect of cure, very few patients are suitable, and the surgical morbidity and mortality remain high. The two operations most widely performed are Whipple's procedure, essentially a radical pancreatico-duodenectomy with anastomosis of the stomach to the proximal small bowel (Fig. 9.22), or total pancreatectomy with preservation of the duodenum, which may be possible depending on the site of the tumour. These are formidable procedures, with high complication rates (fistulae formation, anastomotic leak, local abscess formation), and a

more realistic approach for the majority is simple relief of jaundice by insertion of a semi-rigid stent. This can often be performed percutaneously in view of the grossly dilated bile duct system resulting from the tumour obstruction (Fig. 9.23). This procedure may provide rapid relief of the obstructive jaundice, though the stent is likely to become blocked as the tumour progresses and the period of relief may be short. Where bile salt pruritus is a prominent distressing feature, the relief of obstruction is all the more urgent. If passage of a simple stent is not possible, then a biliary bypass operation is often worth undertaking.

In patients for whom radical surgical resection is suitable, tumours of the ampulla seem to carry a rather better prognosis than other sites.

Radiotherapy is often worth considering, particularly if the site of obstruction can be localized (for example, using ultrasound). A short course of treatment to the porta hepatis area may bring relief of the jaundice and possibly improve the pain. Chemotherapy is not generally regarded as helpful in pancreatic cancer, though short-lived responses are sometimes seen.

In the case of endocrine pancreatic tumours, surgery is again likely to be the cornerstone of treatment, though it may not always be possible. Fortunately these are rare tumours, and in some cases pharmacological blockage may be possible, as with the use of H2 receptor antagonists in patients with the Zollinger–Ellison Syndrome.

The supportive management of patients with pancreatic cancer is particularly important since the symptoms are often extremely distressing, with very few patients cured by surgery or any other means. Attention to pain control and alleviation of pruritus, jaundice and diarrhoea may provide gratifying symptomatic improvement.

WHIPPLE'S PROCEDURE

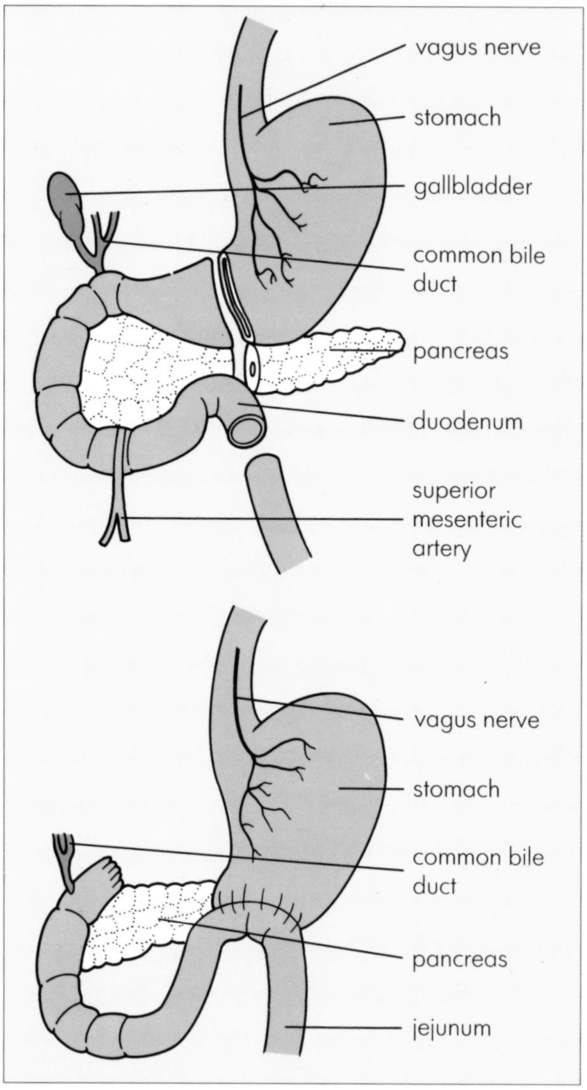

- vagus nerve
- stomach
- gallbladder
- common bile duct
- pancreas
- duodenum
- superior mesenteric artery

- vagus nerve
- stomach
- common bile duct
- pancreas
- jejunum

Fig. 9.22 Schematic representation of radical pancreatico-duodenectomy (Whipple's procedure). The organs removed include the distal stomach, the whole of the duodenum, the first part of the jejunum and the head and part of the body of the pancreas.

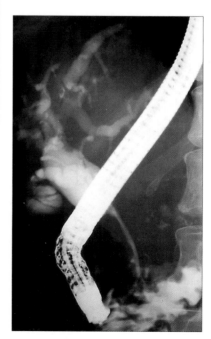

Fig. 9.23 ERCP. This example is from a patient with carcinoma of the common bile duct (CBD). The proximal biliary tree is dilated. A long stricture of the distal CBD is outlined by contrast. Courtesy of Dr W.R. Lees.

Gynaecological Cancer

10

Introduction and Epidemiology

This is an important group of malignancies, accounting for about a quarter of all cancers in women. Indeed, cancer of the cervix is one of the most common of all female cancers. In general, neoplasia of the female reproductive system is amongst the more curable of solid tumours. This is due to a variety of favourable factors which include:

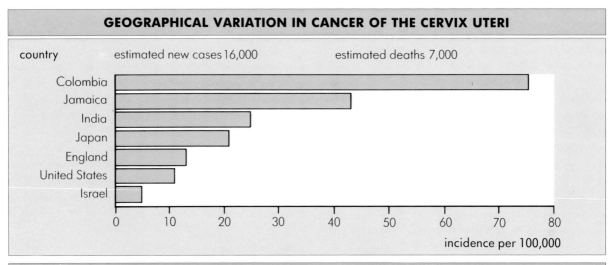

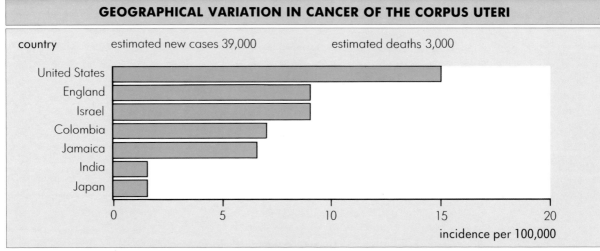

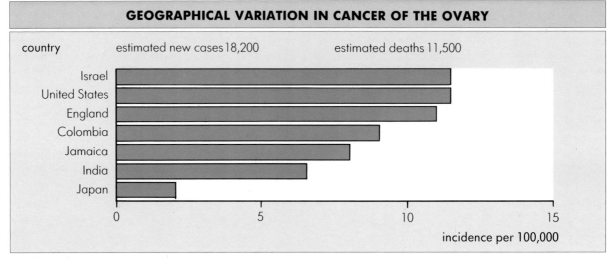

Fig. 10.1 Worldwide incidence of gynaecological cancer.
Geographical variations in incidence of gynaecological cancer throughout the world, showing wide variation in all the major tumour types. Insets show estimated new cases and deaths per year in the USA.

- premalignant changes leading to early definitive therapy (especially cervix);
- loco-regional spread only, at least in the early stages (cervix and endometrium);
- sensitivity to radiotherapy (cervix and endometrium);
- responsiveness to chemotherapy (especially choriocarcinoma and to a lesser extent ovarian cancer).

In invasive carcinoma of the cervix and uterus, mortality rates have fallen dramatically as their incidence has fallen sharply in the past thirty years. Unfortunately ovarian carcinoma is altogether different, its incidence having risen remorselessly this century.

There are major variations in the occurence of this group of tumours around the world, perhaps most particularly in the case of cancer of the cervix (Fig. 10.1). This disease is over 15 times more common in Colombia than in Israel, and though common in prostitutes is virtually unknown in nuns and other celibate women. It is clearly related to early sexual activity, but attempts to isolate the presumed infectious agent have only been partly successful. Recent interest has centred around both the genital herpes and human papilloma viruses, though infections with genital viruses are common and the precise nature of viral causation is far from clear. In many parts of the world (including the UK — particularly the inner cities) there has been a marked increase over the past decade in recognition of abnormal cervical smear patterns indicating a rising incidence of preinvasive cervical cancer. Once again, the natural history of these early lesions is uncertain. Prompt treatment is generally offered to such patients so the frequency of conversion to invasive carcinoma remains unknown. Although in the 1950s invasive carcinoma of the cervix was rarely diagnosed before the age of forty, it is now much more commonly encountered in younger women (Fig. 10.2), and large treatment centres see substantial numbers of patients in their thirties. It is possible that the tumour follows a more aggressive course in this group, though this suggestion remains contentious.

Despite the increase in younger women, invasive carcinoma has become less common in older women, due to the success of cervical screening programmes

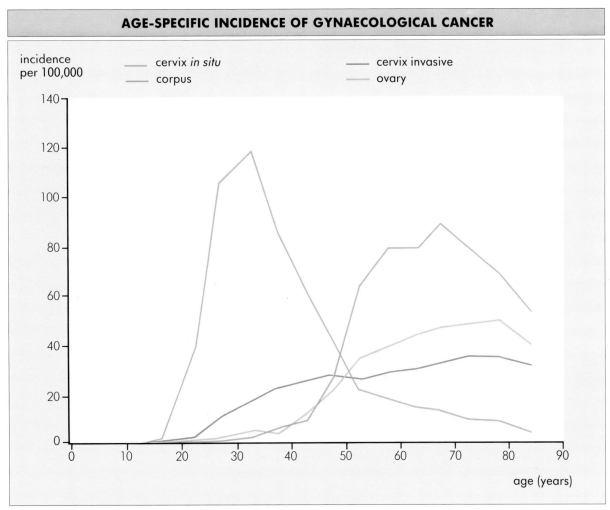

AGE-SPECIFIC INCIDENCE OF GYNAECOLOGICAL CANCER

incidence per 100,000

— cervix *in situ*   — cervix invasive
— corpus   — ovary

age (years)

Fig. 10.2 Age specific incidence of cancers of the cervix, uterine corpus and ovary in white women in the USA. Figures show a high prevalence of *in situ* pre-invasive cervical carcinoma in young women, contrasting with a later age peak for invasive cervical carcinoma.

employing exfoliative cytology techniques (Fig. 10.3). Although this is an easy, convenient and repeatable method of screening it also requires powerful administration and recall services to be effective. The record in the UK is, for these reasons, far less satisfactory than what has been achieved in Scandinavia. Race and social class are also an important epidemiological feature in cancer of the cervix. One study from New York showed that the incidence in Blacks and Hispanics was over five times that of the white population, with even lower incidence amongst white Jewish women.

Less is known about the aetiology of carcinoma of the ovary, although again there are important geographical differences. Japanese women, for example, have a very low rate compared with Europeans and Americans, though Japanese immigrants to the USA develop risk patterns similar to Caucasians within two generations (see Fig. 1.3). Ovarian cancer is also more frequent amongst nulliparous women, and use of an oral contraceptive appears to have protective effects. Although its incidence in the Western World is lower than for cancers of the cervix and endometrium, the death rate from ovarian cancers is the highest of the gynaecological malignancies. Unlike the other tumours, it does not usually produce characteristic symptoms or signs until the cancer has spread beyond the primary site. The incidence in England and Wales is about 5000 cases per annum with 19000 cases per annum in the USA, of whom 70% will die of the disease. Ovarian cancer is now the fourth or fifth commonest cause of death from malignant disease in western countries.

Carcinoma of the corpus uteri, the third major gynaecological site of cancer, is more frequent in the obese, the hypertensive or the diabetic patient, possibly because of a relative inability to metabolize oestrogen in this group. This leads to a prolonged hyperoestrogenic drive causing hyperplasia of the endometrium, and in some cases, neoplasia. Indeed adenomatous endometrial hyperplasia (often associated with prolonged oestrogen administration) appears to behave in a pre-malignant fashion, with about 10% of these lesions progressing to invasive cancer. The disease is commonest in the 50–70 year old age group, with a recent possible slight rise in

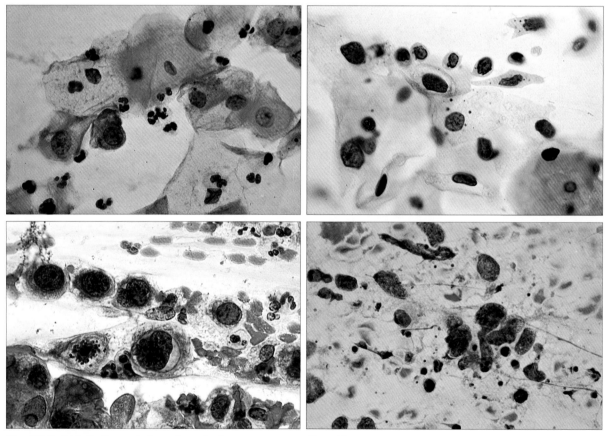

Fig. 10.3 Exfoliative cytology (cervical smear preparations) in carcinoma of the cervix. (a) CIN I showing mild dysplasia, dyskaryosis and slight nuclear atypia. (b) CIN II showing moderate dysplasia, with nuclear hyperchromasia and fine chromatin clumping. (c) CIN III or Cis. The neoplastic cells are larger, with severe dysplasia and marked nuclear atypia. (d) Invasive squamous cell carcinoma, large cell non-keratinizing type. The cells are pleomorphic and there is a necrotic background. Courtesy of Prof C. Gompel.

incidence, leading to fears that hormonal replacement therapy (HRT) may be partly responsible. These anxieties have led to a preference for cyclical types of HRT (i.e. oestrogen/progesterone replacement) rather than continuous oestrogen. Patients who enter their menopause late are also at high risk because of the additional oestrogen exposure at what appears to be a rather sensitive period. Geographical variations are again considerable, with very low rates in Japan and parts of Africa, and a particularly high incidence in the USA — probably due to the prevalence of obesity in North America.

Sarcoma botryoides is a very rare form of genital malignancy (usually vaginal or uterine) which occurs chiefly in children (Fig. 10.4). It is important because of the known aetiology, and is caused by exposure in utero to maternal oestrogen therapy — the most clear cut example of a transplacental carcinogen.

Other gynaecological tumours, such as primary cancers of the vagina, vulva and fallopian tube are far less common. The incidence of the three major tumours is approximately equal, but because treatment for ovarian carcinoma is so unsatisfactory at present the death rate for this tumour now equals the death rates for the other types combined.

▋ Cancer of the Cervix

Worldwide, cancer of the cervix is the commonest of all gynaecological malignancies. However, its mortality rate has fallen dramatically in most western countries in the past 50 years due to a reduction in incidence of invasive cancers, the development of techniques to detect premalignant changes, and improvements in local therapy. The incidence of *in situ* carcinomas has, conversely, risen rapidly in the past 50 years since the introduction of screening programmes (see Fig. 10.2).

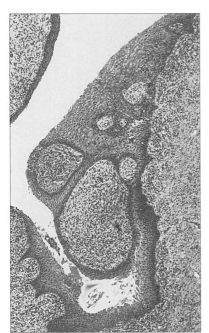

Fig. 10.4 Photomicrograph of sarcoma botyroides. Cellular proliferation is particularly dense immediately beneath the surface epithelium. There is nodular elevation of the surface epithelium, and polypoid masses projected into the vaginal lumen. Courtesy of Prof J.D. Woodruff.

Preinvasive carcinoma is usually recognized at an asymptomatic stage (see Fig. 10.3), by use of Papanicolaou staining ('Pap smear'), which ideally should be carried out regularly in all sexually active women. The current UK government guidelines recommending regular smear examinations only from the age of thirty-five, are widely felt to be inadequate (see below). Carcinoma of the cervix is most common in women in lower socio-economic groups and patients frequently give a history of multiple sexual partners in their teenage years. Ninety-five percent originate in the squamocolumnar junction of the cervix. In prepubertal girls, glandular epithelium covers much of the exocervix but as adolescence progresses, the junction between the glandular and squamous tissues migrates up into the endocervical canal. During this metaplastic progression glandular cells are changed to or are 'overgrown' by squamous epithelium, and it has been suggested that such active tissue may be particularly susceptible to carcinogens, possibly sexually transmitted. The role of males in this process is under investigation, and it may be that use of a condom is protective.

Screening
The spectrum of cytological changes detected by cervical smears is shown in Figure 10.3. Current recommendations for cervical screening programmes vary from country to country but ideal criteria may be summarized as:

- all asymptomatic women over 20 and sexually active women under 20 should have two annual smears;
- if negative, smears should be repeated once every 3 years together with a physical examination;
- cervical smears are generally discontinued at 65 years of age, though some data suggests that older patients may still benefit from screening.

Diagnosis
An increasing proportion of patients are diagnosed by routine cervical smear. The changes of dysplasia leading to carcinoma *in situ* (see Fig. 10.3) are described collectively as 'cervical intraepithelial neoplasia' (CIN). Patients with a persistently abnormal smear (false negative rate 10–20%) should undergo further investigation with colposcopy and biopsy (Fig. 10.5). This will determine the location and extent of 90% of CIN lesions, usually eliminating the need for cone biopsy as a method of investigation.

Symptoms of more advanced invasive carcinoma include dyspareunia, vaginal discharge, sometimes with bleeding and usually offensive in nature, and pelvic pain or discomfort. Low back pain is a very ominous feature suggesting a locally advanced lesion or regional lymphadenopathy. Any of these features should of course lead to prompt vaginal examination, including a careful speculum inspection. A smear should be taken, and many cytologists feel that the use of the cytobrush technique offers superior

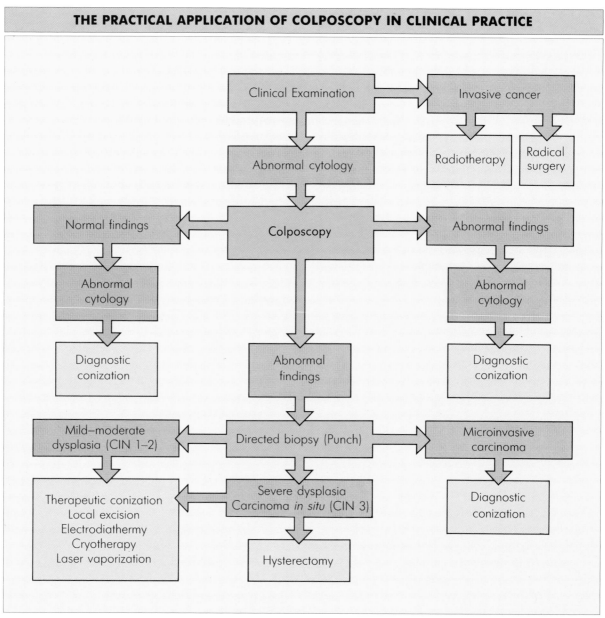

THE PRACTICAL APPLICATION OF COLPOSCOPY IN CLINICAL PRACTICE

Fig. 10.5 Use of colposcopy to direct clinical management.

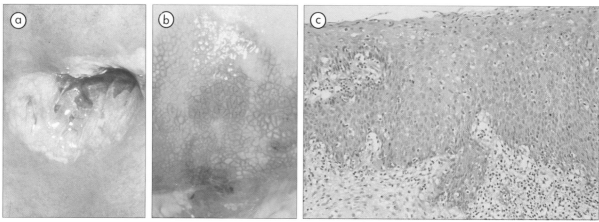

Fig. 10.6 Colposcopic views of the cervix. (a) and (b) Aceto white staining and typical mosaic pattern of pre-invasive carcinoma. Colposcopic techniques give far greater detail than is possible by conventional out-patient examination. Courtesy of Mr A.C. Silverstone. (c) Colposcopic biopsy showing microinvasive carcinoma in a field of CIN III. No tumour was visible to the naked eye.

cytological morphology. Where symptoms persist, urgent gynaecological referral should be undertaken, even if the smear is apparently normal. Colposcopy (Fig. 10.6) gives much more detail of cervical anatomy and early biopsy may be required.

Pathologically invasive carcinomas of the cervix are generally squamous cell cancers, though adeno-carcinoma and mixed tumours are also encountered. The cervix may appear only minimally abnormal, or totally destroyed (Fig. 10.7). The tumour may be exophytic, with cauliflower-like outgrowths, or pre-dominantly ulcerative and excavating.

Staging

Staging is designed to assess the local extent of spread in order to help select appropriate primary manage-ment with surgery and/or radiotherapy. Important staging investigations include, first and foremost, examination under anaesthesia (EUA), at which the anatomy and extent of the tumour can be clearly delineated, and also radiological investigations to give greater detail regarding both the local spread and possible extracervical extension. An IVU is important, but many departments increasingly use CT scanning (Fig. 10.8). Lymphography may also be helpful but is no longer widely used.

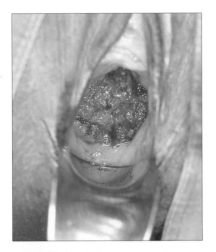

Fig. 10.7 Typical appearance of locally advanced carcinoma of the cervix at EUA. In this case the cervix was almost totally destroyed, and there was obvious involvement of the vaginal fornices.

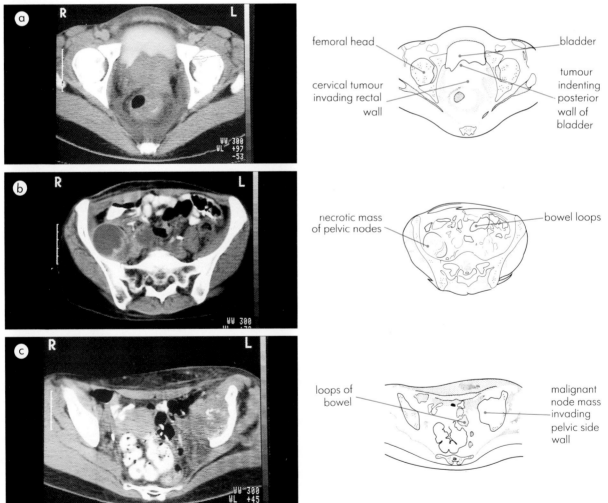

Fig. 10.8 CT scanning in carcinoma of the cervix. (a) Large central tumour with obvious extension posteriorly to the rectal wall, and indenting the bladder anteriorly. (b) Large necrotic mass of iliac nodes adjacent to pelvic side wall. (c) Local pelvic bone erosion from large mass of left sided pelvic nodes.

The incidence of lymph node involvement clearly rises with the stage of the tumour. Even with stage I lesions, pelvic node involvement occurs in up to 20% of cases. With stage III tumours, node involvement occurs in two-thirds of all cases. Some groups recommend laparotomy in order to assess lymphatic involvement. The standard UICC/FIGO staging systems used are shown in Figure 10.9 and survival by stage in Figure 10.10. Although staging is partly subjective it does give a clear guide to prognosis. Patients with stage I carcinomas, for example, where the tumour is confined to the cervix, have an excellent prognosis with an approximate 90% cure rate whereas those with stage IIIb disease, with tumour present within the parametria as far as the pelvic wall, have an overall survival of 30% or less.

The pattern of spread is relatively predictable, initially to adjacent local structures, notably the upper vagina and parametria (spreading from medial to lateral), with progressive involvement of pelvic lymph node groups, and later, the para-aortic nodes (Fig. 10.11). Renal obstruction is a very ominous sign implying gross parametrial involvement and interruption of ureteric patency. Haematogenous metastases are unusual, but the tumour can spread to involve the liver, lungs or other organs.

Treatment
1) Dysplasia.
Patients with cervical dysplasia were traditionally treated by cone biopsy of the cervix. However, with screening of younger populations it has become evident that CIN can start as early as the late teens. The potential hazards of cone biopsy in younger women, with its effects on pregnancy, together with increasing use of colposcopy have led to a change in approach to CIN III. Colposcopy allows accurate visual localization of a lesion, endocervical curettage and biopsy of suspicious areas and these findings are used to plan treatment. If the entire lesion is seen and endocervical curettage is negative several treatment options are available, including excision biopsy, cryosurgery or laser therapy. Lesions of less than 1 cm can be treated by excision whilst larger lesions are best treated by laser or cryosurgery. Following treatment, patients should of course be followed up regularly, and conization of the cervix may be required despite the availability of new techniques.

2) Stage Ia (microinvasive).
This stage is uncommon, accounting for only approximately 5% of cervical carcinomas. Invasion into the stroma is restricted to 5 mm or less, but precise criteria for diagnosis of this stage are unclear. Many of these cases prove on histological review to be CIN (carcinoma *in situ*) or invasive cancer, which has probably led to overtreatment in many cases and makes analysis of results unreliable. A much smaller proportion of patients are probably undertreated by simple hysterectomy, the normal recommended treatment for true stage Ia disease.

Stage	Criteria
	FIGO STAGING SYSTEM FOR CARCINOMA OF THE CERVIX
0	Pre-invasive carcinoma (cervical intraepithelial)
I	Carcinoma confined to the cervix (corpus extension should be disregarded)
Ia	Microinvasive carcinoma
Ib	Occult or clinically invasive carcinoma
II	Carcinoma extending beyond the cervix and involving the vagina (but not the lower third) and/or infiltrating the parametrium (but not reaching the pelvic side wall)
IIa	The carcinoma has involved the vagina
IIb	The carcinoma has infiltrated the parametrium
III	Carcinoma involving the lower third of vagina and/or extending to the pelvic side wall (there is no free space between tumour and the pelvic side wall)
IIIa	Carcinoma involving the lower third of vagina
IIIb	Carcinoma extending to the pelvic wall and/or hydronephrosis or non-functioning kidney due to ureterostenosis caused by tumour
IVa	Carcinoma involving the mucosa of the bladder or rectum and/or extending beyond the true pelvis
IVb	Spread to distant organs

Fig. 10.9 FIGO staging system for carcinoma of the cervix.

3) Stages Ib to IIIb. Radical radiotherapy or surgery are used at this stage of the disease. Although no conclusive randomized trials have been reported the results are probably equivalent for stages Ib and IIa, though radiotherapy is more effective than surgery for stage IIb to IIIb.

Where surgery is considered appropriate, Wertheim's hysterectomy should be undertaken — an operation involving total abdominal hysterectomy, removal of 2–3cm cuff of vagina and all supporting tissues in the pelvis, together with radical pelvic lymphadenectomy. Unexpected lymph node involvement is present in 5–20% of cases. Oophorectomy is optional since spread to the ovaries is uncommon; indeed preservation of ovarian function is one of the major advantages of surgery for early stage disease.

SURVIVAL IN INVASIVE CARCINOMA OF THE CERVIX

Risk group	No. of patients	No. of deaths	Median DFST (months)
—— Good (IIa⁻, IIb⁻)	66	22	92+
—— Intermediate (IIb⁺, IIIa⁻, IIIb⁻)	62	34	31
—— Poor (IIIa⁺, IIIb⁺)	50	35	11

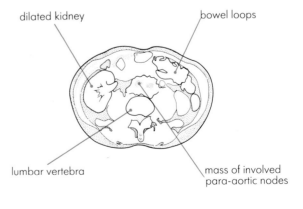

Fig. 10.10 Survival following treatment of invasive carcinoma of the cervix. FIGO staging gives excellent prognostic information, with wide variation in survival largely dependent on tumour stage. Superscripts indicate lymph node status, based on lymphogram findings. [Data from Hammond, J.A. et al. (1981) *Int. J. Rad. Oncol. Biol. Phys.* **7**, 1713–1718.]

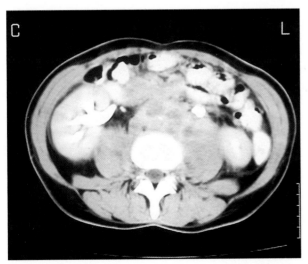

Fig. 10.11 Carcinoma of the cervix. CT scan showing obvious para-aortic node involvement and right sided renal obstruction in carcinoma of the cervix. In this case the node mass is partly necrotic.

Radiotherapy details vary from one instituion to another but usually include intracavitary caesium brachytherapy together with external beam irradiation (Fig. 10.12). Trials of adjuvant chemotherapy (see below) have recently begun, though such treatment cannot at present be accepted as established, and has not yet been shown to give higher survival rates.

4) Recurrent disease. Patients whose disease recurs after surgery alone are generally suitable for radiotherapy if the tumour has remained within the pelvis. Recurrence after irradiation, and distant metastatic disease, can both be treated with chemotherapy. Although encouraging responses are seen, it is not yet clear whether the high response rates of cisplatin based combinations will result in better survival, though symptomatic responses are often impressive, improving the patient's quality of life. A very small proportion of patients — those with central recurrence but no evidence of pelvic node involvement, should be considered for pelvic exenteration.

■ Carcinoma of the Ovary

Clinical Features

Typical symptoms of ovarian carcinoma are shown in Figure 10.13 and are chiefly restricted to patients with advanced disease. In retrospect, between one-third to one-half of patients will admit to having experienced vague epigastric discomfort, often mild and insufficient for the patient to seek medical attention at the earlier stage. These features often appear to develop suddenly and most patients have been symptomatic for a few weeks by the time of presentation. Despite this, many patients have gross physical signs when first seen in hospital (see Fig. 10.13), and the diagnosis is often established prior to surgery. Important investigations in patients with a possible ovarian carcinoma include:

- ultrasound or CT imaging
- cytology of ascitic or pleural fluid
- chest X-ray
- contrast studies of bowel

These tests often reveal a pattern of disease highly suggestive of ovarian neoplasia with or without cytological evidence of malignancy.

Pathology

Functionally the ovary can be regarded as having three elements: the surface epithelium, the germinal cells producing ova and the sex cord, and mesenchymal cells. Each component gives rise to a group of tumours, though the large majority of cancers are derived from the surface epithelium. A thin layer of mesothelium covers the ovary, and is continuous with the peritoneum. Over 90% of ovarian cancers develop from this, either on the ovarian surface or from mesothelium carried into the ovary itself. As they develop, ovarian carcinomas may display cellular characteristics typical of other gynaecological, gastroinestinal or urological tissues, and the pathological classification is based on these appearances (Fig. 10.14).

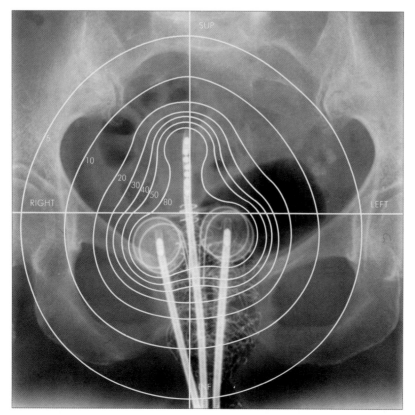

Fig. 10.12 Typical radiation dosimetry following intracavity brachytherapy in carcinoma of the cervix. In this case low dose rate intracavity caesium-137 was used. Central dose is greater than 80 Gy (8000 rad) with a steep fall off to the pelvic side wall. Most radiotherapy centres recommend a combination of intracavity and external beam irradiation for the majority of patients with carcinoma of the cervix. The external beam therapy provides adequate treatment of the parametria and pelvic side wall which cannot be achieved with brachytherapy alone.

Germ cell tumours are uncommon and are generally seen in children or young women. They are divided into dysgerminomas (equivalent to seminoma in males) and ovarian teratomas. Sex cords and stromal tumours of the ovary are also uncommon, most being derived from granulosa cells. Granulosa cell tumours

TYPICAL SYMPTOMS OF OVARIAN CARCINOMA

Pelvic and/or abdominal mass	95%
Non-specific abdominal discomfort	75%
Abdominal bloating	55%
Early satiety	45%
Ascites	40%
Masses in pouch of Douglas	40%
Weight loss	30%
Shortness of breath	20%
Vaginal bleeding	10%
Urinary frequency	10%
Pleural effusion	10%

Fig. 10.13 Symptoms and signs of ovarian cancer.

(about 4% of all ovarian cancers) often produce oestrogen, which in turn can cause breast tenderness and vaginal bleeding.

The following discussion refers principally to epithelial tumours since these make up 95% of ovarian cancers.

Staging
The FIGO system of staging (see Fig. 10.15) is generally used, and is based on the extent of tumour spread at surgery. For adequate staging, the operation should include a careful evaluation of potential metastatic sites. It is worth noting that some patients with stage I ovarian cancer have very large tumours at presentation, often without evidence of spread.

Treatment
Surgery is the mainstay of treatment of ovarian carcinoma. The aims of laparotomy are to perform complete evaluation of tumour extent and then to undertake as complete a surgical clearance as possible. Recommendations include:
- vertical incision for good abdomino-pelvic access;
- careful inspection of abdominal cavity and pelvis, to include sub-diaphragmatic recess, omentum, peritoneal surfaces and other high risk sites;
- total abdominal hysterectomy, bilateral salpingo-oophorectomy and omentectomy. If this is not possible, debulking surgery and pelvic and para-aortic node sampling should be carried out.

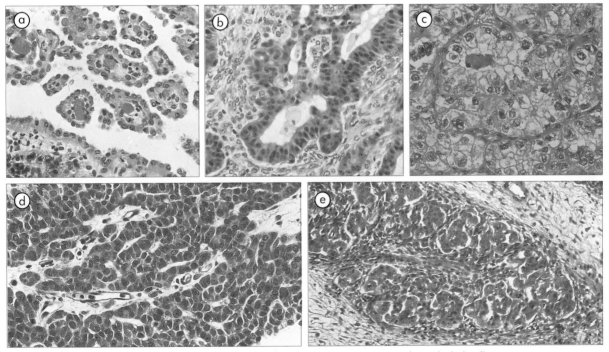

Fig. 10.14 Histological subtypes in ovarian carcinoma. (a) Papillary ovarian carcinoma, well differentiated, showing early invasive features. (b) Ovarian carcinoma with endometrioid features. The glands are not well formed in all areas, and are losing their differentiation. (c) Clear-cell carcinoma showing typical features and a glandular pattern. (d) Granulosa cell carcinoma, with epithelial cells in nests containing small follicular spaces, with solid cords of darkly staining cells. (e) Sertoli–Leydig cell tumour showing nests of epithelial cells forming rudimentary tubules, a potentially malignant tumour of moderate differentiation. Courtesy of Prof J.D. Woodruff.

The prognosis is certainly better if complete clearance is performed and it is highly probable that good debulking also improves survival even if a complete resection cannot be achieved. It is possible that this reflects a better innate survival in cases where surgical debulking is feasible.

Additional post-operative treatment is essential in the majority of patients with ovarian carcinoma. For patients with early stage disease (stages I to IIa), radiotherapy has often been recommended, particularly in the days before chemotherapy had been shown to be effective in this disease. However, pelvic radiotherapy following surgery often fails to prove beneficial due to patients relapsing in the upper abdomen. Because of this, extensive radiation fields treating from the obturator foramen to 1cm above the diaphragm ('whole abdominal irradiation') have sometimes been used. It has been claimed that this treatment significantly improves survival for early ovarian carcinoma though most major groups remain sceptical.

Chemotherapy has been used to treat more advanced stages of ovarian cancer for over 30 years. Initially single oral alkylating agents were used but more recently combinations of drugs (particularly including cisplatin or carboplatin) have been preferred. Although response rates are superior with drug combinations, long term survival is still uncommon. The role of chemotherapy in completely resected early stage (I to IIa) ovarian carcinoma has never been properly tested, though some centres routinely use cisplatin chemotherapy as an alternative to radiotherapy. The most appropriate management for each stage of ovarian carcinoma remains controversial, largely a reflection of the generally unsatisfactory treatment, particularly for advanced stage disease. Current recommendations include: complete surgical clearance if possible; if not, surgical debulking to tumour nodules of less than 1.5cm; bilateral salpingo-oophorectomy and hysterectomy; abdominopelvic radiotherapy after surgery, though chemotherapy using alkylating agents and/or cisplatin is usually preferred, particularly for advanced disease. Although cisplatin combinations produce the highest response rates, it remains unclear whether this approach carries a survival advantage over single agent treatments of lower toxicity. Current treatment recommendations vary from single alkylating agents (especially in unwell or elderly patients) to cisplatin alone or in combination with cyclophosphamide or doxorubicin.

Surgery may also have an important role later in the patient's career since it can be difficult to be certain of the response to treatment, and a 'second look' procedure (laparoscopy or laparotomy) may be necessary for adequate confirmation. Other approaches to management of advanced ovarian cancer are less widely practised but include intraperitoneal injection of cytotoxic drugs, or instillation of radioactive chromic phosphate or gold colloid.

FIGO STAGING OF OVARIAN CANCER	
Stage	**Criteria**
I	Tumour limited to ovaries (26%)
Ia	Tumour limited to one ovary; capsule intact, no tumour on ovarian surface
Ib	Tumour limited to both ovaries; capsules intact, no tumour on ovarian surface
Ic	Tumour limited to one or both ovaries with any of the following: capsule ruptured, tumour on ovarian surface, malignant cells in ascites or peritoneal washing
II	Tumour involves one or both ovaries with pelvic extension (21%)
IIa	Extension and/or implants on uterus and/or tube(s)
IIb	Extension to other pelvic tissues
IIc	Pelvic extension (IIa or IIb) with malignant cells in ascites or peritoneal washing
III	Tumour involves one or both ovaries with microscopically confirmed peritoneal metastasis outside the pelvis and/or regional lymph node metastasis (37%)
IIIa	Microscopic peritoneal metastasis beyond pelvis
IIIb	Macroscopic peritoneal metastasis beyond pelvis, ≤2cm in greatest dimension
IIIc	Peritoneal metastasis beyond pelvis, >2cm in greatest dimension and/or regional lymph node metastasis
IV	Distant metastasis (excludes peritoneal metastasis) (16%)

Fig. 10.15 FIGO staging for carcinoma of the ovary. Figures in brackets refer to proportion of total cases presenting with each particular stage. Although other features such as tumour subtype, grade of differentiation and capsular involvement may also affect survival, the FIGO stage remains the single most important prognostic factor. More recently described features, such as tumour ploidy and oncogene expression, may in the future prove even more predictive.

Recently there has been interest in the use of radio-active iodine linked to antibodies raised to ovarian cancer-related antigens — a so called 'magic bullet'. So far, this approach, though of interest, has not yielded useful results, and it is probable that the antigens are far from specific. Overall the results of treatment are very unsatisfactory (Fig. 10.16), and ovarian cancer represents the most formidable

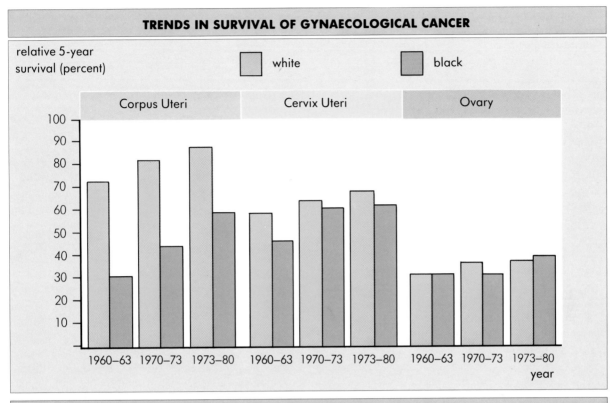

TRENDS IN SURVIVAL OF GYNAECOLOGICAL CANCER

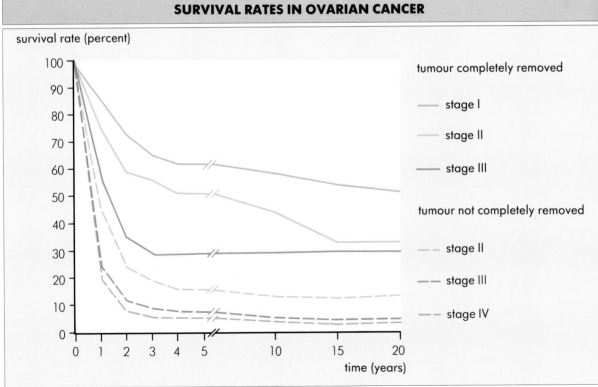

SURVIVAL RATES IN OVARIAN CANCER

Fig. 10.16 Trends in survival by site of cancer and race. (Top) These figures confirm that survival in carcinoma of the ovary has not improved since 1960 though at other sites, particularly the corpus uteri, survival has markedly improved throughout this period. (Data from the Biometry Branch, National Cancer Institute, USA.) (Bottom) Survival rates in carcinoma of the ovary. Although tumour grade and histological subtype are important prognostic factors, FIGO staging remains the most predictive of all.

challenge faced by the gynaecological oncologist. Possible methods for earlier diagnosis include:
- yearly examination and pelvic ultrasound;
- cytological and biochemical testing of fluid from transvaginal aspiration;
- surgical/endoscopic examination of post-meno- pausal women with a palpable ovary;
- testing for ectopic hormones and plasma CEA;
- peritoneoscopy.

None of these techniques has so far proved feasible on a wide scale, though a number of centres are increasingly recommending routine pelvic examina- tion combined with ultrasound techniques.

For granulosa cell tumours (see Fig. 10.14), surgery is the most important method of treatment, though late recurrences are rather characteristic of this tumour, and radiotherapy is then often employ- ed. Even less common are the Sertoli-Leydig cell tumours ('arrhenoblastomas') which are associated with virilization. Overall, survival in ovarian cancer is not only dependent on tumour stage but also pathologic grade. Patients with well differentiated stage Ia tumours have an excellent outlook (5-year survival at least 90%) but the long term prognosis of patients with stage III/IV disease is poor.

Cancer of the fallopian tube, though extremely uncommon, is similar in terms of histology, clinical features and behaviour to ovarian cancer. If cancer within the fallopian tube is encountered at laparo- tomy, it is much more likely to be due to a secondary deposit from a primary ovarian carcinoma rather than a primary malignancy of the tube. Surgical resection is probably the most important part of treatment though, like ovarian cancer, the tumour does show some degree of responsiveness to chemo- therapy.

Cancer of the Body of the Uterus

The incidence of this tumour and aetiological feat- ures are described above. Postmenopausal bleeding is the cardinal symptom, though intermenstrual bleeding or menorrhagia may occur in pre- or peri- menopausal women. Pelvic or lumbar back pain may occur in advanced cases, and occasionally patients present with symptoms and signs of metastatic disease. Cervical smears are of limited value in screening or diagnosis of endometrial cancer.

Pathology
Ninety percent of uterine cancers are adenocarcino- mas, usually arising in the endometrium; occasionally squamous elements are also present (Fig. 10.17). Sarcomas are unusual and generally carry a poor prognosis, though surgical resection may be curative.

Since outcome is closely related to tumour grade in endometrial adenocarcinomas the tumour differ- entiation should be clearly stated by the pathologist. The tumour spreads by direct extension into the endometrium, upper vagina and draining pelvic and para-aortic lymph nodes (Fig. 10.18). Spread via the fallopian tubes into the peritoneal cavity is a late event, though blood borne spread chiefly to the lung, is not uncommon especially in high grade or locally advanced cases.

Staging and Treatment

This tumour is staged using a combination of clinical findings — EUA and uterine sounding, and patho- logical tumour grade. The FIGO system is shown in Figure 10.19.

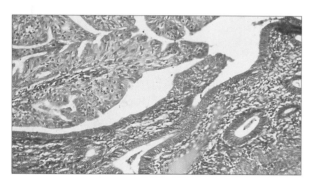

Fig. 10.17 Photomicrograph of typical adenocarcinoma of the endometrium. Tumour (above) is present with normal endometrium (below) in this focus of adenomeiosis. Courtesy of Prof J.D. Woodruff.

Fig. 10.18 Pelvic lymph node involvement in carcinoma of the endometrium. There is a close relationship with depth of myometrial invasion. Figures in brackets refer to the percentage of patients in whom positive nodes were confirmed (140 cases analysed). [Data from Morrow (1980) *Int J Rad Oncol Biol Phys*, 6, 365.]

Depth of myometrial invasion	Histological grade			Total number with positive pelvic lymph nodes	
	I	II	III		
<1/3	1/60	4/42	4/14	9/116	(8%)
>1/3	1/5	2/8	4/11	7/24	(29%)
Total	2/65	6/50	8/25	16/140	(11%)

INCIDENCE OF PELVIC LYMPH NODE METASTASES IN ENDOMETRIAL CANCER

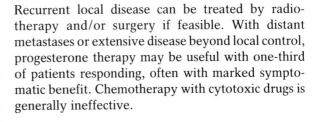

Most patients (75%) have stage I disease, in which the optimum treatment is a total abdominal hysterectomy with bilateral salpingo-oophorectomy. Radiotherapy should only be used as an alternative to surgery if patients are unfit for operation, though post-operative radiotherapy is certainly indicated in the patients with high grade or deeply penetrating lesions which have reached a depth of 50% or more of the myometrium. Survival rates in localized cases are excellent (85–90%).

Stage II disease (about 15% of cases) is usually treated by hysterectomy followed by pre- or post-operative radiotherapy – survival rates are about 50%. Stage III accounts for about 5% of cases and is generally treated by radiotherapy since surgery alone is not totally effective. 5-year survival rates are about 25–30%. Stage IV patients also account for around 5% of all patients. Treatment is individualized and may include radiotherapy and very occasionally exenterative surgery; survival rates are only about 10%.

Stage	Criteria
0	Carcinoma *in situ* (Tis)
I Ia Ib	Carcinoma confined to the corpus uteri (T1) Uterine cavity 8cm or less in length (T1a) Uterine cavity >8cm (T1b)
II	Extension to cervix only (T2)
III	Extension beyond the uterus but disease confined to true pelvis (T3)
IV	Extension beyond true pelvis, or invasion of bladder or rectum (T4)

CLINICAL STAGING IN CARCINOMA OF THE ENDOMETRIUM

Fig. 10.19 Clinical staging in carcinoma of the endometrium. T-stage (from TNM staging system) shown in brackets, but the staging systems are essentially those of FIGO.

Recurrent local disease can be treated by radiotherapy and/or surgery if feasible. With distant metastases or extensive disease beyond local control, progesterone therapy may be useful with one-third of patients responding, often with marked symptomatic benefit. Chemotherapy with cytotoxic drugs is generally ineffective.

Cancer of the Vulva

This unpleasant and uncommon tumour chiefly affects older women and is rarely diagnosed below the age of 55 years. The tumour is a typical squamous cell carcinoma and usually presents as a non-healing ulcer occurring unilaterally on any part of the vulva (Fig. 10.20). It usually produces discomfort, and an offensive slough or crust often forms, though it may reach a surprisingly large size by the time of presentation. The condition of *lichen sclerosus et atrophicus* may co-exist and is often regarded as a predisposing feature. Leucoplakia of the vulva may be present, and there is also a distinct variety of intra-epithelial neoplasia (including carcinoma *in situ*), which is clearly a premalignant lesion, and occurs in carcinoma of the cervix.

In addition to the characteristic vulval ulcer, some patients present with enlarged lymph nodes in the groin (often bilateral since the vulva is essentially a midline structure) or with pruritus vulvae or pelvic discomfort.

Treatment
Despite the advanced age of many of the patients, adequate therapy, usually by surgical resection, is generally recommended both to provide relief of painful and embarrassing symptoms and also to offer any chance of cure. Sites of local extension include the urethra (for anteriorly placed lesions) and anus (Fig. 10.20) for posterior vulval cancers, as well as local lymph nodes, including the linguinal groups and later the deep pelvic nodes including Cloquet's node. Surgery must, therefore, be designed to encompass likely routes of spread, and radical vulvectomy, though undeniably mutilating, can provide excellent

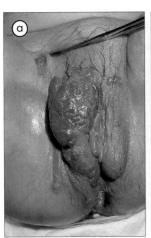
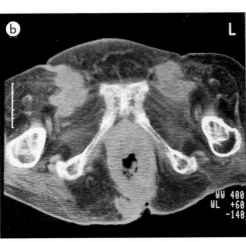

Fig. 10.20 Carcinoma of the vulva. (a) This was a particularly advanced case presenting as a rapidly expanding mass on the anteror part of the right labium majora. The patient then rapidly developed skin satellite nodules, and ipsilateral inguinal nodes. (b) CT scan confirmed massive extension upwards to the perirectal fascia and the rectum itself.

local control with a high probability of cure in node negative patients, and excellent function including normal micturition. Even in more advanced cases where posterior exenteration has to be performed, with loss of the anal sphincter and permanent colostomy, this may be far preferable to leaving a large offensive ulcer with almost inevitable risk of fungation. However, it is often possible to spare the vagina. Clearly, surgery of this type must be accompanied by considerable emotional support, particularly in the younger patient who is sexually active.

Almost half of all patients with carcinoma of the vulva have evidence of local lymph node involvement, and this group of patients cure is much less likely. If there is any doubt about the significance of node enlargement (which may simply be due to local infection), fine needle aspiration cytology is often helpful. CT scanning can sometimes give useful information about local extension and lymphadenopathy which may not be clinically detectable.

Postoperatively, inguinal node irradiation is often given either as prophylaxis if the node areas have not been dissected, or in an attempt to control local disease in patients with positive nodes. Unfortunately, even with postoperative radiotherapy, the patient with node positive vulval cancer may later develop a troublesome and offensive local recurrence and/or disseminated disease. Under these circumstances there is little further that can be done in the way of active treatment, and supportive care remains extremely important. Such patients must be treated with considerable tact and discretion.

Overall, the results of radical vulvectomy are reasonably good, with a 75% 5-year survival rate in node negative patients. The survival figure is much lower, perhaps 40%, in node positive patients where the disease has extended only to the superficial inguinal nodes and is lower still, of the order of 20%, in patients with deep pelvic node involvement.

Carcinoma of the Vagina

This very rare tumour (1% of gynaecological tumours) chiefly affects the older age group (50–70 years) but with a peak age incidence slightly below that of carcinoma of the vulva. Typically a squamous cell carcinoma, it usually presents as an irritating or offensive discharge, often bloodstained and sometimes surprisingly painless. Patients sometimes complain of haematuria and may give a history of prolapse or retention of a vaginal ring pessary for some years. Sarcoma botryoides of childhood (sometimes termed 'clear cell carcinoma') has already been mentioned, but is increasingly rare. In addition to these primary lesions, the vagina is occasionally the site of secondary deposits, notably from carcinoma of the endometrium or occasionally from vulval melanoma.

Local and lymphatic invasion both occur, with direct extension to the parametria, bladder, rectum and pelvic side wall, though this degree of local extension is unusual. FIGO staging is shown in Figure 10.21. Upper vaginal tumours, which represent the majority of vaginal tumours, have a lymphatic spread similar to that for carcinoma of the cervix while those from the lower part and introitus drain more anteriorly to inguinal nodes. Apart from careful vaginal examination a careful inspection of the cervix is essential, where possible, since this is much more likely to be the site of the primary disease. Vaginal smear cytology can be helpful and may point to the correct diagnosis, particularly in cases of vaginal carcinoma *in situ*, where colposcopy has been performed and cervical biopsy proves negative whilst the exfoliative cytology is clearly abnormal.

Treatment

Treatment is by radical surgery or local irradiation. Many favour the latter approach, particularly in

FIGO STAGING SYSTEM FOR CARCINOMA OF THE VAGINA		
Stage	Criteria	5-year survival rates (with radiation therapy)
0	Intraepithelial	—
I	Limited to vaginal wall	80%
II	Extends to subvaginal tissue but not to pelvic side wall	50%
III	Extends to pelvic side wall	30%
IV	Extends beyond true pelvis or involves mucosa of bladder or rectum	5%
IVa	Adjacent organs	—
IVb	Distant organs	—

Fig. 10.21 FIGO staging of vaginal carcinoma. As the vaginal wall is very thin, even small vaginal cancers may rapidly develop into stage II cases, in contrast to cervical tumours of comparable size. As with other gynaecological cancers, FIGO staging is the best single predictor for survival presently available.

elder patients, since radical vaginectomy, abdominal hysterectomy and node dissection are required for surgical success, and should probably only be considered in patients with early lesions. Although radiotherapy is generally preferred, the proximity of the rectum and bladder makes these organs susceptible to radiation damage. Considerable thought is required in the planning of the external irradiation and possible intravaginal implant therapy. Nonetheless, in localized cases the five year survival rate (generally a cure) is of the order of 75% though with more advanced tumours, the success rate falls off sharply.

Choriocarcinoma

This extremely unusual tumour (Fig. 10.22) is of great importance since it is a malignant tumour of young patients and is highly curable by chemotherapy, even when advanced. Moreover it was recognized many years ago that the trophoblastic cells secrete a tumour marker 'human chorionic gonadotrophin' (HCG) which gives a quantitative estimate of the amount of tumour still left after treatment, well beyond the point at which other tests could demonstrate persisting disease. This not only allows for the possibility of treatment tailored to the requirement of the patient, but provides an important demonstration of the value of tumour markers, now increasingly widely used.

Typically, the tumour occurs following pregnancies which have themselves resulted in a hydatidiform mole (1 in every 1500 normal pregnancies), though choriocarcinoma may very rarely follow an apparently normal pregnancy. The tumour is usually diagnosed when patients present with persistent vaginal bleeding just after pregnancy, particularly if the baby had appeared 'large for dates' or if the patient was generally unwell thoughout pregnancy.

These problems, coupled with any suggestion of retention of placental products or evacuation of a mole, should at least raise suspicion about a possible diagnosis of choriocarcinoma, and ultrasound examination will usually provide the answer, generally before delivery. A molar pregnancy or persistent elevation of HCG levels should routinely lead to careful surveillance of the patient with further investigations of the HCG level and CT or ultrasound scanning.

Treatment

Patients with early or low risk disease (i.e. no evidence of distant metastases, young age, relatively modest HCG level and rapid identification from pregnancy to treatment) usually do well with simple chemotherapy (single agent methotrexate) or hysterectomy, or a combination of both. Indications for treatment with chemotherapy are shown in Figure 10.23. More advanced cases, with higher HCG level

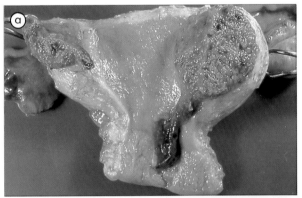

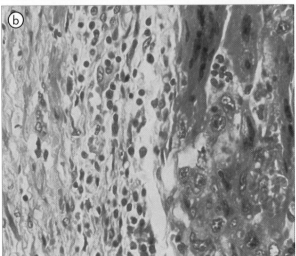

Fig. 10.22 Choriocarcinoma. (a) This large mass of choriocarcinoma was attached to the fundus producing a prolapsing polyp. (b) Histologically, myometrium (left) is being destroyed by malignant cytotrophoblast and syncitiotrophoblast to the right. Courtesy of Prof J.D. Woodruff.

INDICATIONS FOR CHEMOTHERAPY

Serum HCG above 20,000iu/l more than 4 weeks after evacuation, because of the risk of uterine perforation

Histological evidence of choriocarcinoma

Evidence of metastases in brain, liver or gastrointestinal tract, or radiological opacities >2cm on chest X-ray

Long-lasting uterine haemorrhage

Rising HCG values

HCG in body fluids 4–6 months after evacuation

Fig. 10.23 Indications for chemotherapy in choriocarcinoma.

or distant metastases, will require combination chemotherapy, but are still usually curable. This is among the most chemosensitive of tumours, and very few deaths are now recorded. In general, even intensive treatment does not appear to deprive a patient of her fertility, and it is important to reassure patients that further pregnancies should be safe and are very likely to result in the successful delivery of a normal infant.

Genito-Urinary Cancer

Introduction

This large group of tumours includes major primary sites of which two, bladder and prostate, are amongst the commoner tumours, whilst two others, the kidney and testis, are far less frequently encountered.

Cancer of the prostate is amongst the commonest among all cancers in males, third only to malignancy of the lung and large intestine. Despite its often slow and insidious course, the mortality rate is high, particularly in blacks (according to data from the USA). Incidence is closely related to increasing age, which may account for the slightly higher death rates from this tumour seen since the Second World War. Carcinoma of the bladder is often preceded by years or decades of benign bladder neoplasm, usually in the form of bladder papillomas, which can be repeatedly resected cystoscopically. Aetiologically, it has long been linked with industrial exposure to aniline dyes, such as beta-naphthylamine, an active carcinogen. Other important groups affected include a second group of industrial workers in the rubber and cable industries; those previously infected with bilharzia which causes fibrosis of the bladder, and later, increased incidence of bladder tumours, particularly squamous cell cancers; and lastly those who smoke cigarettes, presumably as a result of a persistently high level of excreted urinary carcinogens from tobacco smoke.

Testicular tumours, which are increasing rapidly in incidence, occur much more commonly in men with a history of testicular maldescent; the tumour may be on the side of the undescended testis or on the contralateral side. The testicular tumour typically does not arise until the age of 15–35 years, and there is considerable interest in the effect of changes in the hormonal environment of the testis in the fetus and in early life. These changes may result in later tumour development, with maldescent being an epiphenomenon. Overall, the incidence of testicular tumours has increased considerably over the

last 25 years, as has maldescent; the only other known aetiological factor is that a patient with one testicular tumour, nowadays usually cured by surgery or chemotherapy, has a higher than expected risk of a second primary testicular tumour in the remaining testis.

Very little is known about the aetiology of adult renal carcinoma, an unusual tumour (about 2% of all cancers), with an incidence 3 times higher in men than in women. It is certainly more common in smokers, again presumably because of persistent exposure to products of inhaled carcinogens. As with testicular tumours, there is some evidence that patients who have been cured of renal carcinoma by surgery have a higher than expected incidence of a tumour in the remaining kidney. In children, Wilms' tumour (nephroblastoma) is one of the more common solid malignancies (see chapter 16). Apart from the numerical importance of this group of tumours, there are other important features of interest, notably the unusual relationship in the bladder between benign conditions (papillomas) and their tendency to local recurrence and malignant change (not a common pattern of behaviour of other sites of the body); the curious clinical behaviour of cancers of the kidney; the remarkable endocrine dependence of prostatic carcinomas; and finally, the extraordinary change in prognosis of testicular tumours since the advent of highly effective chemotherapy.

Cancer of the Bladder

This relatively common tumour arises from the mucosal surface of the bladder, sometimes at a single abnormal site, often at multiple sites. There is often a lengthy history of bladder papillomas, and the commonest cell type is, not surprisingly, transitional cell carcinoma (Fig. 11.1). A typical benign bladder papilloma has an obviously pedunculated appearance,

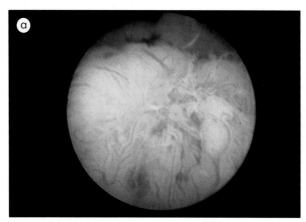

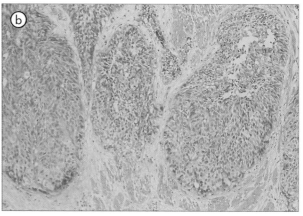

Fig. 11.1 Bladder cancer. (a) Cystoscopic appearance of a carcinoma of the bladder. Nodules of transitional cell carcinoma can be seen within the mucosa. Courtesy of Mr C. Smart. (b) Histological appearance of transitional cell carcinoma of the bladder. Courtesy of Dr J. Theaker.

whereas the frankly malignant ones are generally more flattened, erosive and wart-like in appearance. They are locally invasive, tending to infiltrate deeply into the mucosa, submucosa and muscular layers of the bladder (Figs 11.2 and 11.3), allowing relatively easy staging of these tumours (Fig. 11.4). Local extension may progress widely prior to diagnosis, with the tumour advancing through to the serosa of the bladder exterior, thence to local organs such as the rectum or pelvic side wall. Local pelvic node involvement is common with these more advanced tumours.

The majority of non-transitional cell bladder cancers, which make up 10% of bladder cancers, are squamous carcinomas, particularly in areas of bilharzia infection (notably Egypt and the Middle East). Exposure to aluminium products has also been suggested as a possible cause of bladder tumours.

Clinical Presentation

Symptomatically, the commonest presenting feature is painless haematuria, although clot retention, frequency of micturition, and incomplete emptying of the bladder may also be important features – the latter two particularly with cancers of the bladder base or neck. Patients with a lengthy recurrent history of bladder papillomas should already be under close surveillance with regular cytoscopy, so many bladder cancers are recognized before specific clinical features have developed.

Patients with painless haematuria should always be investigated further, though a reddish discolouration of the urine is occasionally caused by something other than blood, for example, rifampicin treatment for tuberculosis, beetroot ingestion or treatment with the anti-tumour antibiotic doxorubicin. In females, a particularly careful history needs to be taken,

DEPTH OF INVASION AND STAGING IN BLADDER CANCER

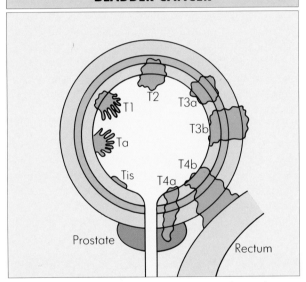

Fig. 11.2 Staging of bladder cancer. Relationship between depth of invasion and T stage for bladder cancer.

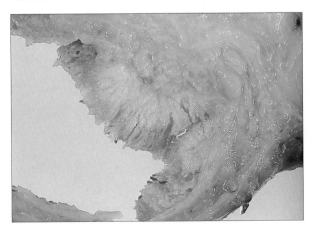

Fig. 11.3 Local invasion of bladder cancer.
Cystectomy specimen showing a typical exophytic transitional cell carcinoma invading through the mucosa to the deep muscle. Courtesy of Dr J. Theaker.

TNM STAGING FOR BLADDER CANCER

Stage	Criteria
Tis	Pre-invasive carcinoma (carcinoma *in situ*)
Ta	Papillary non-invasive carcinoma
T0	No evidence of primary tumour
T1	Tumour limited to the lamina propria. Bimanual examination may reveal a mobile mass which cannot be felt after TUR.
T2	Tumour limited to superficial muscle. Mobile induration of the bladder wall may be present, but should be impalpable following TUR.
T3	Invasion of deep muscle layer of the bladder wall. On bimanual palpation a mobile mass is felt which persists after TUR.
T3a	Deep muscle invasion.
T3b	Invasion through the muscle wall.
T4	Invasion of prostate or other local structures; tumour fixed or locally extensive.
T4a	Tumour infiltrates prostate, uterus or vagina.
T4b	Tumour fixed to pelvic and/or abdominal wall.
N0	No regional lymph node involvement.
N1	Involvement of a single ipsilateral regional node group.
N2	Contralateral, bilateral or multiple regional node involvement.
N3	Fixed regional lymphadenopathy (i.e. a fixed space between this and the tumour).
N4	Involvement of juxta-regional nodes.
M0	No distant metastases.
M1	Distant metastases.

Fig. 11.4 TNM staging classification for bladder cancer.

since it can sometimes be difficult to distinguish between a blood-stained vaginal discharge and true haematuria.

Investigation should include an intravenous urogram (Fig. 11.5), cystoscopy by an experienced urologist, and, in most modern centres, a CT scan (Fig. 11.6). A scan can give particularly useful information on the likely extravesical spread of the tumour, which clearly cannot be assessed cystoscopically. Bimanual palpation under EUA will help determine the fixity of the bladder, an important surgical consideration. A cystoscopic biopsy should give adequate tissue for both the histological examination and tumour grading, an important prognostic feature.

Treatment

Like many other solid cancers, treatment of bladder cancer requires close cooperation between surgeon, radiotherapist, chemotherapist and pathologist; increasingly, a combination of treatment, surgery, radiotherapy and sometimes chemotherapy will be necessary.

For bladder papillomas and pre-invasive tumours of doubtful or borderline malignancy, a local excision is usually sufficient. This is generally performed cystoscopically, using diathermy or fulguration. Because of the ease of repeat cystoscopic examination, it is generally easy to follow up the progress of such tumours. In frail patients, or those with multiple superficial bladder tumours, many urologists will continue to use this method of treatment successfully, even when the tumour has clearly become malignant. The most important point of tumour progression lies between the T2 and T3 tumour stage (i.e. between tumour limited to superficial muscle and still bimanually mobile, to a tumour with deep

muscular invasion and clearly beyond the level of resectability by the transurethral route) (see Fig. 11.3). At this point, either a more substantial operation, or a course of radical radiotherapy are necessary to provide adequate control and any prospect of cure.

It can be difficult for a surgeon to decide between these two alternatives. If the tumour is sufficiently localized, and the bladder capacity adequate, a partial cystectomy may be possible, leaving a satisfactory residual bladder despite removal of the tumour and an adequate margin. If necessary, the ureter can be re-implanted. This type of operation is less suitable for tumours of the bladder base, since the reconstructive surgery would be considerably more complex. More often, radical bladder surgery effectively means complete removal – total cystectomy – which is a major procedure since it clearly requires an alternative means of urinary collection and discharge, and a period of rehabilitation for the patient. A bladder reconstruction with normal transurethral voiding is not yet possible, and the most popular type of surgical diversion performed in the UK is the ileal conduit procedure, in which the total cystectomy is followed by resection of a length of ileum, with bowel anastomosis, the ureters are sutured to one end of the ileum conduit and the other end is implanted into the abdominal wall as a permanent stoma. For most patients, this surgical restoration is acceptable and serves very well.

Nonetheless, the problems of living with a stoma, which include bag leakage, local irritation, discomfort or eversion of the ileal mucosa, are considerable. It is fortunate, therefore, that local irradiation has an increasingly important role in the management of bladder cancers, and may give results similar to

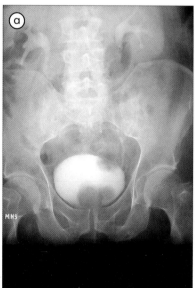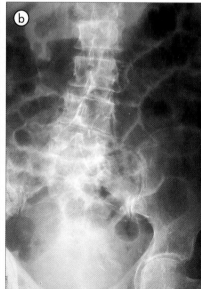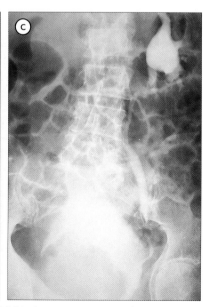

Fig. 11.5 IVU in bladder cancer. (a) Multiple malignant papillomata of the bladder demonstrated by IVU (20 mins after injection of contrast). Courtesy of Dr S. Birch. (b) Plain film showing a calcified carcinoma of the bladder. (c) IVU shows a corresponding mass in the bladder with a non-functioning right kidney and left hydronephrosis.

surgery. High doses of radiotherapy are required, and treatments are generally given over a six week period, initially to the whole of the pelvis to include the pelvic lymph node drainage sites, and finally, as a boost or 'top-up' to the bladder itself. There is good evidence that microscopic nodal disease, often present in the pelvic node areas, can be sterilized by modest doses of radiotherapy, an important point since the presence or absence of obvious lymphadenopathy is probably the most important prognostic feature in bladder cancer. It is important to recognize though, that radiation side effects are likely to occur in virtually every case, and may be quite troublesome and slow to resolve. These include frequency of micturition, often with local pain, despite repeatedly negative urinalysis, diarrhoea, proctitis, and a brisk skin reaction. Since many of the patients are elderly, these problems cannot be taken lightly, particularly where the patient lives some distance from the local radiotherapy centre and may have to be admitted to hospital for a prolonged period.

Despite these disadvantages, radiotherapy is increasingly preferred to total cystectomy. Patients with haematuria can confidently be reassured that the radiotherapy is an extremely effective means of control, usually within a fortnight or so from the start of treatment. Other symptoms may be more difficult to control, and painful urinary frequency may even get worse during treatment.

Potassium citrate, urinary antiseptics and bladder antispasmodics may be helpful symptomatically during the radiotherapy, though many patients experience a great deal of discomfort before symptoms improve. In elderly frail men, it is usually better to confine the radiotherapy to the bladder itself, rather than attempting a wider field of irradiation, since the bowel-related radiation side-effects in many cases outweigh the potential advantage.

Combinations of pre-operative radiotherapy and total cystectomy are often used (particularly in the USA) and local control rates are probably rather

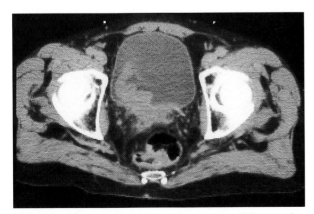

Fig. 11.6 CT imaging in bladder cancer. CT scan of the pelvis showing extensive tumour within the bladder and posteriorly on the rectum. Courtesy of Dr R. Blaquire.

higher than with total cystectomy alone. A recent study comparing radical radiotherapy with total cystectomy and postoperative irradiation suggested a slight advantage in the group undergoing surgery, with a five-year survival rate of just under 40% compared with 29% in patients who were treated without a cystectomy. Since total cystectomy is generally still possible after radical irradiation, this rather small difference in outcome has tended to support the view that total cystectomy with permanent ileostomy should be withheld in favour of radical radiotherapy, particularly for younger patients who would particularly wish to avoid a permanent stoma.

Once the patient has overcome the acute radiation effects, permanent damage from radiotherapy is fortunately not common, though the proximity of the rectum is always a worry for the radiotherapist. Since this is a sensitive part of the bowel, rectal bleeding in a patient irradiated some years before for a carcinoma of the bladder is most likely to be due to long-term mucosal telangiectasia in the rectum rather than a tumour recurrence. Chronic diarrhoea is fortunately not common, and if it does occur can generally be managed by regular codeine phosphate or diphenoxylate taken by mouth.

Modern stoma appliances are very much better than they used to be, so problems of general hygiene, spillage and odour are correspondingly less troublesome. Nonetheless, many patients need prolonged counselling and reassurance, particularly about body image and sexuality. A skilled stoma therapist is not only aware of the difficulties but can judge which patients will benefit from self-help groups. Overall, the outlook for patients with bladder cancer is reasonably good, particularly for those without evidence of nodal disease or extravesical extension. Early (T1) carcinomas are curable in about three-quarters of all patients, whereas the outlook for T2/T3 tumours drops sharply to 50% alive, presumably cured after 5 years. Where nodal involvement has already occurred, the survival rate is under 10%.

Substantial advances have been made in the use of chemotherapy, particularly for patients with advanced disease, and both intravesical and systemic chemotherapy are used. The most commonly used agents are methotrexate and cisplatin. A combination of these two agents yields response rates of 30–50%, often with very useful symptomatic benefits, particularly where patients are no longer suitable for surgical or radiotherapeutic treatment. At present, a number of studies are assessing the use of chemotherapy as an adjuvant to primary treatment. However, it is too early to say whether the side effects, particularly important in the elderly group, will prove acceptable in the face of what is likely to be a rather small advantage in quality and length of survival. For patients with multiple superficial bladder tumours, without deep invasion, intravesical chemotherapy has become an integral part of the standard approach to management.

Long-term follow-up is extremely important, particularly since the bladder is so easy to inspect. Most authorities feel that such patients should be examined cystoscopically, at least on an annual basis, for life, since recurrent bladder tumours are common, and the outcome of treatment depends closely on vigilant detection of low-grade and early stage tumours. A 20-minute general anaesthetic once or twice a year should be regarded as time well spent.

Cancer of the Prostate

Prostatic cancer has a particular historic significance, since it has now been known for over 50 years that this form of cancer is usually hormone-dependent, thus allowing for relatively non-toxic and widely applicable treatment, even in frail elderly patients with widespread disease.

The cause of the tumour is not known, though testosterone is clearly essential to its pathogenesis – prostate cancers never occur in castrated males. It is also known that prostatic cancer can be present for many years without becoming clinically detectable,

and its clinical course for many patients is remarkably benign. Estimates of its incidence are difficult to judge, since postmortem studies of elderly men often show evidence of occult disease.

Clinical Presentation

Apart from chance finding in a specimen from an operation for benign hypertrophy, the other important symptoms are similar to benign disease or relate to secondary deposits in bone, an extremely common finding in prostatic cancer. Typically, the metastases are located in the lumber spine and pelvis (Fig. 11.7), though any part of the skeleton can be involved, and the patient can present with widespread bone pain or even a pathological fracture. The third type of presentation is by diagnosis of the asymptomatic patient during an annual routine examination, provided of course that this includes a rectal examination. Typically, the prostate feels hard and craggy and irregular, whereas patients with benign hypertrophy have a distended, firm but smooth glandular enlargement, of varying degree. Carcinomas tend to arise from the peripheral or capsular area of the gland,

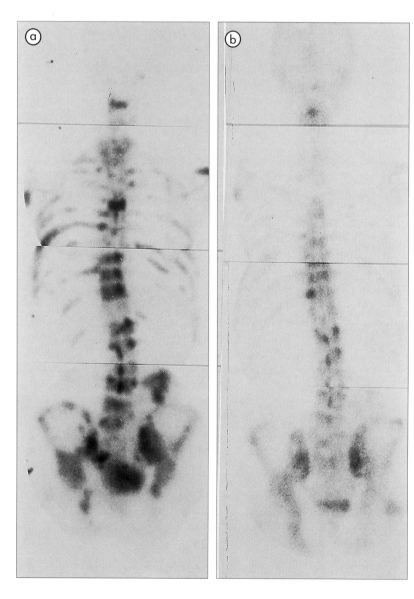

Fig. 11.7 Bone imaging in prostate cancer. (a) Image shows extensive bony involvement of the spine and pelvis prior to treatment; (b) Image shows marked improvement 8 months after hormone therapy. The patient remained well for 18 months then developed more bone pain. Further hormone manipulation proved increasingly unsuccessful but he responded to palliative radiotherapy, surviving three years from diagnosis of metastatic disease.

which has often been depressed by the presence of benign prostatic hyperplasia, though these tumours can also be truly multicentric throughout the gland. The great majority are adenocarcinomas and if diagnosis is delayed there may be extensive local infiltration (Fig. 11.8). Transitional cell carcinomas of the prostate are also occasionally encountered.

Prostatic biopsy is always worthwhile, even in patients with obvious bone metastases, since it is important not only to make a diagnosis but also to assess the tumour grade, as this may well determine the likely outcome. Apart from the dissemination to bone, other important routes of spread are via the pelvic lymph nodes, and also, uncommonly, directly to local structures including the rectum and pelvic side wall. The propensity for local bone involvement is a particularly odd feature of prostatic carcinoma, not found in other tumours which disseminate to bone, and is thought to be due specifically to invasion of venous channels between the prostate and pelvis, possibly in relation to the initial lymphatic sites of involvement, namely the obturator and pelvic lymph nodes.

Staging

Staging in prostatic cancer, which is rather unsatisfactory, is essentially based on local extent. A stage I tumour is not only confined to the prostate, but consists of microscopic disease only – often the type of cancer discovered unexpectedly following histological examination of curettings obtained at a transurethral resection for benign disease. Stage II tumours are still confined to the prostate, but produce a well-defined nodule, and in stage III carcinoma, there is local extension beyond the gland itself, but without evidence of distant metastases, which would put the patient into stage IV.

Staging investigations should include a chest X-ray and bone scan in every case, since asymptomatic bone metastases are not uncommon. The bone lesions are typically sclerotic, and this is thought to reflect their rather slow clinical evolution with time for osteoblastic healing (Fig. 11.9). This type of radiological appearance in elderly males is virtually pathognomonic of prostatic cancer. It is also important to measure acid phosphatase and alkaline phosphatase levels in the blood; one or other will

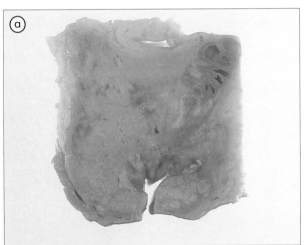
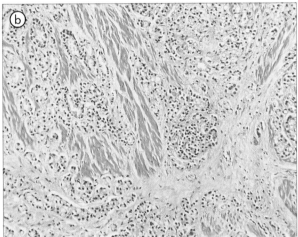

Fig. 11.8 Local invasion and histology of prostate cancer. (a) Gross specimen showing the extent of local invasion of a large prostatic carcinoma into the bladder and rectum. Courtesy of Dr J. Theaker. (b) The typical histological appearance of adenocarcinoma of the prostate.

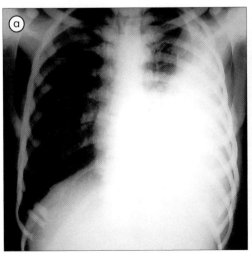
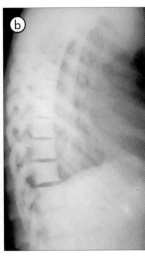

Fig. 11.9 Bone metastases from prostate cancer. Extensive osteosclerotic bone metastasis from prostate cancer. Nearly all the skeleton is grossly involved producing a marked increase in bone density (lateral and antero-posterior chest X-ray). There is also a large left pleural effusion. Courtesy of Dr S. Birch.

certainly be raised in the majority of patients, even without evidence of dissemination beyond the primary site. The IVU is often revealing, with a typical large defect at the bladder base, though it may be difficult to distinguish from benign hypertrophy. Occasionally, the IVU reveals unilateral or bilateral hydronephrosis, from ureteric obstruction (Fig. 11.10). CT scanning is also worthwhile as a means of demonstrating tumour anatomy, but ultrasound investigation, using a transrectal probe, gives better pictures in longitudinal view (Fig. 11.11) and is more easily repeatable (and cheaper) than CT scanning. It is, therefore, particularly helpful when monitoring the response of a primary prostate cancer to treatment with radiotherapy or hormone manipulation. It is usually possible with ultrasound, to visualize the prostatic carcinoma within the hypertrophied gland, as well as its relation to the seminal vesicles and other local structures.

Treatment

It is difficult to be dogmatic about the management of patients with prostate cancer since considerable confusion exists as to what forms of treatment are most appropriate for each stage. For patients with localized disease (stages I–III) the choice for local management with curative intent lies between a radical surgical excision and local irradiation. Most surgeons have now moved away from radical surgery as a primary manoeuvre since the radical operation is demanding for the patient, resulting in impotence and long-term urinary difficulties in a very high proportion of patients. Radical irradiation is generally

well-tolerated, and the side effects of treatment are essentially similar to those of carcinoma of the bladder, with urinary frequency and the ever present danger of rectal problems both short and long term. Local implantation of radioactive seeds is now possible, using an ultrasound guided direct implant

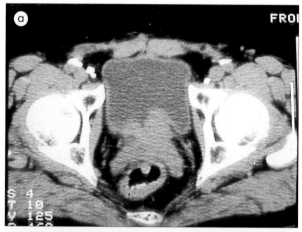

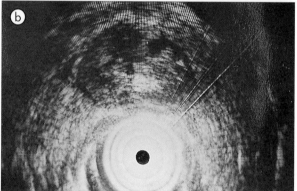

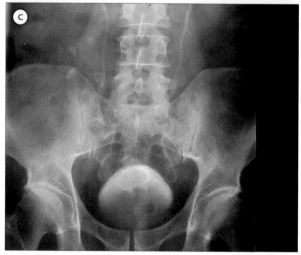

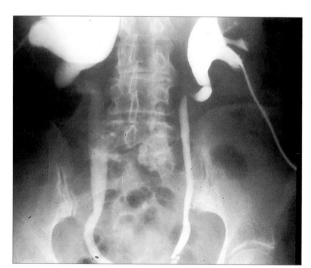

Fig. 11.10 Urinary obstruction from prostate cancer. Bilateral hydronephrosis caused by obstruction of the ureters due to carcinoma of the prostate. Stents have been used to relieve the obstruction.

Fig. 11.11 Prostatic carcinoma. (a) CT image of the pelvis showing carcinoma of the prostate involving the seminal vesicles and bladder. Courtesy of Dr R. Blaquire. (b) Transrectal ultrasound. The prostatic carcinoma appears as an echo-poor area just anterior and to the left of an area of midline calcification. Courtesy of Dr K. Dewbury. (c)IVU showing gross prostatic hypertrophy elevating the bladder and indenting the bladder base. This apparently benign lesion contained adenocarcinoma.

technique, giving a high local dosage to the prostate bed itself, without over-irradiation of adjacent tissues or the pelvic side wall. Although expensive, this form of treatment is gaining ground, and the side effects are impressively low.

For more advanced tumours, any attempt at local treatment is bound to fail. Oestrogen produces responses in at least three-quarters of patients, though with troublesome side effects including venous thromboses and unwanted breast enlargement in many cases. Indeed, this form of treatment in the early days led to a sufficiently high mortality, from cardiac and pulmonary episodes, to have brought it into disrepute. More recently, smaller doses of oestrogen have been used which still maintain the therapeutic advantage without the unwanted treatment morbidity. Bilateral subcapsular orchidectomy is simple, effective and with few physiological side effects. Newer agents are often now preferred, including goserelin (Zoladex), an LHRH agonist, which probably works by interfering with pituitary gonadotrophin release and thence causing a reduction in circulating testosterone.

The advantage of these agents is their improved tolerance over oestrogen, coupled with their ability to reduce testosterone to castrate levels without the need for orchidectomy, which is often considered an effective alternative. Indeed, for the patient who has no personal objection to orchidectomy, this form of treatment could be extremely successful in producing symptomatic relief of metastatic pain, and responses are often remarkably durable. Testicular prostheses can be placed in the scrotum if desired by the patient.

Some authorities believe that local treatment has no place in the management of prostatic cancer, preferring to rely entirely on one or other of the hormone measures. One of the reasons for the controversy is the slow course of prostatic cancer, particularly when first diagnosed as early stage disease. Under these circumstances, it is possible that treatment with low dose hormone therapy can, in the hormone sensitive group (i.e. the majority) achieve similar results to surgery or radiotherapy, but with fewer side effects. The debate continues, but in the younger fit patient who might benefit from a local therapy (generally irradiation), most urologists or radiotherapists would feel that local treatment is still worthwhile.

Figure 11.12 shows the outcome of treatment following local irradiation. There is a strong indication that adequate treatment of early stage disease may yield 10-year survival rates which, bearing in mind the relatively high death rate in this group of elderly patients, is surprisingly similar to men without prostate cancer; these results, however, from Stanford University in California, have been difficult to duplicate in other centres.

When primary hormone therapy fails, other hormonal agents of value include cyproterone acetate, aminoglutethinide and tamoxifen.

Apart from hormone therapy, the other important treatment modality for metastatic disease is palliative radiotherapy. Although the dose does not generally have to be high, it is often both possible and necessary to deliver a wide-field (or so-called 'hemibody') radiation if there is widespread bone pain. This is

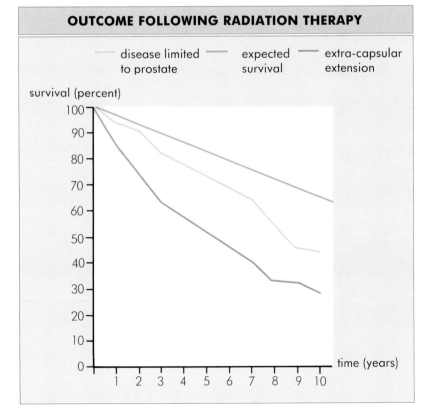

OUTCOME FOLLOWING RADIATION THERAPY

— disease limited to prostate — expected survival — extra-capsular extension

Fig. 11.12 Outcome following irradiation for prostatic carcinoma.

often the most simple effective means of providing pain relief. Long bones are not generally affected so orthopaedic fixation is rarely necessary. Skeletal metastases from prostate cancer are often not as destructive as metastases from other primary sites.

It is sometimes worth considering a hypophysectomy, which is a less dramatic procedure than it sounds, and is sometimes capable, at minimal morbidity to the patient, of producing long-lasting symptomatic relief, even with widespread metastases no longer responsive to conventional hormone treatment.

Because of the advanced age of most patients, coupled with the high probability of hormone responsiveness and lack of very active cytotoxic drugs, chemotherapy is not often used in this group. One final use of radiotherapy is for prevention of gynaecomastia in patients given Stilboestrol, a useful psychological boost for the patients, which is unfortunately often forgotten about.

The small group of patients with hormone resistant prostate cancer on the whole do very poorly, often complaining bitterly of widespread bone pain. Interestingly, radiotherapy can prove remarkably unhelpful in this group, and it is extremely important to consider all aspects of pain control and supportive care, and to be on guard for additional spinal problems, including cord compression and vertebral collapse. Recently systemic therapy with Strontium-90 has proven useful in some patients resistant to conventional therapy. The isotope is concentrated in bone, thus providing moderately high local doses to bone whilst relatively sparing bone marrow.

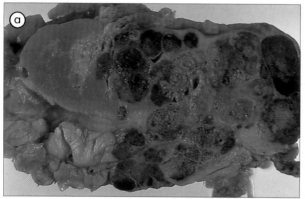
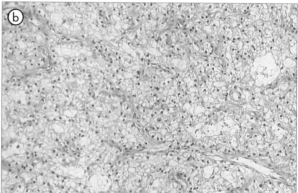

Fig. 11.13 Local invasion and histology of renal cell cancer. (a) Gross specimen of renal cell carcinoma of the lower pole of the kidney. There is extensive spread to perinephric fat. (b) Histological appearance of renal cell carcinoma, showing typical clear cells. Courtesy of Dr J. Theaker.

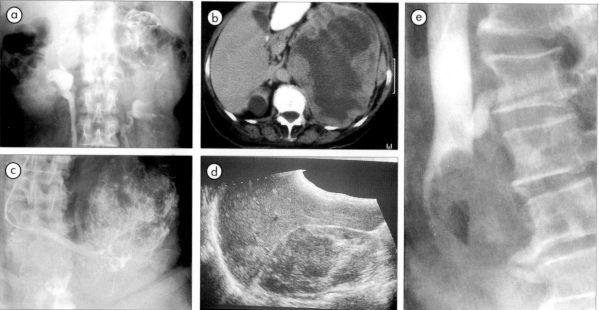

Fig. 11.14 Calcified renal cancer and tumour imaging. (a) IVU showing a grossly calcified renal cell carcinoma of the upper pole of the left kidney. The calyceal pattern on that side is distorted. (b) CT image of the abdomen showing a massive left renal cell carcinoma filling most of the left side of the abdomen. The renal vein remains patent. Courtesy of Dr R. Blaquire. (c) Arteriogram showing the extensive pathological circulation within a large renal cell carcinoma. (d) Ultrasound image showing a typical renal cell carcinoma of the right kidney. Courtesy of Dr K. Dewbury. (e) Venogram showing extensive tumour thrombus occluding the inferior vena cava (same case as in c).

Cancer of the Kidney

Renal cancers in children are nearly always nephroblastomas (Wilms' tumours), discussed in chapter 16. The commonest malignant kidney tumour in adults is the hypernephroma (renal cell carcinoma) which accounts for more than 85% of renal cancers. Overall kidney cancers form 2–3% of human malignancy.

Aetiology

Most cases of kidney cancer are sporadic though some familial tumours have been reported. The incidence of this tumour is three-times greater in men than in women, and its incidence is increasing in both sexes. There is evidence suggesting a five-fold increase in risk amongst men who are heavy cigarette and cigar smokers. Obesity and a diet rich in fat also seem to increase risk.

Up to 30% of people with von Hippel-Lindau disease (haemangioblastoma in the cerebellum and retina with phaeochromocytoma) develop renal cell carcinoma. A reciprocal translocation between chromosomes 3 and 8 (t[3;8][p14;q24]) has been described in a family with bilateral renal cancer in three generations. In general, inconsistent karyotypic changes are seen.

Pathology

Grawitz originally thought that this tumour arose from cell rests in adrenal tissue and the term hypernephroma was used. Current studies have shown that renal cell carcinoma develops from the epithelium of the renal tubules (Fig. 11.13).

Local invasion, and lymphatic and blood-borne spread are important. Spread to perinephric fat is present in 45% of cases and beyond Gerota's fascia in 10%. Renal vein invasion occurs in 30% of cases and extends into the inferior vena cava in 10%. Regional lymph node involvement is found in 20% of patients. Distant metastases are seen in a variety of sites: lung (40%); bone (28%); kidney (6%); spinal cord (5%); liver (5%); nodes (5%); brain (5%).

Clinical Presentation

Three quarters of patients present with urological symptoms, most of the rest having metastatic disease which is symptomatic. Common symptoms are haematuria (50%); flank or abdominal pain (40%); palpable mass (35%); classical triad of all three (10%). Non-specific symptoms are common; these include non-haemolytic anaemia (25%), weight loss (20%), fever (20%), hypertension (10–15%), hypercalcaemia (5%) and liver dysfunction without hepatic metastases (20–30%). These symptoms usually remit following nephrectomy.

Investigation (Fig. 11.14) includes intravenous pyelography and, if necessary, CT imaging. Arteriography is rarely required, though ultrasound can be useful in differentiating solid from cystic lesions. Venography may be indicated if extensive renal vein invasion is suspected. Chest X-ray is mandatory before surgery and some centres use preoperative CT to exclude lung metastases. Isotopic bone imaging is the most sensitive way of detecting bone involvement. Survival is clearly related to stage; staging is by the TNM system (Fig. 11.15).

Treatment

Surgery is the treatment of choice, although up to 25% of patients have tumours which are inoperable at presentation. Radical excision has been recommended for advanced stage disease though it remains controversial. Some centres undertake lymphadenectomy even if the tumour is localized to the kidney (stage I/II) whilst others will use partial nephrectomy for selected stage I cases.

Some surgeons have advocated nephrectomy when there are distant metastases in the belief that this may induce a spontaneous regression. In general it seems highly likely that the morbidity and mortality of nephrectomy outweigh the chances of a spontaneous regression – which is likely to be of short duration and rarely prolongs life.

TNM STAGING FOR RENAL CANCER	
Classification	Criteria
T1	Small tumour (<2.5cm) no enlargement of kidney
T2	Large tumour (>2.5cm) cortex not broken
T3	Perinephric or hilar extension Venous involvement
T4	Extension to neighbouring organs
N1	Single homolateral regional (<2cm)
N2	Contra- or bilateral/multiple regional
N3	Fixed regional
N4	Juxtaregional
M0	No metastasis
M1	Distant metastasis

Stage	Grouping			5-year survival rate
Stage I	T1	N0	M0	75%
Stage II	T2	N0	M0	60%
Stage III	T3	N0	M0	40%
Stage IV	T4	N0	M0	5%
	Any T	N1,2,3,4	M0	
	Any T	Any N	M1	

Fig. 11.15 TNM staging classification for renal cancer. 5-year survival is clearly related to stage.

Embolization is sometimes used as a palliative measure in disseminated disease though its efficiency is doubtful. Radiotherapy, given pre- or post-operatively, does not improve survival. Its major role is in the palliation of bone and CNS metastases (Fig. 11.16).

Chemotherapy has proven to be remarkably in-effective with no single cytotoxic drug achieving a 20% response rate. Progesterone therapy, despite early enthusiasm, has a low response rate. Recently, interleukin-2 has been reported to induce responses in up to 25% of patients, though treatment remains relatively toxic.

Cancer of the Adrenal Glands

Tumours of the adrenal cortex and medulla are un-common but present a fascinating challenge because of their propensity to produce hormones. It is also important to remember that adrenal cancer may be part of the 'Multiple Endocrine Neoplasia' (MEN) syndrome (see Fig. 9.6).

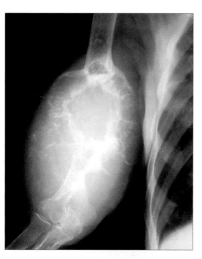

Fig. 11.16 Gross destructive bone metastasis from renal cell carcinoma.

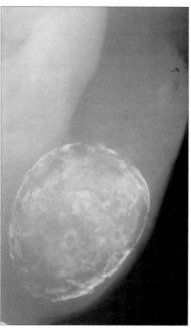

Fig. 11.17 Late presentation of testicular tumours. X-ray of scrotum showing a large calcified testicular tumour. The patient had been aware of the lump for many years and it only came to light on routine physical examination – it was benign.

Adrenocortical Cancer

These tumours are difficult to diagnose early and because of this are rarely curable. In one series they accounted for only 0.04% of all cancers referred to a large centre. They are seen at all ages but most patients are middle aged.

They may be steroid or non-steroid producing. Steroid production, where present, is often inefficient and uncoordinated, with abnormal hormones being produced together with an excess of precursors. Despite this the C_{19} steroid pathway is usually intact so that there is high urinary output of 17-ketosteroids. The syndromes associated with these tumours include Cushings syndrome, virilization, feminization, pre-cocious puberty, sodium retention and hypokalaemic alkalosis and hypoglycaemia.

Diagnosis is generally based on CT scanning though angiography can be used, but is generally not required if CT imaging is used. Urinary excretion of steroids may be helpful in establishing the diagnosis and for monitoring response.

Histopathologically these tumours are often quite large (over 100g). The cut surface is tan to yellow in colour and there is pseudoencapsulation. Micro-scopically it may be difficult to differentiate between carcinoma and an adenoma. Capsular and blood vessel invasion are the most useful indications of malignancy.

Management

Surgery can be undertaken in about one-half of all patients and it has been claimed that aggressive resection of metastatic disease, particularly in the liver, may extend survival. Such radical *en bloc* operations demand a thoracoabdominal approach.

Radiotherapy can be useful palliatively but the high dose required for tumour eradication can rarely be delivered. Chemotherapy is generally used for

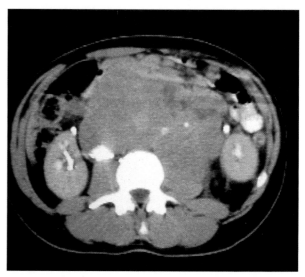

Fig. 11.18 Gross para-aortic malignant teratoma metastatic from the testicle. There is invasion of the psoas muscle causing severe back pain (see Fig. 2.4). Courtesy of Dr G. Mead.

advanced or recurrent disease, though, as with radio-therapy, it may be used as an adjuvant after surgical resection. The drug mitotane (ortho-para prime DDD or $O_1P'DDD$) can produce objective responses in metastatic disease. The drug is taken orally and after ingestion up to 50% is absorbed and is deposited in fat, liver, brain and adrenal tissues. Tissue levels are detectable for up to one year later. Gluco- and mineralocorticoid replacement is usually required. The main dose limiting side effect is nausea and vomiting; diarrhoea is also seen though CNS symptoms and skin rash are uncommon.

The results of therapy are closely related to stage at presentation. Small well differentiated tumours are highly curable with surgery, whereas cure is rare in advanced cases. Chemotherapy produces objective responses in one-third of cases and may, in appropriate cases, prolong life. Median survival in reported series varies from 3 months to 2 years.

Adrenal Medullary Cancer

The cells of the adrenal medulla are embryologically distinct from those of the cortex. Ten to fifteen per cent of phaeochromocytoma are malignant, though criteria to establish malignancy are difficult to define. Pleomorphism and excess mitoses may be seen in benign lesions as may capsular invasion, so that the diagnosis of malignancy may have to be based on biological behaviour. Tumours may be functional or non-functional. Functional tumours secrete similar hormones to benign tumours so that there is a similar risk of hypertension, stroke, cardiovascular and renal disease due to excessive adrenaline and noradrenaline.

Urinary metanephrines are useful in establishing the diagnosis but may give false negatives, and plasma catecholamines (with or without clonidine) are also useful. CT imaging has largely superceded angiography.

Malignant phaeochromocytomas may metastasize to lung, bone and brain, but disease progression is often slow and life-threatening complications are usually due to secreted hormones.

Management

Surgery requires preparation with blockade of α-adrenergic receptors with phentolamine. Beta-adrenergic blockade may also be helpful but should only be undertaken after full α-adrenergic blockade. Surgery is generally palliative as is radiotherapy. Chemotherapy with streptozotocin or drug combinations is generally only partially effective. Radio-labelled MIBG (meta-iodobenzylguanidine) may be used for tumour localization and recently has been tested as a therapeutic modality. If ^{131}I-MIBG uptake is good, it is possible to deliver doses of several thousand cGy with modest tumour response. Life-threatening hypertensive crisis following systemic therapy has been reported but this complication can be avoided by α-adrenergic blockade.

Testicular Cancer

Testicular tumours are increasing in frequency in Western countries and are now the commonest malignancy in the age group 15–35 years. Although the reasons for the rise in incidence (see Fig. 1.7) are unclear, it seems likely that hormonal effects on the developing fetus at least play a part in causation of this tumour. They are amongst the most curable of cancers even when disseminated, as a result of their extreme sensitivity to modern chemotherapy (see below). For this reason, testicular tumours have an importance which far outweighs their numerical incidence.

There are two established aetiological factors. Maldescent of the testis substantially increases the risk of testicular neoplasia, emphasizing the importance of early orchidopexy (preferably well below the age of 10 years) even if the testis has spontaneously descended as far as the inguinal canal but not into the scrotum itself. In young men with unilateral testicular maldescent the contralateral testis is also at increased risk of neoplasia, suggesting that it is more than simply the local environment of the undescended testis that is the cause of neoplastic change. The second known risk factor is of relevance only in patients who have already been diagnosed and treated for a testicular tumour. In this group the incidence of a second primary tumour, in the contralateral testis, is far higher than in the normal population. It has also been suggested that both maldescent and testicular neoplasia are more common in young men who were exposed to high levels of oestrogens *in utero*. Research into this theory is currently underway and there is some evidence that the mothers of men who develop testicular tumours and/or maldescent were of higher weight at the time of the birth than mothers of men who did not develop these problems – the implication being that obesity may result in higher than normal levels of maternal oestrogen during pregnancy.

Most patients present with a lump in the testis which may or may not be painful. Unfortunately, diagnosis is often delayed (Fig. 11.17). This is sometimes due to reluctance on the part of the patient to see their doctor with a testicular mass, but delay may also occur because of the erroneous assumption that the mass is an epididymo-orchitis, which should be treated by antibiotic therapy. Any patient with a lump in the testis, painful or not, should be referred urgently to a urologist. Some patients present with symptoms of metastatic disease, the commonest symptom apart from testicular swelling being backache caused by retroperitoneal tumour involving the psoas muscles (Fig. 11.18). Rarely tumour may invade through vertebral foramina and cause spinal cord compression. Extensive disease in the lungs may cause shortness of breath and rarely haemoptysis (see Fig. 11.19), whilst occasionally patients may present with symptoms and signs of brain

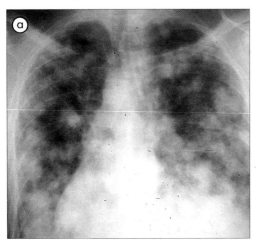
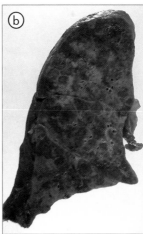

Fig. 11.19 Lung metastasis from testicular cancer. (a) Diffuse lung involvement by metastatic choriocarcinoma of the testis. The patient presented with dyspnoea and haemoptysis and was unaware of a testicular mass (see also Fig. 2.4). Courtesy of Dr G. Mead. (b) Post mortem appearance of the lung of a patient with extensive choriocarcinoma of the testis. The patient died shortly after the first cycle of chemotherapy – all the lung nodules sampled showed necrosis without viable malignant teratoma. Courtesy of Dr J. Theaker.

metastasis (Fig. 11.20).

If a testicular tumour is clinically suspected, ultrasound may be helpful in confirming the diagnosis. Tumour markers (AFP and ß-HCG) are useful if their levels are raised (see below). If the mass is thought to be a testicular tumour the appropriate surgical procedure is a radical orchidectomy through an inguinal incision. This approach allows the testis to be examined directly, and if there is a neoplasm the cord and vessels can be clamped and the tumour removed, allowing for histological inspection of the complete specimen, including the testis, its coverings, and the cord and vessels. Involvement of these more proximal tissues, particularly the cord or vessels, is critically important since it may represent the only evidence in marker-negative cases of spread beyond the testis. Scrotal incision or aspiration of masses should not be undertaken since the risk of local spread complicates further management.

Histologically, most testicular tumours are malignant (Fig. 11.21), the commonest being malignant teratomas of various subtypes (Fig. 11.22) and seminoma. Here, seminoma and teratoma will be discussed separately since their behaviour and treatment are different.

Seminoma

This tumour accounts for nearly one-half of testicular tumours and is seen in a slightly older age group (25–45 years, median 35 years) than are teratomas. The tumour spreads in a predictable pattern from the testis to the retroperitoneal nodes via the thoracic duct to the supraclavicular and mediastinal nodes. Blood-borne spread is generally a very late feature. At presentation, most patients have tumour confined to the testis (stage I) or limited spread to the para-aortic lymph nodes. Because of this predictable mode of spread and its exquisite radiosensitivity, radiotherapy has become a standard part of management. Following surgery, a chest X-ray and CT scan of the abdomen (and, if indicated, thorax) should be done and tumour markers should be measured. A raised AFP or ß-HCG of >100i.u. suggest a teratoma

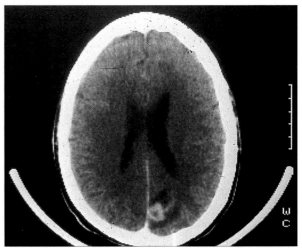

Fig. 11.20 Brain metastasis from testicular teratoma. Posterior fossa brain metastasis in a man with a testicular teratoma. This was asymptomatic, being found when he was noted to have a raised beta-HCG in the absence of active disease at other sites. The finding of unexplained raised marker should prompt a search for sanctuary sites (CNS and testes). Courtesy of Dr G. Mead.

and these patients should be treated as such. Levels of placental alkaline phosphatase (PLAP) may also be raised in seminoma. Patients with normal markers and X-rays or those with minimal retroperitoneal lymph node involvement are treated with radiotherapy. Patients with bulky retroperitoneal lymph node involvement (Fig. 11.24) or more extensive disease are treated with platinum based combination chemotherapy, with excellent results; seminoma seems to be as chemoresponsive as teratoma. In the case of extensive retroperitoneal disease some centres still use large field radiotherapy with good results, though such an approach will reduce tolerance to chemotherapy should it be needed for relapse. Surgery (see below) for residual masses on CT scan after chemotherapy is extremely difficult as these tumours are very adherent to blood vessels and other neighbouring structures which they envelope

HISTOPATHOLOGICAL CLASSIFICATION OF TESTICULAR GERM CELL MALIGNANCIES AND THEIR FREQUENCIES

Classification		Frequency
British testicular tumour panel	Dixon and Moore (USA)	
Seminoma	Pure seminoma	40%
Malignant teratoma undifferentiated	Embryonal carcinoma	25%
Malignant teratoma intermediate	Teratoma with malignant areas	25%
Malignant teratoma trophoblastic	Choriocarcinoma	2%
Teratoma differentiated	Teratoma	6%

Fig. 11.21 Histological classification of testicular tumours and their frequencies. Comparison of British and American classifications.

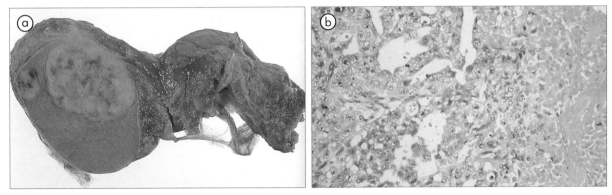

Fig. 11.22 Macroscopic and microscopic appearance of testicular teratoma. (a) Macroscopic appearance showing two nodules of teratoma within the testis. (b) Microscopic appearance of typical malignant teratoma intermediate. Courtesy of Dr J. Theaker.

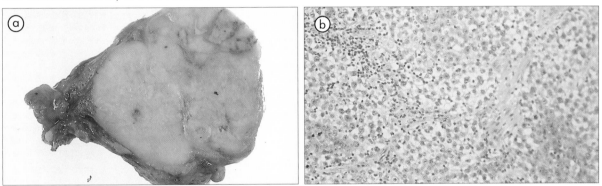

Fig. 11.23 Macroscopic and microscopic appearance of testicular seminoma. (a) Macroscopically there are small areas of necrosis which are commonly seen in large seminomas. (b) Classic microscopic appearance of seminoma.

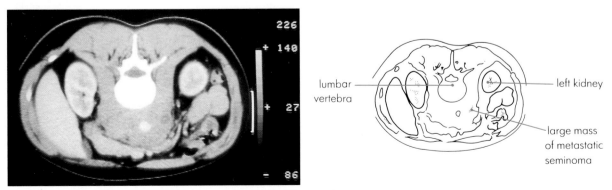

Fig. 11.24 Metastasis from testicular seminoma. CT scan showing massive retroperitoneal involvement. Courtesy of Dr R. Blaquire.

in sheets. In contrast to teratoma, such operations to remove residual masses are rarely indicated – serial CT showing gradual disappearance of the remaining masses.

The majority of patients have early stage disease which is treated surgically and with simple radiotherapy – the relapse rate for these patients is only 1–2%. For patients with bulky advanced disease, chemotherapy results in long-term survival in 85% of cases. Overall, this is one of the most curable of all malignancies.

Teratoma

This tumour also spreads in an orderly fashion to retroperitoneal lymph nodes (Fig. 11.25), but blood borne spread occurs more commonly and at an earlier stage than for seminoma (15–35 years, median 25 years). Initial staging should include:
- careful physical examination;
- chest X-ray;
- CT scan of abdomen and thorax;
- repeated monitoring of AFP and ß-HCG levels after surgery to observe rate of fall.

The management of early and advanced teratoma has changed dramatically in the past 15 years with the advent of highly effective therapy for advanced disease.

Patients are staged according to the sites of disease spread and its bulk. There are several classifications in use. Patients with stage I disease (50% of cases) have a relapse rate of 20–25%. The Medical Research Council have identified certain histological features

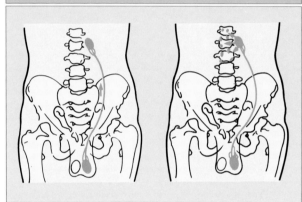
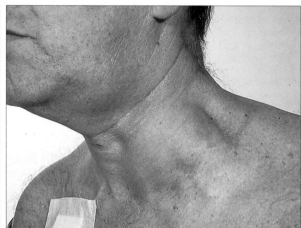

LYMPHATIC SPREAD IN TESTICULAR CANCER

Fig. 11.25 Lymphatic spread of testicular cancer. Testicular tumours spread from the testicular lymphatics centrally to the paraortic nodes (left) and thence via the thoracic duct to the left supraclavicular fossa (right). Courtesy of Dr G. Mead.

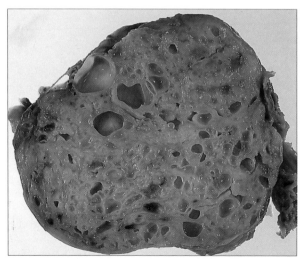

Fig. 11.26 Mass of teratoma differentiated removed from the retroperitoneum following chemotherapy. Such masses may increase in size during chemotherapy whilst tumour markers fall. This is due to increasing distention of the cystic areas. Persistent masses after chemotherapy for teratoma should always be considered for surgical excision. Courtesy of Dr J. Theaker.

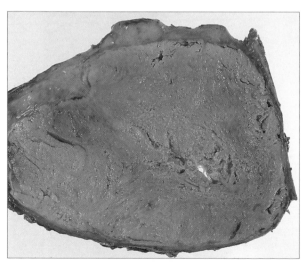

Fig. 11.27 Resected mediastinal teratoma. This surgical specimen shows a solid mass of differentiated mediastinal teratoma. Tumour markers were just beginning to rise at the time of surgery and there is a small focus of malignant teratoma at the very top of the specimen. Courtesy of Dr J. Theaker.

which indicate a high likelihood (50–60%) of relapse. These include:

- invasion of testicular veins;
- invasion of testicular lymphatics;
- absence of yolk-sac elements;
- presence of undifferentiated tumour.

Patients with stage I disease with less than 3 of the above risk factors have a low rate of relapse (10–15%) and may be monitored carefully (chest X-ray, CT and markers). Patients who have progression are detected early and virtually 100% should be cured with chemotherapy. An alternative approach is to undertake a radical lymphadenectomy, as is used in some centres in the USA. Such surgery requires a high level of skill, does not necessarily deal with all disease since 50% relapse at distant sites and is not without long-term complications. Stage I patients with 3 or more risk factors should probably undergo chemotherapy. These patients and those with detectable spread of disease should be treated with cisplatin based chemotherapy. The most commonly used regime also includes etoposide and bleomycin. Using such an approach, more than 85% of patients treated in specialist centres should be cured.

Despite chemotherapy, many patients with bulky disease are left with residual masses after chemotherapy. These may be composed of differentiated teratoma (Fig. 11.26), malignant teratoma (Fig. 11.27) or fibrous and necrotic tissues. In addition to CT, markers (AFP and ß-HCG) are very useful in estimating disease activity. One or both are raised in 85% of cases of advanced testicular teratoma and the serum level reflects disease activity well. Where there are residual masses after chemotherapy, with normal markers, surgical excision even of multiple sites is often indicated (Fig. 11.28). Even in cases where there are raised markers, surgery may be curative if the disease is localized. The optimal use of chemotherapy and surgery requires a high degree of experience and testicular teratomas should always be treated in specialist centres. Radiotherapy may be used as an adjunct to surgery in carefully selected cases. They are amongst the most curable of neoplasms though some patients will require very intensive and complicated therapies.

Cancer of the Penis

This is an uncommon cancer, which accounts for about 0.1% of male cancer deaths in the West. It is commoner in parts of Asia and Africa. Early circumcision appears to be protective and poor hygiene increases the risk of developing this cancer. There appears to be an increased incidence of cervical cancer in the partners of men with cancer of the penis.

There are several premalignant conditions which should be locally excised. These include:

- Intra-epithelial carcinoma (Bowen's disease);
- Leukoplakia;
- Paget's disease;
- Erythroplasia of Queyrat.

Cancer of the penis generally presents as an exophytic or ulcerating lesion in the glans penis or the inner surface of the prepuce (see Fig. 11.29). A wide area of the surface may become involved before there is deep penetration which may extend into the corpora cavernosa and eventually the urethra. Extension to inguinal lymph nodes is common though nodal enlargement may also be due to infection of

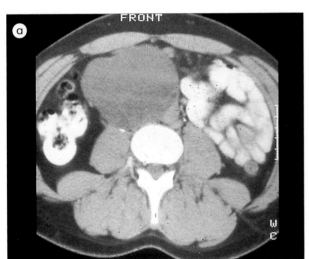
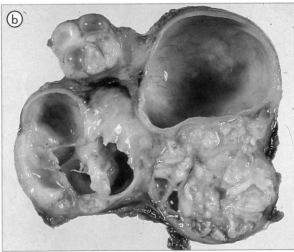

Fig. 11.28 Resected residual teratoma. (a) CT image of an extensive residual mass after chemotherapy for testicular teratoma. (b) Surgical specimen of resected mass – teratoma differentiated. Left *in situ* such benign tumours may continue to grow or may transform into malignant phenotypes – carcinoma and/or sarcoma. Courtesy of Dr G. Mead.

the ulcerating tumour. Biopsy is essential to differentiate the tumour from benign conditions that may mimic this tumour, such as penile condylomata, leucoplakia or lymphogranuloma venereum. Staging uses a TNM system (Fig. 11.30), but assessment of lymph node extension may be difficult because of the problem of infection.

In the past, surgical amputation was the prime mode of management with excellent results in patients with early stage disease. Because of failure in more advanced stages some surgeons have recently advocated lymphadenectomy. An alternative approach has been to use radiation therapy, with surgery held in reserve for failure. Both external beam and brachytherapy has been used. Results have been good in selected patients. Patients with T1 or T2 N0 M0 disease are usually cured, with 4-year disease-free survival rates of 75% or better achieved with either surgery or radiotherapy.

■ Summary

Urological malignancy has been the focus of much attention, with marked improvement in the survival

of testicular teratomas. This has followed the introduction of cisplatin based chemotherapy. Bladder cancer is also responsive to similar chemotherapy and use of this modality together with irradiation or surgery may improve survival. Prostate and kidney cancer remain largely incurable if not detected at an early stage.

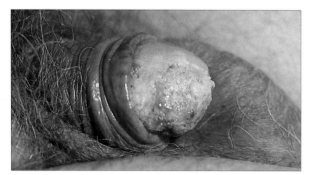

Fig. 11.29 Carcinoma of the penis. This was a tumour of the glans and distal shaft, treated by local excision and radiotherapy. Courtesy of Dr P. Hopkins.

TNM STAGING FOR PENILE CANCER

Stage	Criteria
Tis	Carcinoma *in situ* (Bowen's and Erythroplasia of Queyrat are included)
T1	Tumour invades subepithelial connective tissue
T2	Tumour invades corpus spongiosum or cavernosum
T3	Tumour invades urethra or prostate
T4	Tumour invades other adjacent structures
N0	No regional lymph nodes
N1	Metastasis in a single superficial inguinal lymph node
N2	Metastasis in multiple or bilateral superficial inguinal lymph nodes
N3	Metastasis in deep inguinal or pelvic lymph nodes
M0	No distant metastasis
M1	Distant metastasis

Fig. 11.30 TNM staging classification for penile cancer.

Lymphoma

12

Introduction

The lymphomas are a diverse group of malignancies derived from the lymphoreticular cells. They usually arise in the lymphoid tissue of lymph nodes, bone marrow and spleen but may arise in almost any tissue in the body. Hodgkin's disease has traditionally been viewed separately from the other lymphomas, referred to collectively as non-Hodgkin's lymphoma, though there is recent evidence suggesting that this division may be artificial – at least in certain subtypes of Hodgkin's disease. For reasons of convenience, this chapter will stick with tradition and discuss Hodgkin's disease separately from the rest of the lymphomas.

Hodgkin's Disease

This condition was first reported by Thomas Hodgkin in 1832 when he described seven cases based on their particular clinical and gross morphological appearance. Although four of these cases would not now be considered as Hodgkin's disease, the lymph nodes of three have been shown to contain Reed–Sternberg cells – an essential histological feature of the disease.

Hodgkin's disease is one of the commonest neoplasms in young adults. Its incidence rises steeply from 15 years, and falls between 35 to 60 years,

with a second peak of high incidence at about 70 years of age. There is a slight predominance in males (ratio 1.5:1). Familial factors appear to operate in some cases, so that the sibling of a patient with Hodgkin's disease has a five-fold increase in risk of developing the disease. If the sibling is of the same sex, the risk is increased to nine-fold that of an individual without a sibling with Hodgkin's disease. Preliminary data has suggested that a region near the dR locus may be associated with familial cases. Despite numerous attempts to link Hodgkin's disease with an infectious agent, none have so far fulfilled Koch's postulates.

Pathologically, the diagnosis of Hodgkin's disease is made on the basis of the presence of Reed–Sternberg cells (or one of its mononuclear variants) in a particular stromal setting. Reed–Sternberg cells are characterized by large inclusion-like nucleoli and double or multiple nuclei of large size (Fig. 12.1). Mononuclear variants are typical of some varieties of Hodgkin's disease, though they are less reliable diagnostically. They are often surrounded by a clear zone (lacunar), have a large nucleolus which is spherical and homogenous eosinophilic or amphophilic cytoplasm. The surrounding infiltrate may vary greatly depending on the subtype but includes lymphocytes, eosinophils, histiocytes and plasma

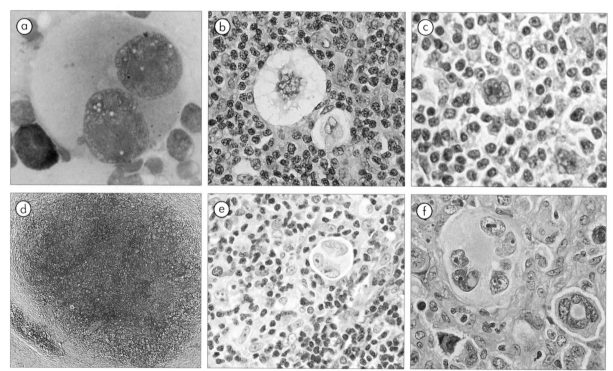

Fig. 12.1 Cytological appearance of Hodgkin's disease. (a) Cytological appearance of a Reed–Sternberg cell (touch preparation). (b) Typical lacunar cell in nodular sclerosing Hodgkin's disease.
(c) Lymphocyte predominant Hodgkin's disease with abundant lymphocytes and two 'popcorn' cells.
(d) Nodular sclerosing Hodgkin's disease: nodule of tumour surrounded by marked sclerosis. (e) Mixed cellularity Hodgkin's disease with Reed–Sternberg cells and a mixed population of background cells including eosinophils. (f) Lymphocyte depleted Hodgkin's disease with bizarre Reed–Sternberg cells and few lymphocytes. Courtesy of Prof D.H. Wright.

cells. There may also be infiltration with bands of fibrosis and necrosis occurs occasionally (see Fig. 12.1).

The Lukes and Butler classification (Fig. 12.2) divides Hodgkin's disease into four main subtypes, based on the histological characteristics of the Reed–Sternberg cells and surrounding infiltration. Using this classification, 80–90% of cases fall into the category of nodular sclerosis (60–70%) or mixed cellularity (20–30%). Prognosis is related to cell type, survival being best in lymphocyte predominant and worsening through to lymphocyte depleted.

Clinical Features

In the great majority of cases, patients present with a painless enlarging mass, most often in the neck (Fig. 12.3). On examination this is found to be a discrete, rubbery lymph gland or group of lymph nodes. The other common sites of presentation are shown in Fig. 12.4. Occasionally, respiratory symptoms

LUKES AND BUTLER CLASSIFICATION FOR HODGKIN'S LYMPHOMA
Lymphocyte predominant
Reed–Sternberg cells are rare. There are abundant normal-looking lymphocytes with or without histiocytes.
Nodular sclerosis
Nodules of lymphoid infiltration separated by bands of collagen. Numerous Reed–Sternberg cells (lacunar cells).
Mixed cellularity
Pleomorphic infiltrate with eosinophils, plasma cells, histiocytes and lymphocytes. Numerous Reed–Sternberg cells.
Lymphocyte depleted
Few lymphocytes with numerous and often bizarre Reed–Sternberg cells.

Fig. 12.2 Classification of Hodgkin's disease.

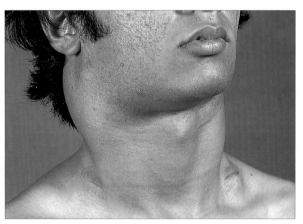

Fig. 12.3 Adenopathy in Hodgkin's disease.
Cervical lymphadenopathy in Hodgkin's disease. Note previous biopsy scars in both supraclavicular fossae. Courtesy of Prof J.M.A. Whitehouse.

Fig. 12.4 Common sites of presentation of Hodgkin's disease.

SITES OF PRESENTATION IN HODGKIN'S DISEASE

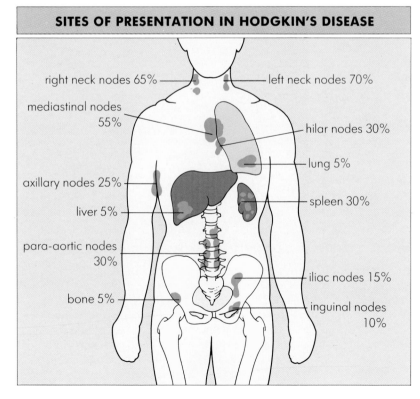

right neck nodes 65%
left neck nodes 70%
mediastinal nodes 55%
hilar nodes 30%
lung 5%
axillary nodes 25%
spleen 30%
liver 5%
para-aortic nodes 30%
iliac nodes 15%
bone 5%
inguinal nodes 10%

caused by extensive mediastinal lymphadenopathy (Fig. 12.5) are the presenting feature.

Some patients have unexplained fevers and night sweats or itching as their first symptom. Fatigue and weight loss are also fairly common. Such patients tend to be older and to have more extensive disease on staging. Rarely, patients complain of pain in enlarged glands soon after drinking alcohol – such a finding is very suggestive of Hodgkin's disease. Its aetiology is unexplained. Presentation due to the effects of compression of organs or nerves by enlarged lymph nodes involved by Hodgkin's disease

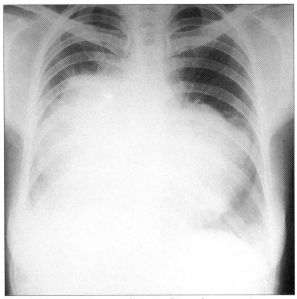

Fig. 12.5 Massive mediastinal involvement in Hodgkin's disease. Tracheal or bronchial compression may occur even when mediastinal involvement is much less obvious.

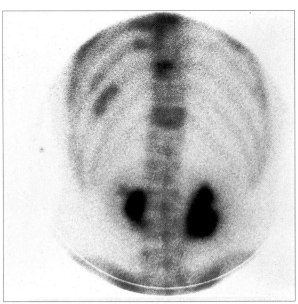

Fig. 12.6 Bone involvement in Hodgkin's disease. Isotopic bone image showing involvement of vertebrae and ribs. Courtesy of Prof J.M.A. Whitehouse.

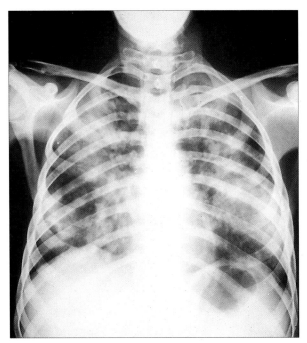

Fig. 12.7 Pulmonary infiltration with Hodgkin's disease. Usually a feature of recurrent disease. Courtesy of Prof J.M.A. Whitehouse.

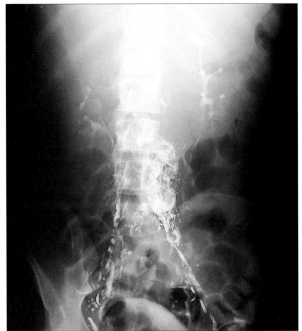

Fig. 12.8 Lymphangiography and IVU showing enlarged foamy para-aortic lymph nodes involved with Hodgkin's disease. The left kidney is displaced laterally by a mass of unfilled involved lymph nodes. CT imaging provides information on upper abdominal nodes, mesenteric nodes and organs, whilst lymphangiography provides detailed information on the size and architecture of para-aortic and pelvic lymph nodes.

or infiltration of bone (Fig. 12.6) are relatively un-common. Pulmonary infiltration at presentation is uncommon but becomes increasingly frequent with relapse (Fig. 12.7). Infiltration may appear to extend out from enlarged hilar nodes or may take on the form of patchy multiple discrete pulmonary nodules.

Initial Evaluation

All patients with Hodgkin's disease should be expertly evaluated in order to ascertain the extent of spread of the disease. This includes a careful history, with special attention to the presence of unexplained systemic symptoms (fever, night sweats and pruritis) which suggest a worse prognosis. On examination particular attention should be paid to node bearing areas (preauricular, cervical, supra- and infraclavi-cular, axillary, epitrochlear, iliac, inguinal, femoral and popliteal). The liver and spleen are examined for enlargement, though an enlarged spleen does not necessarily indicate Hodgkin's disease.

CT imaging is used to assess the thorax and abdomen. Lymphangiography is also useful in asses-sing para-aortic lymph nodes and may occasionally be complimentary to CT scanning (Fig. 12.8). The addition of routine biochemistry, full blood count and ESR, and bone marrow aspirate and trephine provides sufficient information for staging. However, in selected situations some centres recommend a staging laparotomy. This operation was introduced in the late 1960's as the most accurate way of defining the extent of intra-abdominal disease. Multiple lymph nodes are sampled, the spleen removed and biopsies of the liver taken. Perhaps the most import-ant information to come from this procedure is the state of the spleen, which is of major prognostic significance. Non-invasive tests are notoriously poor at assessing splenic involvement (half of patients with a clinically or radiologically enlarged spleen do not have involvement whilst one-quarter of normal sized spleens are involved with Hodgkin's disease), so that the only reliable way of assessing its state is by surgery When used to select patients for different patterns of radiotherapy, chemotherapy or combined therapy staging laparotomy serves a useful function. However, recent trends towards combined therapy or primary chemotherapy means that it is used less often. In addition, some groups use radiotherapy fields which include the spleen (without causing renal problems, as used to be feared), thus avoiding the need for splenectomy.

Staging

The commonly used staging classification (Fig. 12.9) is named after Ann Arbor (the site of the conference which introduced it) and provides useful prognostic information; prognosis worsens with increasing stage and the presence of systemic symptoms ('B' symptoms).

Fig. 12.9 The Ann Arbor staging system for Hodgkin's disease.

ANN ARBOR STAGING CLASSIFICATION FOR HODGKIN'S DISEASE	
Staging Classification*	Criteria
Stage I	Involvement of a single lymph node region or of a single extralymphatic site (IE).
Stage II	Involvement of two or more node regions on the same side of the diaphragm, or of a localized extranodal involvement and one or more lymph node regions on the same side of the diaphragm (IIE).
Stage III†	Involvement of lymph nodes on both sides of the diaphragm, which may include the spleen (IIIS) or a localized extranodal site (IIIE) or both (IIISE).
Stage IV	Diffuse involvement of one or more extralymphatic organs.

* Suffix A = no constitutional symptoms. Suffix B = constitutional symptoms present. These are fevers, night sweats and/or loss of 10% or more of body weight over 6 months. Pruritus is not included. Suffix E = localized extra-nodal involvement.

† Stage III disease can be subdivided according to the extent of intra-abdominal node involvement. Stage III_1 = involvement of spleen, splenic, coeliac or portal nodes or any combinations of these. Stage III_2 = involvement of para-aortic, iliac or mesenteric nodes with or without upper abdominal disease.

Treatment

The first successful treatment for Hodgkin's disease, radiotherapy, was developed in the 1950's and 1960's. The treatment relied on accurate definition of the sites of disease and the use of moderately high doses of irradiation delivered to all known areas of disease as well as lymph node areas considered to be at risk of involvement. The introduction of mega-voltage equipment at this time greatly improved the ability to deliver the type of radiation therapy needed. Because there was no effective chemotherapy, radiation fields were often very extensive in an attempt to treat all disease at the outset – such fields were described as total lymphoid irradiation (Fig. 12.10). This approach produced a rapid improvement in results in patients with stages I to IIIa disease. However, such extensive irradiation is, not surprisingly, associated with a wide variety of side effects. These include:

- acute effects such as nausea and vomiting, diarrhoea, pancytopenia and hair loss in irradiated sites;
- pneumonitis;
- pericarditis;
- hypothyroidism;
- L'hermitte syndrome ('electric' sensation on flexing neck);
- amenorrhoea;
- cardiac dysfunction;
- secondary malignancy.

More recently, with the development of highly effective chemotherapy, there has been a trend towards reducing the extent of radiation fields. Thus some of the centres who pioneered extensive radiation are now testing involved-field irradiation with simple chemotherapy regimes in patients with limited disease at presentation. Current results are encouraging.

Chemotherapy

Hodgkin's disease is highly sensitive to a wide variety of cytotoxic agents but it was not until the late

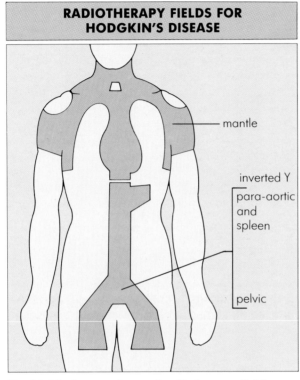

RADIOTHERAPY FIELDS FOR HODGKIN'S DISEASE

— mantle

inverted Y
para-aortic and spleen

pelvic

Fig. 12.10 Commonly used radiotherapy fields used to treat Hodgkin's disease. The upper field is called a mantle, the lower an inverted Y. When both are used together it is called 'total nodal irradiation'. If the iliac fields of the inverted Y are omitted, and the para-aortic and mantle fields only are given, this is called 'sub-total irradiation'.

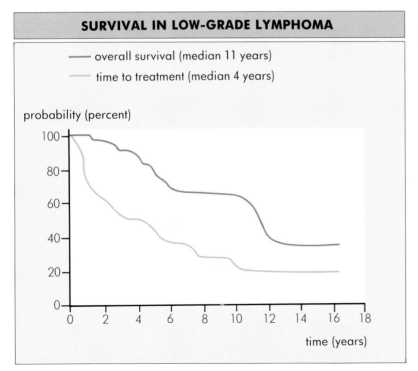

SURVIVAL IN LOW-GRADE LYMPHOMA

—— overall survival (median 11 years)
—— time to treatment (median 4 years)

probability (percent)

time (years)

Fig. 12.11 Survival in low-grade lymphoma. Survival and time to treatment of patients with low-grade lymphoma – treatment was delayed until required (90% had stage IV disease).

1960's that potentially curative combinations were derived. The first of these used nitrogen mustard, vincristine, procarbazine and prednisolone (MOPP) and produced an 80% complete remission rate in patients with stage III and IV disease. Long-term survival was achieved in over 50% of patients. Since then a variety of other drug combinations have been developed which seem to be as effective as MOPP but which may have less severe side effects. MOPP causes severe emesis because of the inclusion of nitrogen mustard and also causes sterility (especially in males) and induces leukaemia. For these reasons other combinations have been extensively tested

in an attempt to lessen toxicity whilst maintaining or improving the therapeutic results. A number of regimes (such as ABVD – adriamycin, bleomycin, vinblastine, DTIC) appear to be as effective as MOPP whilst not causing secondary malignancy or infertility.

Recommended Treatment by Stage

There have been continuous subtle changes in the management of Hodgkin's disease in the past 20 years. Absolute recommendations, therefore, are not possible as there is still controversy regarding the exact therapy for each situation and substage. However, it is clear that for accurately staged patients with stage I and II disease there is a 90% probability of cure with extensive irradiation (the exact extent required is still debatable). Selected patients at high risk of relapse, such as those with large mediastinal masses, should also receive chemotherapy. Some centres use less extensive radiation with simple chemotherapy for early stage disease. Patients with stage IIIa disease can be divided by the extent of their abdominal involvement (number and sites of disease) into those with a good outlook with irradiation alone and those requiring additional chemotherapy. Stages IIIb and IV are treated primarily with chemotherapy with moderately good results.

Relapse of Hodgkin's disease following radiotherapy is often successfully treated with chemotherapy. However, relapse after chemotherapy is much more difficult to salvage. Recently, high-dose chemotherapy supported with autologous bone marrow transplantation has been shown to produce long-term survival in about 20% of cases. The introduction of haemopoietic growth factors may simplify the use of the new generation of dose intensive cytotoxic drug regimes with further improvement in cure rates.

WORKING FORMULATION FOR NON-HODGKIN'S LYMPHOMA

Low grade

A. Small lymphocytic
B. Follicular, predominantly small cleaved†
C. Follicular, mixed small cleaved and large cells†

Intermediate grade

D. Follicular, predominantly large cell†
E. Diffuse, small cleaved cell
F. Diffuse, mixed small and large cells
G. Diffuse, large cell cleaved or non-cleaved cell

High grade

H. Large cell, immunoblastic†
I. Lymphoblastic, convoluted or non-convoluted
J. Small, non-cleaved cell Burkitt or non-Burkitt

* May be plasmacytoid
† May have diffuse areas

Fig. 12.12 Working formulation for the histopathological classification of non-Hodgkin's disease.

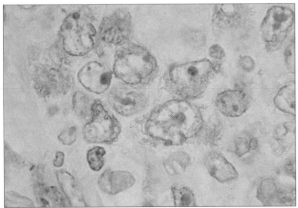

Fig. 12.13 Immunocytochemistry of lymphoma. The nature of the tumour can be confirmed by use of monoclonal antibodies directed against epitopes in specific tissues. In this case the tumour is common leucocyte antigen positive and antibodies for lambda are also positive with brown peroxidase pigment. Kappa staining was negative confirming that this is a monoclonal lambda B cell neoplasm.

Non-Hodgkin's Lymphoma

These represent one of the most diverse groups of all malignancies. At one end of the spectrum they may be very indolent, patients living many years without treatment (Fig. 12.11), whilst at the other extreme they may be the most rapidly growing of all cancers (Burkitt's lymphoma). Thus the grouping of all types of lymphoma together is completely artificial and many workers have devised histopathological classifications dividing tumours by cytological appearance and immunological characteristics. Because of the confusion of multiple classifications, the National Cancer Institute organized an international panel of experts to devise a classification for use in reporting studies. This is known as the 'Working Formulation' – although not universally used it provides the best compromise at present (Fig. 12.12).

Lymphomas are generally monoclonal tumours – all tumour cells being derived from a single clone. Because of this, immunological methods are useful in defining subtypes (Fig. 12.13).

AGE AND SEX RATIOS FOR NON-HODGKIN'S LYMPHOMA

Subtype	Median age (years)	Sex ratio (M:F)
Small lymphocytic	60.5	1.2:1
Follicular, small cleaved cell	54.3	1.3:1
Follicular, mixed	56.1	0.8:1
Follicular, large cell	55.4	1.8:1
Diffuse, small cleaved cell	57.9	2.0:1
Diffuse, mixed	58.0	1.1:1
Diffuse, large cell	56.8	1.0:1
Immunoblastic	51.3	1.5:1
Lymphoblastic	16.9	1.9:1
Diffuse, small non-cleaved	29.8	2.6:1

Fig. 12.14 Age and sex ratio of non-Hodgkin's lymphoma: Working formulation.

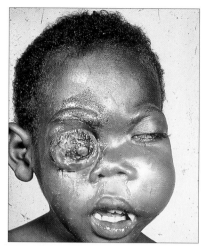

Fig. 12.15 African Burkitt's lymphoma affecting the maxilla. Courtesy of Prof D.H. Wright.

Fig. 12.16 Adenopathy in non-Hodgkin's lymphoma. Massive lymphadenopathy in the neck (a) and axillae (b) in two cases of high-grade lymphoma.

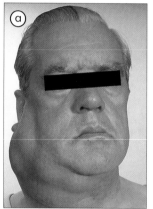

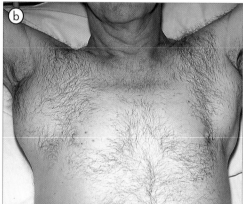

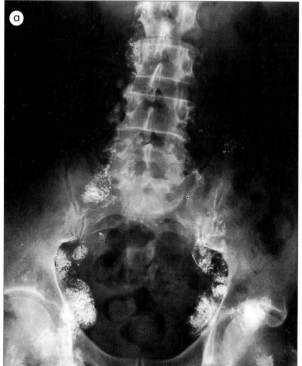

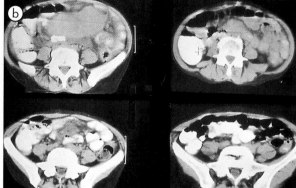

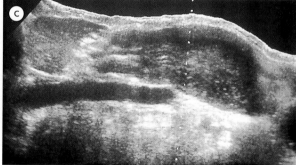

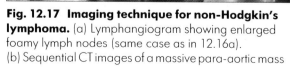

Fig. 12.17 Imaging technique for non-Hodgkin's lymphoma. (a) Lymphangiogram showing enlarged foamy lymph nodes (same case as in 12.16a).
(b) Sequential CT images of a massive para-aortic mass of lymph glands rapidly regressing with chemotherapy over 6 months. Courtesy of Dr R. Blaquire.
(c) Ultrasound image (sagittal) showing an enormous mass of para-aortic glands involved with lymphoma.

With so many subtypes, useful discussion of incidence, epidemiology and aetiology are difficult (Fig. 12.14 gives some simple data). Age of onset and sex ratios are very variable and some types of lymphoma have very particular characteristics. For instance, Burkitt's lymphoma (Fig. 12.15) is especially common in parts of Africa and New Guinea and is found only sporadically in other parts of the world. A specific high-grade lymphoma of the bowel (heavy chain disease) is also restricted geographically and is common in certain racial groups; similarly a type of T-cell lymphoma has been found in parts of Japan and the Caribbean. It is clear from these data that there are likely to be many different factors associated with the causes of lymphoma. Animal and *in vitro* models, however, suggest that there may be an association with viruses. Data suggests a link between HTLV-1 and Epstein–Barr virus and certain lymphomas. Acquired and congenital immunodeficiencies predispose to lymphoma and lymphoma is sometimes seen following treatment for Hodgkin's disease. Characteristic chromosomal abnormalities have been identified in some lymphomas but the relationship between the genetic abnormality and causation of the lymphoma remains speculative.

Initial Evaluation

Nodal disease in non-Hodgkin's lymphoma is often indistinguishable from Hodgkin's disease but occasionally may be very bulky, especially in high-grade lymphoma (Fig. 12.16). Evaluation is, in general, very similar to that used for Hodgkin's disease (Fig. 12.17) with the exceptions that extranodal disease is much more common and that staging laparotomy is not done. The sites of likely involvement vary according to the histological subtype of lymphoma. Extra nodal sites include:

- bone marrow (Fig. 12.18);
- gastrointestinal tract (Fig. 12.19);
- meninges;
- skin, with varying characteristics (Fig. 12.20);
- testes/ovaries;
- other unusual sites (see Figs 12.21 and 4.7).

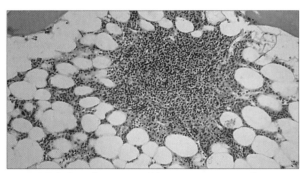

Fig. 12.18 Involvement of bone marrow with a nodule of low-grade lymphoma.

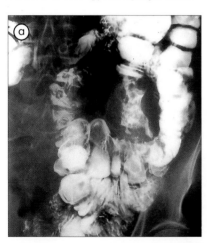
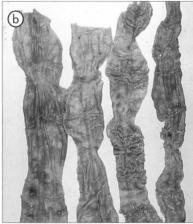

Fig. 12.19 Gastrointestinal tract involvement in non-Hodgkin's lymphoma. (a) Upper gastrointestinal tract contrast studies showing multiple filling defects in the small bowel. (b) Pathological specimen showing diffuse involvement of the small bowel with lymphoma. Courtesy of Prof J.M.A. Whitehouse.

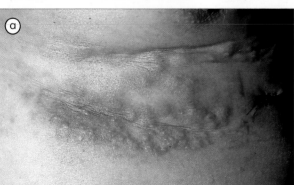
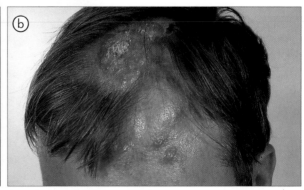

Fig. 12.20 Skin involvement in non-Hodgkin's lymphoma. (a) Nodular skin recurrence of high-grade lymphoma. (b) Gross exophytic recurrence of high-grade lymphoma on the scalp.

Staging

This also uses the Ann Arbor classification (see Fig. 12.9) developed for Hodgkin's disease. Because of the variation within lymphoma, and because the pattern of disease seen in non-Hodgkin's disease is different from Hodgkin's disease, the system is far from ideal and alternatives have been developed for some subtypes.

Treatment

Because of the diversity in natural history of the different subtypes of non-Hodgkin's lymphoma it is difficult to generalize about treatment. The situation is made all the more difficult as there are rapid developments in therapy for these diseases. Lymphomas are, in general, highly sensitive to radiotherapy and chemotherapy (Fig. 12.22). A good proportion can be cured and even when cure is not possible the great majority of patients benefit from treatment.

It is a conundrum that so called low-grade lymphomas are generally incurable whilst intermediate and high-grade lymphomas may be cured. Because of this, simple palliative therapy is usually indicated for low-grade lymphoma whilst intensive chemotherapy is appropriate for many patients with lymphoma of a higher grade.

Radiotherapy is less useful curatively in non-Hodgkin's lymphoma than in Hodgkin's disease. Some patients with localized low-grade lymphomas may be cured by local field irradiation. Similarly, occasional patients with high-grade stage I bone lymphoma can be cured with radiotherapy. Radiation may also be used as part of CNS prophylaxis in high-grade lymphoma and in combination with chemotherapy to treat bulky disease. It is also useful as palliation in selected patients with recurrent disease.

Chemotherapy is the most important modality in this disease. Most lymphomas are very responsive to a wide variety of cytotoxic drugs, regardless of their grade. Since low-grade lymphomas are not cured, simple oral alkylating agent therapy is often used for these patients. This may be delayed in some centres until the patient is symptomatic or demands therapy. Higher grade tumours are usually treated with combinations of drugs. The most commonly used regime of cyclophosphamide, doxorubicin, vincristine and prednisolone (CHOP) produces complete remissions in 60–80% of patients, these being durable in over half. Despite the development of more complex multidrug regimes there is no reliable data to show that these are significantly more likely to produce long-term survival than CHOP. The introduction of haemopoietic growth factors may allow the development of more dose-intensive schedules which could improve cure rates though this awaits testing in properly designed trials. Intrathecal chemotherapy is given as CNS prophylaxis in selected patients with high-grade lymphoma where the risk of meningeal lymphoma is high.

Overall, a reasonable proportion of patients with intermediate and high-grade lymphoma can be cured with intensive chemotherapy, the remainder being palliated. For low-grade lymphoma therapy is essentially palliative and simple treatment is used wherever possible.

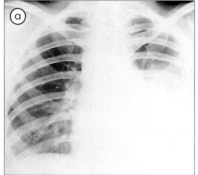
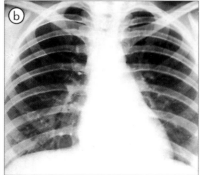

Fig. 12.21 Unusual sites of involvement in non-Hodgkin's lymphoma. (a) Gross bilateral breast infiltration with high-grade lymphoma. Courtesy of Dr J.W. Sweetenham. (b) Gross tonsillar involvement with an intermediate-grade lymphoma compromising the patient's airway.

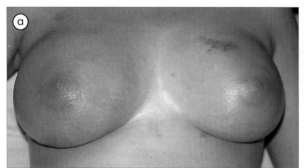
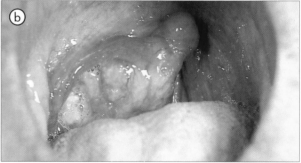

Fig. 12.22 Response to chemotherapy. Rapid and complete response of a high-grade lymphoma to single agent cyclophosphamide. Courtesy of Prof J.M.A. Whitehouse.

Leukaemia and Myeloma

13

Introduction

The incidence and frequency of the different types of leukaemias varies according to age, sex and race. Simplistically, acute lymphoblastic leukaemia (ALL) is a disease of childhood, acute myelogenous leukaemia (AML) is seen at all ages, chronic myelogenous leukaemia (CML) is generally a disease of the middle ages and chronic lymphocytic leukaemia (CLL) is a disease of old age. Myeloma is seen with increasing frequency in the years after age 40, the median age of onset being 65–70 years.

Aetiology of Leukaemia

Ionizing radiation has been shown to be an important environmental factor. Studies of persons exposed to irradiation after the atomic bombs in Hiroshima and Nagasaki give conclusive evidence of this – cases of leukaemia (usually AML) peaked 5–10 years after exposure. Studies of the incidence of cancer after irradiation for diagnostic purposes or for benign conditions have confirmed these data.

A number of industrial chemicals, such as benzene and arsenic, carry a risk of inducing leukaemia. Certain pharmaceutical drugs also apparently increase the risk, principally of AML, including alkylating cytotoxic drugs, chloramphenicol and phenylbutazone.

Genetic conditions resulting in an increased frequency of leukaemia include Down's syndrome, Bloom's syndrome, Fanconi's aplasia, Klinefelter's syndrome and congenital aneuploidy. The increased occurence of leukaemogenesis in these syndromes suggests a chromosomal mechanism for the causation of some or even all leukaemias.

There is firm evidence that RNA viruses are implicated in the causation of a variety of animal leukaemias. Current evidence suggests that retroviruses may play a role in human leukaemias as well, though conclusive data is still lacking.

The leukaemias are classified into a large number of subtypes according to their cytochemical and immunological characteristics, pattern of differentiation and natural history. This classification is summarized in Fig. 13.1

The diagnosis is established by morphological, histochemical and immunological studies of cytological preparations of cells from peripheral blood and bone marrow.

MORPHOLOGICAL CHARACTERISTICS OF ACUTE AND CHRONIC LEUKAEMIAS	
Acute (poorly differentiated) leukaemia – incompletely differentiated cells predominate	Chronic (well differentiated) leukaemia – cells similar to normal population
Myelogenous	Myelogenous
FAB classification M_1 Myeloblastic without maturation M_2 Myeloblastic with differentiation M_3 Promyelocytic M_4 Myelomonocytic M_5 Monocytic/poorly or well differentiated M_6 Erythroleukaemia	Chronic myelogenous leukaemia (CML) Philadelphia chromosome (Ph_1) positive Ph_1 negative Chronic myelomonocytic leukaemia Chronic monocytic leukaemia
Lymphoblastic	Lymphocytic
Common type (cALLa positive) Null cell T cell B cell	B cell chronic lymphocytic leukaemia (B-CLL) T-CLL Prolymphocytic leukaemia Hairy cell leukaemia

Fig. 13.1 The classification of leukaemia. cALLa, common acute lymphocytic leukaemia antigen.

Acute Lymphoblastic Leukaemia (ALL)

Leukaemia is the leading cause of death from malignant disease in children, and nearly all cases of leukaemia are of the acute lymphoblastic type; incidence peaks at 4 years after which it rapidly declines, so that after the age of 16 years it is an uncommon cancer. The symptoms of ALL, in common with other leukaemias, are due mainly to the reduction of normal haemopoietic cells.

Diagnosis

Symptoms of ALL include malaise and tiredness which are very common and may have been present for some weeks or a little longer. Loss of appetite and weight, abdominal pain and headache are also relatively common. Fever and bleeding from gums and nose occur in up to one-half of patients. Bone pain may be severe in a few patients.

Signs include pallor, purpura, enlargement of the liver or spleen, or testicular swelling (Fig. 13.2). Lymphadenopathy is also fairly common.

The diagnosis is made by examining blood and bone marrow. Features include:

- anaemia;
- thrombocytopenia;
- abnormal white cell count (high or low) with peripheral blast cells;
- marrow replacement by lymphoblasts;
- marked decrease in erythroid, granulocytic and megakaryocyte cells;
- presence of periodic acid Schiff (PAS) material in the cells (stains glycogen);
- metabolic abnormalities, including hyperuricaemia.

Prognostic Factors

ALL has been divided morphologically into three types (FAB classification; see Fig. 13.3). L$_1$ (85% of cases) has small cells with little cytoplasm and indistinct nucleoli. L$_2$ (15%) has large cells with more cytoplasm and prominent nucleoli. L$_3$ is very uncommon, the cells are large with deep blue cytoplasm

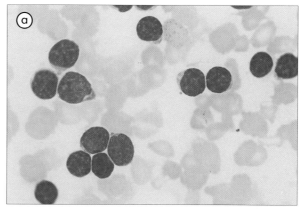

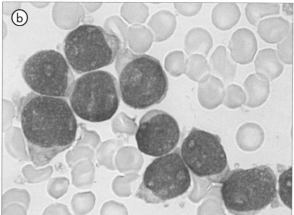

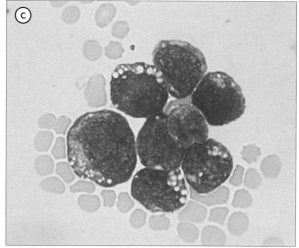

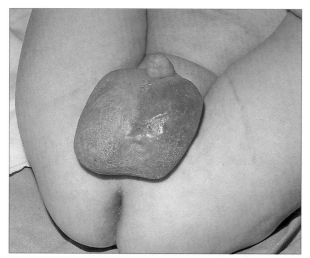

Fig. 13.2 Testicular involvement in a child with acute lymphoblastic leukaemia. Courtesy of Dr J. Kohler.

Fig. 13.3 Classification of acute lymphoblastic leukaemia. (a) L$_1$ subtype. Predominantly small cells with high nucleo-cytoplasmic ratio and few nuclei and sometimes azurophilic granules. Courtesy of Dr B.J. Bain. (b) L$_2$ subtype. Blast cells vary greatly in size and in the amount of cytoplasm. There are often numerous nucleoli. (c) L$_3$ subtype. Blast cells have a deeply staining blue cytoplasm with many small perinuclear vacuoles. Courtesy of Prof A.V. Hoffbrand.

IMMUNOLOGICAL MARKERS AND GENE REARRANGEMENTS IN ACUTE LEUKAEMIA

	c-ALL	T-ALL	AML
'stem cell'			
terminal deoxynucleotidyl transferase (TdT)	+	+	−
HLA–DR	+	−	±
CD34 (e.g. My10, 3C5)	±	−	+
B cell-associated:			
CD10 (e.g. J5)	+	−	−
CD19 (e.g. B4)	+	−	−
CD20 (e.g. B1)	+	−	−
CD22 (e.g. RFB4)	+	−	−
T cell-associated:			
CD2 (e.g. T11)	−	+	−
CD3 (e.g. T3)	−	+	−
CD5 (e.g. T1)	−	+	+
CD7 (e.g. 3A1)	−	+	−
myeloid/monocytic-associated:			
CD11 (e.g. Mo1)	−	−	+
CD13 (e.g. My7, MCS2)	−	−	+
CD14 (e.g. FMC17, UCHM1)	−	−	+ (especially M_4, M_5)
CD33 (e.g. My9)	−	−	+
megakaryoblastic (platelet gpIIb/IIIa)			
CDW41 (e.g. J15)	−	−	+ (M_7)
glycophorin	−	−	+ (M_6)
immunoglobulin genes	rearranged	germline	germline
T cell receptor genes	germline	rearranged	germline

Fig. 13.4 Immunological markers and gene rearrangements in acute leukaemia. [Modified from Hoffbrand and Pettit, *Sandoz Atlas of Clinical Haematology*, Gower Medical Publishing, London.]

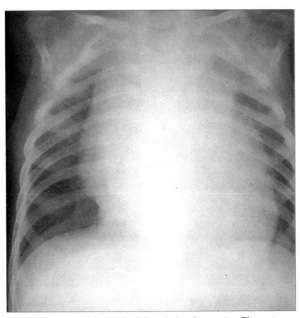

Fig. 13.5 T-cell lymphoblastic leukaemia. There is a typical large mediastinal mass in this one-year-old child with lymphoblastic leukaemia. Courtesy of Dr A. Smith.

and vacuoles (Burkitt like). Patients with L_1 disease have a better outlook than L_2 patients. Alternatively, patients may be classified immunologically (Fig. 13.4). A quarter of cases of ALL have T cell markers (T-ALL), 5% are B or pre-B cell (B-ALL) and the remainder have neither B or T markers (null cell). Three-quarters of null cell patients have leukaemic cells which react to an antibody from a panel of patients with null cell ALL. These cases are called 'common ALL antigen (cALLa) positive' (c-ALL).

The group with the most favourable outlook is those patients between the ages of 4–7 years with common type ALL, with a white cell count of less than 10000×10^9/l. Patients with T cell ALL (often with a high white blood cell count and mediastinal mass; Fig. 13.5) have a poor outlook. In general males have a worse prognosis than females. The rare B cell ALLs also have a poor outlook.

Treatment

The aim of therapy is the eradication of all leukaemic lymphoblasts, with regeneration of normal marrow

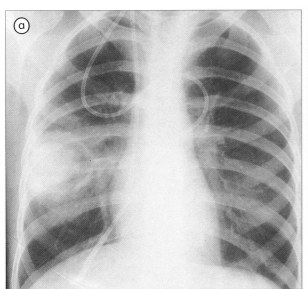

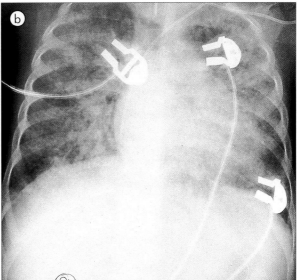

Fig. 13.6 Infection in childhood acute lymphoblastic leukaemia. (a) Aspergillosis in a child undergoing intensification therapy for ALL. (b) Measles pneumonia in an infant undergoing maintenance therapy. Courtesy of Dr J. Kohler.

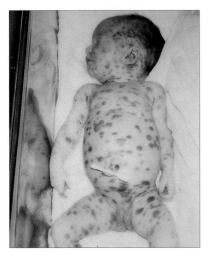

Fig. 13.7 Acute myelogenous leukaemia in a newborn infant. Courtesy of Dr A. Smith.

elements to repopulate the peripheral blood. The principles of treatment are similar to AML (see below), though less intensive therapy is generally given since ALL cells are more sensitive than AML cells to cytotoxic therapy.

Chemotherapy is used in three distinct phases:
- induction therapy – the principal drugs (vincristine, prednisone, doxorubicin or L-asparaginase) result in a complete remission rate of over 90%;
- intensification – although induction produces apparent complete remission it is assumed that up to 10^9 blast cells remain. Further chemotherapy (including cytosine arabinoside) is given;
- maintenance therapy – methotrexate and mercaptopurine are usually given in chronic low dose to maintain remission and to rid the patient of a low burden of persisting disease.

Use of such a therapeutic regime 20 years ago led to much improved results but it soon became evident that many patients were relapsing with central nervous system disease. Because of this, CNS prophylaxis is given – radiation to the brain combined with intrathecal methotrexate. The gonads are another sanctuary site, but prophylactic therapy does not seem to be helpful.

Supportive Therapy

As with all leukaemias an essential element of therapy is support of the patient. Since therapy is less intensive than that for AML, fewer problems are encountered during induction. However, red cell and platelet transfusions may be required along with appropriate antibiotics. Care must also be taken with patients receiving intensification and maintenance therapy since common bacterial, fungal and viral infections, such as chicken pox and measles, may be lethal (Fig. 13.6).

Outcome

Prognosis is radically different for children than for adults, with up to one-half of all children with ALL surviving without relapse for 3 years. If maintenance therapy is stopped in those in continued remission, about 75% remain disease free. Patients relapsing after an initial remission are generally very responsive to further chemotherapy though remission duration is shorter with each subsequent treatment. Bone marrow transplantation after high-dose therapy may be curative in up to one-third of patients if undertaken following remission reinduction. Testicular relapse is a particular problem and some groups use testicular biopsy to monitor disease status and others use prophylactic radiation.

Patients over 15 years of age fare much worse, with few, if any, patients surviving disease-free for prolonged periods. Remission rates are lower and complete remissions only last on average for about 18 months. Mean overall survival is less than two years, despite aggressive induction therapy, CNS prophylaxis and maintenance therapy.

Acute Myelogenous Leukaemia (AML)

Although most common in middle and late life, AML is seen at all ages (see Fig. 13.7), though in children it is proportionately less important than ALL.

Diagnosis
The symptoms of AML are due to a lack of normal elements in the blood and extension of haemopoiesis to abnormal sites (Fig. 13.8). They include: anaemia – tiredness, dyspnoea, pallor and palpitations; neutropenia – local or systemic infection (Fig. 13.9);

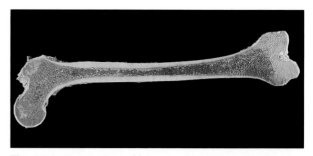

Fig. 13.8 Extension of haemopoiesis to abnormal sites. In this case, marrow in the whole length of the femur is packed with AML cells. Courtesy of Dr A. Smith.

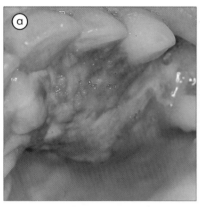
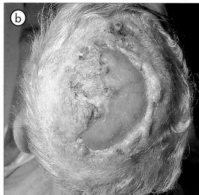
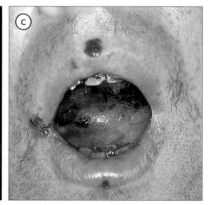

Fig. 13.9 Infection in acute myelogenous leukaemia induction. In addition to bacterial infections, fungal, viral and opportunistic infections are common. (a) Severe oral candidiasis in AML. Courtesy of Dr A. Smith. (b) Pyoderma gangrenosum. Bacterial infections may be severe and unusual in their behaviour. (c) Severe oral mucositis due to neutropenia. Such mucosal damage provides an easy portal of entry for pathogenic organisms. Courtesy of Prof J. Whitehouse.

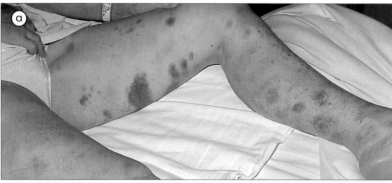

Fig. 13.10 Consequences of thrombocytopenia. (a) Multiple bruises on the legs of a patient with AML. (b) Intramuscular injection should always be avoided in the presence of thrombocytopenia. This slide illustrates the consequences of a single 1ml injection. (c) Antibiotic rash with purpura in a patient with AML.

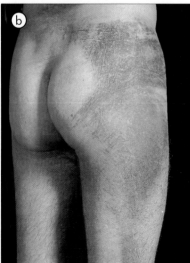
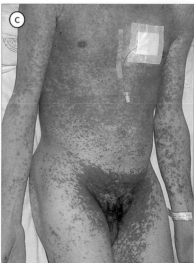

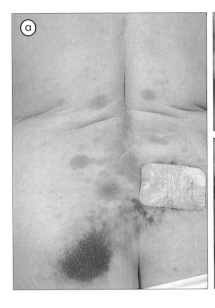

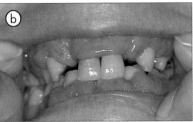

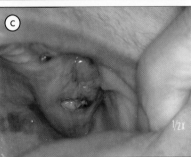

Fig. 13.11 Sites of presentation in acute myelogenous leukaemia. (a) AML presenting as subcutaneous masses. Bruising is from the biopsy site under the plaster. (b) Gum involvement is common in myelomonocytic leukaemia (M_4), with resulting hypertrophy. (c) Similar gum hypertrophy is occasionally seen in other subtypes (in this case M_2 disease). Courtesy of Dr A. Smith.

and thrombocytopenia – petechiae, purpura, bleeding from the nose, and gums and gastrointestinal or genitourinary tract (Fig. 13.10). Splenomegaly is seen in 30–40% of patients but lymphadenopathy and/or hepatomegaly is uncommon. Occasionally leukaemic masses (chloromas) present at a wide variety of sites (Fig. 13.11). CNS involvement is rare.

Prognostic Factors

Various studies have examined the prognostic significance of a number of factors. Survival is related to:
- attaining a complete remission with induction chemotherapy;
- age – prognosis worsens with increasing age;
- preceding myelodysplasia, indicating a poor outlook. Similarly patients with AML secondary to prior cytotoxic therapy do poorly;
- prolonged preceding symptoms or pancytopenia. These are adverse features;
- documented pretreatment fever or hepatosplenomegaly. These correlate with poor response to therapy.

The relationship between the FAB classification (see Figs 13.1 and 13.12) and prognosis is not clear cut, partly due to improvements in induction therapy and support. For instance, M_3 (promyelocytic leukaemia) carried a grave prognosis in the past because of the severe bleeding associated with this variety of AML. However, improved supportive care and management of the associated clotting disorders have led to this subtype having among the most favourable outlooks of the various subtypes of AML. In general M_5 and M_6 leukaemia have, at present, the poorest prognosis.

As well as the morphological characteristics used in the FAB classification, biological markers are useful prognostically. These include:
- chromosomal abnormalities – ploidy and specific chromosomal defects (see Fig. 13.13);
- labelling index/DNA histogram, though correlation is inconsistent;
- rapidity with which peripheral blasts are cleared from the blood after induction therapy;
- use of monoclonal antibodies to identify cells possessing specific epitopes (Fig. 13.14).

Treatment

The initial decision in AML is whether active therapy is indicated. Evidence suggests that if cytotoxic therapy is used it should be used intensively. Lesser therapy induces marked myelosuppression which may be longer lasting than that induced by a short course of intensive therapy. Since the elderly have a worse outlook, aged and feeble patients are probably best served by supportive therapy alone. For the majority of patients who are deemed suitable for chemotherapy the initial aim is the induction of marrow aplasia and eradication of the clone of leukaemic cells. This initial treatment is thus known as 'induction therapy'.

Induction therapy

There are two principles behind induction therapy. First, there are two clones of haemopoietic cells – normal and leukaemic cells. This is supported by chromosomal studies. Second, eradication of the leukaemic clone can only be achieved with intensive cytotoxic therapy which severely affects the normal haemopoietic cells. This results in a period of profound neutropenia and thrombocytopenia.

A variety of regimes are available but the most commonly used drugs are daunorubicin, cytosine arabinoside and thioguanine. These, and/or other drugs, are used intensively over about seven days and then therapy is stopped and the patient's general condition supported. Response to therapy is judged by findings in the peripheral blood and bone marrow. Between 60 and 80% of patients will achieve an apparently normal bone marrow within 1–3 cycles

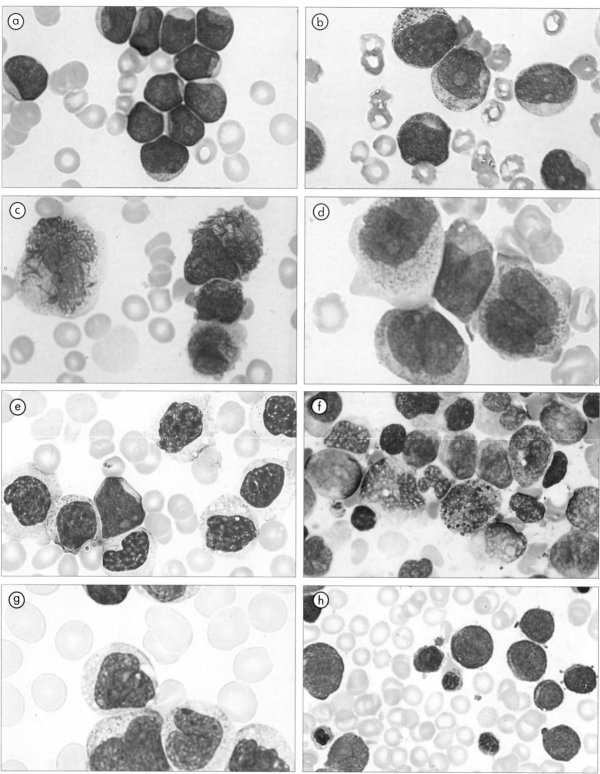

Fig. 13.12 Classification of acute myelogenous leukaemia. (a) M$_1$ subtype. Blast cells have large irregular nuclei with one or more nucleoli. The cytoplasm is often placed eccentrically. Auer rods are uncommon. (b) M$_2$ subtype. Blast cells are often folded with several nucleoli and azurophilic granules and occasional Auer rods. (c) M$_3$ subtype. Promyelocytes contain coarse azurophilic granules and so called 'faggots' or Sultan bodies made up of aggregates of granules. (d) M$_3$ subtype (microgranular type). These promyelocytes contain many small azurophilic granules. (e) M$_4$ subtype (myelomonocytic leukaemia) showing blasts with cytoplasmic granules (myelo- and promyeloblasts) together with blasts with cytoplasmic vacuoles and folded nuclei (microblasts). (f) M$_4$ subtype (myeloblastic leukaemia). Blast cells are myelomonocytic. There is one eosinophil with basophilic granules. (g) M$_5$ subtype (monoblastic leukaemia). Blast cells have pale cytoplasm and cytoplasmic vacuoles. Central nuclei may be folded or kidney shaped. (h) M$_6$ subtype (erythroleukaemia). The predominant cells are erythroid and are at all stages of development. Courtesy of Prof A.V. Hoffbrand.

CYTOGENETIC ABNORMALITIES IN ACUTE LEUKAEMIAS

Acute Lymphoblastic Leukaemia	Acute Myelogenous Leukaemia
L_1 and/or L_2 (c-ALL or null-ALL) t(9;22)(q34;q11) t(4;11)(q21;q23) t(1;19)(q22;p13) del(6)(9) t(11;14)(q13;q32) t or del(12)(p12) 9p− +21 B-ALL t(8;14)(q24;q32) t(8;22)(q24;q11) t(2;8)(p11−13;q24) T-ALL 14q+(q32) or 14q−(q11) t(11;14)(p13;q11) 9p−	Relatively specific M_2t(8;21)(q22;q22) M_3t(15;17)(q22;q11) M_4inv(16)(p13;q22) or del(16)(q22)* M_5t(9;11)(p21;q23) Others t(9;22)(p22;q11) t(6;9)(p22;q34) t(3;3)(q21;q29) inv(3)(q21;q26)** +8 +21 5q−/−5 7q−/−7 12p11 −p13(del or t)***

```
  *  associated with abnormal eosinophils
 **  associated with thrombocytosis
***  associated with increased basophils
```

Fig. 13.13 Cytogenetic abnormalities in acute leukaemias. [Modified from Hoffbrand and Pettit, *Sandoz Atlas of Clinical Haematology*, Gower Medical Publishing, London.]

CYTOCHEMISTRY IN ACUTE LEUKAEMIA

	c-ALL	T-ALL	AML
myeloperoxidase	−	−	+
Sudan black	−	−	+
non-specific esterase	−	−	+ (M_4, M_5)
periodic acid-Schiff	+ (coarse)	−	−
acid phosphatase	−	+	+ (fine except in M_6)

Fig. 13.14 Cytochemistry in acute leukaemia.

of such induction chemotherapy. Supportive care is essential and is one of the major reasons for improved results in the past two decades. Areas requiring attention include treatment of infections and bleeding as well as management of a variety of metabolic complications including hyperuricaemia.

Consolidation therapy

Most patients achieving an apparently normal bone marrow (a complete remission) will be treated with additional courses of chemotherapy similar to their induction schedule. Such treatment appears to increase the chances of long-term disease control or at least to delay recurrence. Since the patient has relatively normal haematological parameters when they receive such treatment, the period and depth of

pancytopenia is usually less severe so that this phase of treatment is better tolerated.

Maintenance therapy (see ALL) is little used in this type of leukaemia.

Bone marrow transplantation

High-dose chemotherapy and/or whole body irradiation with allogeneic bone marrow transplantation (or, in the rare instance of an identical twin, syngeneic) may be used in selected younger patients. Such an approach is complicated and there is a relatively high early mortality rate. Failure may be due to: graft versus host (GVH) disease (the engrafted cells attack host cells immunologically), uncontrolled infection or recurrent leukaemia. Early deaths are usually due to infection and GVH disease. Patients

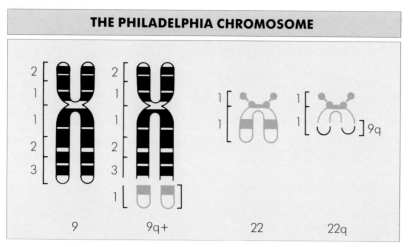

THE PHILADELPHIA CHROMOSOME

9   9q+   22   22q

Fig. 13.15 The Philadelphia chromosome in chronic myelogenous leukaemia.

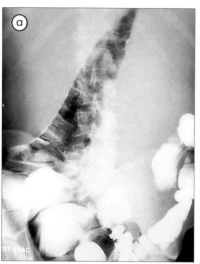
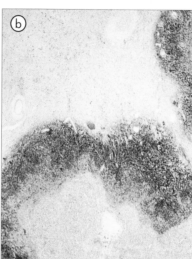

Fig. 13.16 Clinical features in chronic myelogenous leukaemia. (a) Massive hepatosplenomegaly shown during a barium enema. (b) Histological appearance of splenic infarct, showing necrosis (top), iron deposition (Perl's stain) and splenic tissue infiltrated by CML (bottom). Courtesy of Dr A. Smith.

surviving the first year have a lower rate of leukaemic relapse than patients simply completing induction and consolidation therapy. Patients having a syngeneic transplantation have a higher leukaemic relapse rate than those receiving allogeneic marrow, suggesting that a degree of GVH disease may aid the eradication of persistent leukaemic cells.

Bone marrow transplantation is most successful in first remission but may be useful in patients responding to re-induction therapy (see below).

Recently autologous bone marrow transplantation has been tried, using marrow taken from the patient during complete remission. Clearly marrow obtained in this way may contain leukaemic cells. However, even such marrow may buy time, and manipulation in the laboratory (with or without purging) may damage the cells. This relatively new technique is still at the stage of assessment and remains, ideally, experimental.

Re-induction therapy
Patients relapsing after a prolonged remission stand a good chance of a further remission if similar chemotherapy to the original induction therapy is used. Second remissions, however, are generally of shorter duration. For patients relapsing soon after induction chemotherapy or those failing to achieve an initial complete remission, second-line therapy generally produces poor results. In such patients the potential benefits of therapy must be carefully weighed against the prolonged hospitalization and toxicity of further induction treatment.

Therapeutic results
Untreated, the median survival of AML is only two months. In trials of cytotoxic therapy this is increased to 14 to 24 months, depending on the selection criteria used. A proportion of patients (up to 10%) survive several years without relapse. Use of high-dose chemotherapy and/or whole body irradiation with bone marrow transplantation produces prolonged survival in about half of those patients suitable for such an approach.

Chronic Myelogenous Leukaemia (CML)

This disease is uncommon before 10 years of age, but gradually increases in frequency after this time. The condition is due to a disorder in haemopoietic stem cells which causes a marked increase in proliferation of granulocytic cells and megakaryocytes.

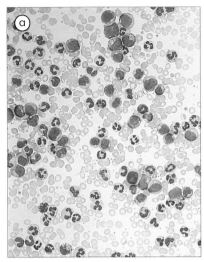
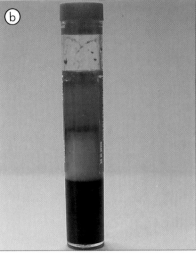
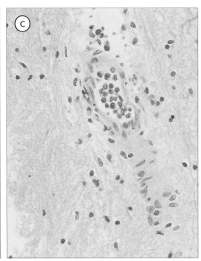

Fig. 13.17 Blood changes in chronic myelogenous leukaemia. (a) Peripheral blood film in CML, showing cells at all stages of granulopoiesis. Courtesy of Prof A.V. Hoffbrand. (b) Blood sample from a patient with CML. On standing, the red and white cells have separated from the plasma, revealing the gross excess of white cells. (c) Leucostasis in the brain of a patient with CML. 'Sludging' of CML cells in a blood vessel can be seen. Courtesy of Dr S. Roath.

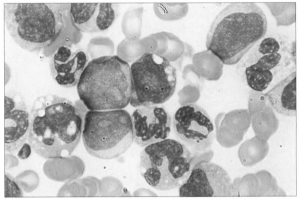

Fig. 13.18 Juvenile chronic myelogenous leukaemia. Peripheral blood film showing occasional blasts, myelomonocytic cells, atypical agranular band and segmented neutrophils. Courtesy of Prof A.V. Hoffbrand.

Maturation of cells is not as severely disordered as in AML and erythropoiesis is less impaired. Since maturation continues, cells in the peripheral blood mainly consist of segmented neutrophils or myelocytes. Neutrophils and platelets may be functionally impaired but this is usually not severe enough to lead to infection or bleeding.

The Philadelphia chromosome (Ph_1), a translocation of the long arms of chromosome 22 to another chromosome (most often number 9), is usually found in the marrow (Fig. 13.15). Studies of identical twins have shown that the Ph_1 chromosome is an acquired defect. It is present in over 90% of patients with typical CML. Since it is also present in other haemopoietic cells this has been taken as evidence that the defect in CML lies in a common stem cell.

Diagnosis

Non-specific initial symptoms mean that CML initially has an insidious course, indeed some cases are only discovered on routine medical examination or investigations. The common symptoms and signs include fatigue and malaise, abdominal discomfort, easy bruising, sweating, enlarged spleen (in more than 90% of cases; Fig. 13.16), purpura or bleeding from gums and lymphadenopathy and hepatomegaly, though they are uncommon.

Diagnosis rests on examination of the peripheral blood and bone marrow and demonstration of the Ph_1 chromosome.

The peripheral blood generally shows a mild to moderate anaemia with leucocytosis, which may reach markedly elevated levels (more than $500 \times 10^9/l$) causing viscosity changes and leucostasis (Fig. 13.17). In most cases the white cell count exceeds $50 \times 10^9/l$. Myeloblasts, promyelocytes and nucleated red cells are present, though segmented neutrophils and myelocytes predominate. Increased basophils and eosinophils are a regular feature. Platelets are usually normal or at elevated levels at presentation.

The marrow shows granulocytic and megakaryocytic hyperplasia; maturation generally appears fairly normal, but there may be some increase in reticulin fibres in the marrow. Ph_1 chromosome is present in virtually all of the metaphase cells in the marrow.

Such cases of typical CML need to be distinguished from other variations of CML as well as from other similar conditions.

Such conditions include CML in which eosinophils or basophils predominate (absence of Ph_1 distinguishes this condition from eosinophilic leukaemia); CML in very young and elderly patients which may be clinically atypical and occasionally lacks Ph_1 (Fig. 13.18); and myelomonocytic leukaemia, which generally has a higher proportion of blast cells and also lacks Ph_1. Additionally, the borders between

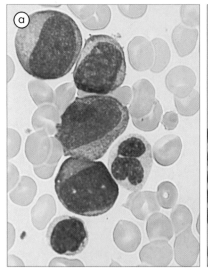
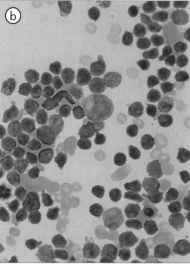

Fig. 13.19 Accelerated phase chronic myelogenous leukaemia. (a) Myeloid blast cell transformation. Courtesy of Prof A.V. Hoffbrand. (b) Lymphoid blast cell transformation (Ph₁ positive).

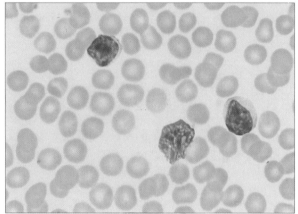

Fig. 13.20 Chronic lymphocytic leukaemia. PB film showing two mature lymphocytes and a single smear cell. Nuclear chromatin is condensed and nucleoli are barely detectable.

CML and polycythemia rubra vera, haemorrhagic thrombocythemia and myelofibrosis are often blurred. Ph₁ is absent.

Although CML starts as a chronic leukaemia, progression to an acute illness is inevitable. This 'accelerated phase' of CML is the result of a Ph₁-bearing clone evolving into a more malignant phenotype. At this stage the CML dyshaemopoietic changes worsen with increasing anaemia and thrombocytopenia. Immature cells become more frequent and the spleen enlarges further. Fever and bone pain increase and the condition rapidly transforms into an acute leukaemic-like phase. Alternatively, blast crisis may occur. This is a very rapid evolution to an acute leukaemia of AML type. However, in 15% of cases immunological studies show lymphoblasts, usually of T cell type (Fig. 13.19). Progressive fibrosis of the bone marrow may also occur, with resultant pancytopenia.

Treatment

Therapy is designed to reduce the rate of excessive haemopoiesis in the bone marrow and spleen. The aim is to keep the blood count relatively near normal and to shrink the spleen. This improves the patient's well being and reduces symptoms. There is no attempt to eradicate the abnormal clone.

Chemotherapy with drugs such as busulfan or hydroxyurea given by mouth produce good control in most patients. Intensive therapy should be avoided as it may be hazardous. When using busulfan or hydroxyurea care should be taken not to reduce the blood count unduly. Patients may be maintained on low doses of chemotherapy though some clinicians prefer to stop treatment and only to re-treat when the patient's condition warrants it.

In recent years syngeneic and allogeneic bone marrow transplantation have been used successfully, after intensive chemotherapy and radiotherapy. Eradication of the Ph₁ clone can sometimes be achieved by this means. Such treatment is, however, best reserved for selected patients with chronic phase disease since results in accelerated phase disease have been very poor.

When the accelerated phase disease does develop, results of any treatment are generally very poor. Regimes similar to those used to treat AML are rarely helpful, though for patients with blast crisis of lymphatic type, remission of short duration is possible.

Outlook

The median survival of CML is 3.5 years; chemotherapy has made little difference but is very helpful in reducing morbidity. Once patients develop accelerated phase disease survival is extremely poor – median survival is only 3 months. The introduction of high-dose therapy with bone marrow support in selected patients is the first therapy to have a significant effect on outcome.

Chronic Lymphocytic Leukaemia (CLL)

This form of leukaemia is rare below the age of 30 years and increases in frequency in subsequent decades. The cause is unknown. Genetic factors

IMMUNOLOGICAL MARKERS OF CLL		
	B-CLL	T-CLL
Surface Ig	± (IgM ± IgD)	−
M–RBC rosettes	+ +	−
S–RBC rosettes (CD2)	−	+
Surface Antigens		
HLA–DR	+	
CD19 (B4)	+	−
CD20 (B1)	+	−
CD5 (T1)	+	−
CD3 (T3)	−	+
CD25	−	−
FMC7	−	−
Gene Rearrangement		
IgH	+	−
TCR$_\beta$	−	+

IgH, immunoglobulin heavy chain; TCR, T-cell receptor; M, mouse RBC; S, sheep RBC; CD25, IL-2 receptor

Fig. 13.21 Immunological markers for chronic lymphocytic leukaemia.

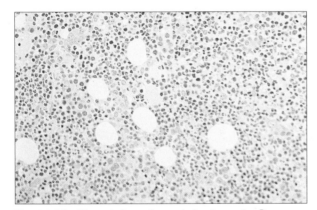

Fig. 13.22 Chronic lymphocytic leukaemia. Bone marrow trephine showing an increase in lymphocytes, diffusely infiltrating the marrow.

have been identified and familial cases (some with consistent chromosomal abnormalities) have been described. CLL is a disorder in which there is a progressive accumulation of immunologically defective lymphocytes. It is usually a B cell clonal disorder though T cell CLL also occurs in about 5% of patients. There is a male preponderance (ratio 25:1), the median age of onset being 65 years.

Clonality is established by showing that the abnormal lymphocytes all carry one light chain (kappa or lambda). Glucose-6-phosphate dehydrogenase studies also support the monoclonal nature of the condition. Acquired abnormalities of T cell function occur later in the course of the disease and exaggerated delayed hypersensitivity reactions and production of autoantibodies to red cells or platelets are a common feature.

Diagnosis

Many patients are asymptomatic at the time of diagnosis, the condition being revealed by a routine full blood count or on medical examination. Symptoms and signs of active CLL include malaise and fatigue, weight loss, fevers and sweats, abdominal pain, pathological enlargement of lymph nodes, splenomegaly/hepatomegaly, cutaneous infiltration and, in the case of very advanced disease, infection and bleeding.

Diagnosis is based on cytological (and histological) examination of peripheral blood, bone marrow or lymph nodes. Mild anaemia with or without thrombocytopenia is not uncommon. Severe anaemia and thrombocytopenia on diagnosis is a very poor prognostic variable. There is always an absolute lymphocytosis. The involved lymphocytes are small with scant cytoplasm (Fig. 13.20) and are difficult to distinguish from normal lymphocytes. In 95% of cases the cells express monoclonal surface immunoglobulin (mainly IgM or IgD) as well as other B cell markers (Fig. 13.21). The bone marrow shows diffuse infiltration with small, differentiated lymphocytes. The diagnosis, however, can usually be made on the peripheral blood appearance together with immunocytochemistry (Fig. 13.22). Red cell autoantibodies (positive Coombs' test) and haemolytic anaemia may occur, but immune thrombocytopenia is rare. As the disease progresses, immunoglobulin levels fall progressively to very low levels.

Staging

CLL can be subclassified according to its phenotype, T cell CLL having a much worse prognosis than B cell CLL. Extent of disease is based on the blood count and sites of disease at presentation (Fig. 13.23). Prolymphocytic leukaemia, sometimes grouped with CLL, has a poor prognosis (Fig. 13.24) while hairy cell leukaemia, another indolent lymphoma, responds to interferon and/or splenectomy (Fig. 13.25). In some patients with CLL, extensive lymph node or soft tissue involvement is seen (Fig. 13.26).

REVISED INTERNATIONAL CLASSIFICATION OF CLL	
Group A (good prognosis)	haemoglobin >10g/dl; platelets >100 × 10⁹/l; <3 sites of palpable organ enlargement
Group B (intermediate prognosis)	haemoglobin >10g/dl; platelets >100 × 10⁹/l; ≥3 sites of palpable organ enlargement
Group C (bad prognosis)	haemoglobin <10g/dl; platelets <100 × 10⁹/l

Fig. 13.23 Stage grouping in chronic lymphocytic leukaemia. One site = spleen or liver, or lymph nodes in the neck, axillae or groin.

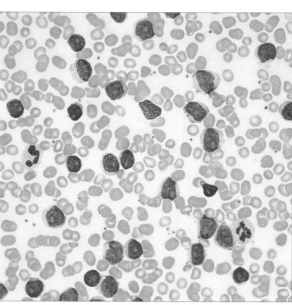

Fig. 13.24 Prolymphocytic leukaemia. Blood film showing prolymphocytes with prominent pale, central nucleoli and abundant pale cytoplasm. Courtesy of Dr A. Smith.

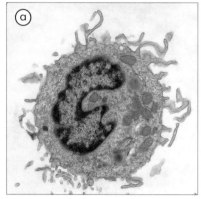 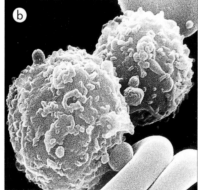

Fig. 13.25 Hairy cell leukaemia. (a) Low-power electron micrograph showing red cells and cells of hairy cell leukaemia. There is abundant cytoplasm and numerous villi giving the cell its characteristic hairy appearance. (b) Scanning electron microscopy of hairy cell leukaemia showing typical ruffles. Courtesy of Dr S. Roath.

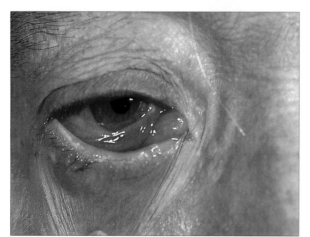

Fig. 13.26 Scleral involvement in B cell chronic lymphocytic leukaemia. Courtesy of Dr A. Smith.

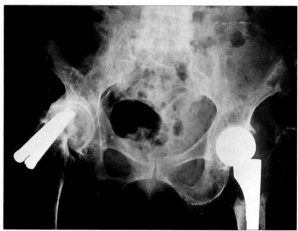

Fig. 13.27 Pathological fracture in multiple myeloma. This patient with gross bony destruction has had surgery for bilateral fractures of the neck of the femur. Courtesy of Prof J. Whitehouse.

Treatment

None of the available treatments is curative so that the first decision is 'at what point chemotherapy or other treatment is justified'. Many patients with minimal symptoms and signs of disease may live a normal life for years. Such patients probably do not benefit from treatment during this phase of their disease. In patients with anaemia, thrombocytopenia, gross lymphadenopathy or splenomegaly an attempt to reduce disease bulk and activity is justified.

Alkylating agent chemotherapy with or without steroids has been the mainstay of treatment. Combinations including other drugs have not been shown to produce superior results and current approaches favour simple treatment with minimal side effects used palliatively to reduce symptoms for as long as possible. Steroids are useful in the treatment of immune haemolytic anaemia or thrombocytopenia.

Whole body irradiation can also be useful, though complete responses are not seen. Splenectomy may help when there is an autoimmune anaemia or thrombocytopenia.

Outlook

Most patients die of their condition, usually from the effects of immunosuppression with recurrent infections. There may be an excess of other types of cancer. Occasionally the disease appears to change in character resulting in an accelerated phase similar to that seen in CML. Such blast crisis, with poorly differentiated blast cells in the peripheral blood and marrow, is known as 'Richter's syndrome'.

Multiple Myeloma

This is a malignant proliferation of plasma cells, characterized by elevation of serum and/or monoclonal immunoglobulins, lytic bone lesions and anaemia. Incidence is roughly equal among the sexes, with an increasing rate after the age of 40 years.

The aetiology of this disease is unknown, but the monoclonality of the abnormal immunoglobulin suggests a clonal origin.

Diagnosis

The commonest symptom is bone pain, usually in the back. This may be due to uncomplicated lytic lesions or to pathological fracture (Fig. 13.27). Normochromic, normocytic anaemia with tiredness may be the presenting feature. Repeated infections often occur because of poor antibody production. Renal failure may develop due to a variety of factors, including hypercalcaemia, infection and amyloid deposits associated with Bence Jones proteinuria (free light chains).

Diagnosis is based on finding two or three of the following features:
- lytic bone disease (Fig. 13.28);
- marrow infiltration with plasma cells (involving more than 10% of marrow cells; Fig. 13.29);
- monoclonal increase in serum immunoglobulin (raised IgG in 54% of patients, IgA in 22% of patients;
- Bence Jones proteinuria (45% of cases).

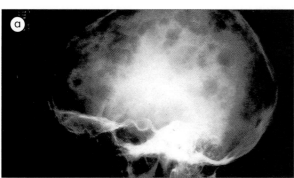

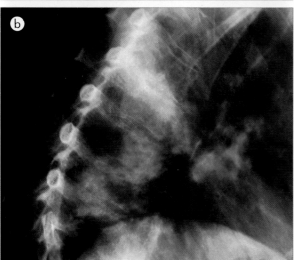

Fig. 13.28 Lytic bone metastasis in multiple myeloma. (a) Radiograph of multiple lytic lesions of the skull. (b) Radiograph of the spine showing typical severe demineralization with vertebral collapse.

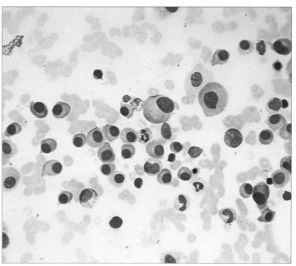

Fig. 13.29 Infiltration of bone marrow with plasma cells.

Other features include amyloid deposition (Fig. 13.30) and hyperviscosity due to very high immunoglobulin levels (Fig. 13.31).

Treatment

Progressive symptomatic myeloma is treated with chemotherapy. Melphalan and prednisone have been the mainstay of treatment for some 30 years. Treatment is given until the abnormal immunoglobulins fall to a stable level (plateau phase) and is then stopped until the disease later becomes active once again. More recently combinations made up of 3 or 4 of the following drugs – an alkylating agent, vincristine, cyclophosphamide, dexamethasone/prednisone, doxorubicin and a nitrosurea – have been reported to be more active than melphalan/prednisone. Further studies are ongoing, but such an approach seems warranted in selected younger fitter patients.

Radiotherapy is extremely useful as palliative therapy for localized bone pain. When there is diffuse painful lytic disease, uncontrolled by chemotherapy, hemibody irradiation may be useful. Radiotherapy is also used for isolated plasmacytomas.

Care must be taken to treat hypercalcaemia adequately. Infection may be a problem requiring, where appropriate, vigorous antibiotic therapy. Atypical infections, including fungal and viral infections, are relatively common.

Outcome

Despite an objective response to chemotherapy in two-thirds of patients the disease always becomes active again and median survival is about 3 years.

Summary

The haematological malignancies are a disparate collection of neoplasms with widely varying biological behaviour. Most are very sensitive to cytotoxic agents though cure is only likely in childhood acute lymphatic leukaemia. In the other haematological cancers the disease may be controlled and lifespan increased by treatment. Use of high-dose therapy in AML results in some patients surviving long term and very intensive therapy with bone marrow support may improve on this.

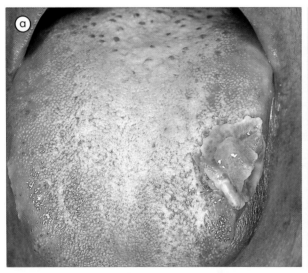
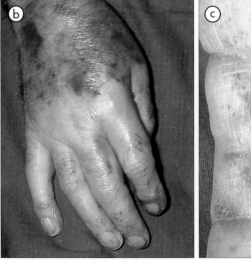

Fig. 13.30 Amyloid deposition in multiple myeloma. (a) Tongue infiltrated with amyloid showing macroglossia and ulceration. The waxy appearance is typical of amyloid deposition. (b) Amyloid infiltration of skin of the hands (left). The skin is waxy and there is purpura (right). Courtesy of Prof A.V. Hoffbrand.

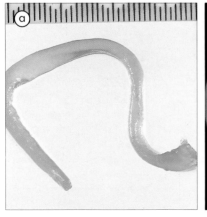
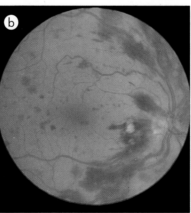

Fig. 13.31 Hyperviscosity in multiple myeloma. (a) Post mortem cast (from a blood vessel) of IgM protein in a patient with hyperviscosity. (b) Appearance of the retina in a patient with IgM hyperviscosity. Courtesy of Dr S. Roath.

Skin Cancer

Introduction

Skin cancers are the commonest of all malignant tumours in Western nations, but are much less frequent in countries where the population is chiefly black or coloured. In India, for example, most types of skin cancer are very rare.

The skin is the largest organ in the body, continuously exposed to a variety of carcinogens including sunlight, the most important aetiological factor (Fig. 14.1). It is probably the ultraviolet component which is most damaging. In certain parts of the world (including the UK and Australia) skin tumours have recently increased in frequency; this is probably related to our increased thirst for sun-drenched holidays, the encouragement of artificial tanning aids (such as ultraviolet light and solar couches) and, very likely, to a reduced ultraviolet filtration by an impaired ozone layer. In Australia the incidence of melanoma, the most virulent form of skin cancer, directly relates to geographical location – the closer to the equator, the higher the incidence (see chapter 1). Those with fair skin and red hair (typical Celtic colouring) seem at most risk. In basal cell carcinoma, the commonest of skin cancers in Britain, it is the exposed sites such as the face and the backs of the hands which are most frequently affected.

Other carcinogens of importance include those which are directly applied to the skin. This group of substances has particular historical interest, since the first known example, a carcinoma of the scrotal skin of boys who clambered up chimneys to clean them, was probably also the first clear-cut example of a direct carcinogen. In this case the offending material was the soot in the chimney flue. Later on many additional industrial examples were identified, such as arsenical compounds (in sheep dips), croton oil (an industrial lubricant) and naphthylamine compounds (used in a variety of industrial processes).

Radiation is another well documented cause of skin cancer, one of the many reasons for limiting the use of radiotherapy to malignant conditions. In the past, when radiotherapy was used more frequently for diseases such as ringworm of the scalp, childhood thymic enlargement or ankylosing spondylitis, skin cancers would sometimes occur in the previously treated areas (Fig. 14.2). Previously irradiated skin is probably more likely to undergo neoplastic change if the dose has been relatively low, characteristically the case when treating benign conditions. Immune suppression may also result in skin cancer, for example in renal transplant patients or those with AIDS, and there are one or two inherited conditions in which the skin's ability to protect itself from

KNOWN CARCINOGENIC FACTORS IN SKIN CANCER		
Chemical		
Arsenical compounds, polycyclic aromatic hydrocarbons (PAHs), quinolones, nitrogen mustard, psoralens, phenol, anthralin, phorbol esters, benzoyl peroxide, topical cytotoxic drugs		
Radiation related		
UV (including background solar) Ionizing radiation Occupational – in early radiation workers		
Immunosuppression		
AIDS and HIV related disease Renal transplantation Other immunosuppressive therapy		
Inherited disorders		
Xeroderma pigmentosum, Gorlin's syndrome, Albinism, von Recklinghausen's syndrome		

Fig. 14.1 Known carcinogenic factors in the aetiology of skin cancer.

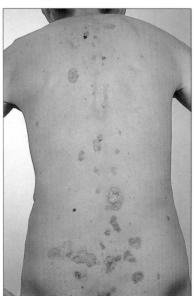

Fig. 14.2 Radiation-induced multiple skin cancers. This patient underwent treatment 20 years previously for ankylosing spondylitis. The lesions are mostly basal cell carcinomas, but some are squamous carcinomas. This first appeared 12 years after radiotherapy.

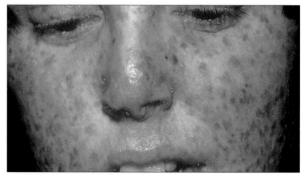

Fig. 14.3 Xeroderma pigmentosum. An autosomal recessive disease characterized by a remarkable sensitivity to ultraviolet light. This leads to multiple premalignant and frankly malignant skin lesions on exposed surfaces. These are generally squamous or basal cell cancers. The defect in this lesion appears to be due to ultraviolet-induced DNA damage. Courtesy of Dr A. du Vivier.

harmful ultraviolet or ionizing radiation is reduced – albinism and xeroderma pigmentosum are good examples (Fig. 14.3).

Malignant change can also occur at the edges of long-standing chronic ulcers, such as those resulting from burns or osteomyelitis (Fig. 14.4), and skin tumours can of course form part of a more wide-spread disease, as in the case of skin lymphoma. Mycosis fungoides is a specific form of skin lymphoma in which the disease process is initiated in the skin and only much later progresses to involve lymph nodes and other typical lymphoma sites (Fig. 14.5 – see also chapter 12). Multiple skin cancers are also found in Gorlin's syndrome, which consists of multiple basal cell carcinomas together with skeletal abnormalities including bifid ribs, frontal bossing and mandibular cyst formation (Fig. 14.6).

Secondary deposits from other primary sites (chiefly lung) are not infrequently diagnosed in the skin (see Figs 14.7 & 8.9). Some of the primary soft tissue sarcomas may also present as skin tumours, for example lymphosarcoma, dermatofibrosarcoma protruberans or neurofibrosarcoma, a particular feature of Recklinghausen's syndrome (Fig. 14.8).

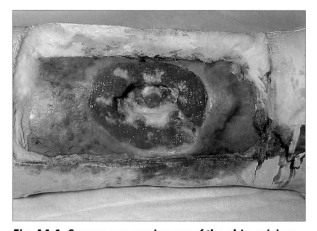

Fig. 14.4 Squamous carcinoma of the skin arising in a chronic osteomyelitic leg ulcer. Local excision and graft repair proved impossible, and the limb was eventually amputated.

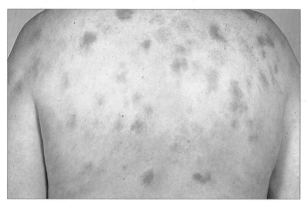

Fig. 14.5 Mycosis fungoides. One of several types of skin lymphoma. There is often an erythematous or pre-tumour stage, but this patient exhibits the classical features of infiltrative or plaque-type disease. Later these lesions often enlarge and ulcerate; internal organ involvement may occur.

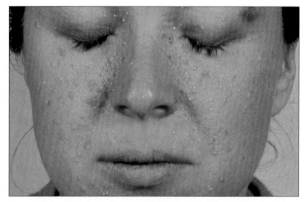

Fig. 14.6 Gorlin's (naevoid basal cell carcinoma) syndrome. Multiple basal cell carcinomas are common in this syndrome. The disease is inherited as an autosomal dominant; this patient is typical in that the lesions often develop in young adult life. Courtesy of Dr A.C. Pembroke.

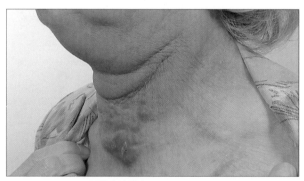

Fig. 14.7 Secondary deposits in the skin from a squamous carcinoma of the bronchus. This patient had a number of small nodules in the anterior part of the neck which eventually coalesced.

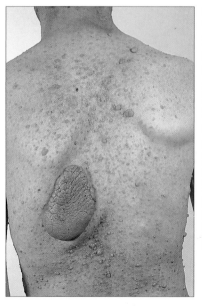

Fig. 14.8 Von Recklinghausen's syndrome. This case shows multiple small benign skin lesions and a single large saccular plexiform neurofibroma beneath the left scapula. Biopsy later confirmed a low-grade neuro-fibrosarcoma.

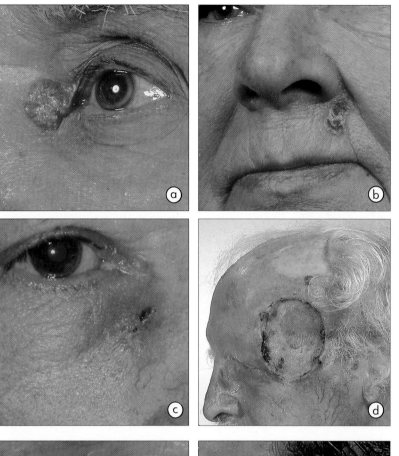

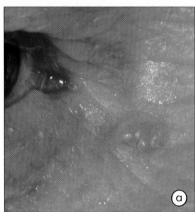

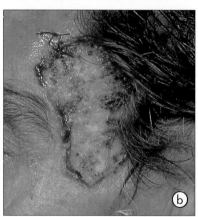

Fig. 14.9 Basal cell carcinomas.
(a) A typical lesion situated at the inner canthus with clearly defined margins and a typical pearly edge. Courtesy of Dr A. du Vivier.
(b) Ulcerating basal cell carcinoma situated beneath the left columella.
(c) Recurrent squamous carcinoma at the inner canthus following radiotherapy which had apparently been given successfully 5 years before. (d) Large destructive basal cell carcinoma recently excised. This patient has had multiple tumours and has previously undergone surgery and grafting for a lesion situated at the vertex. He has also lost the left external ear from a separate basal cell carcinoma of the pinna.

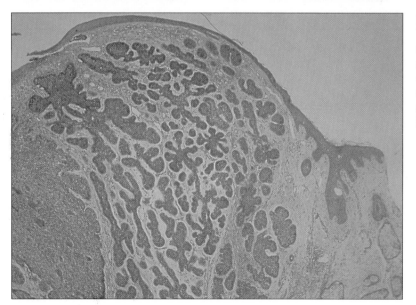

Fig. 14.10 Variants of basal cell carcinoma. (a) Cystic type.
(b) Pigmented type. Note the striking pigmentation at the edge of the lesion. Courtesy of Dr A. du Vivier.

Fig. 14.11 Basal cell carcinoma. This low power view shows the characteristic appearance of a nodular basal cell carcinoma. The dermis is extensively invaded by discrete islands of small, darkly-staining uniform cells. Courtesy of Dr A. du Vivier.

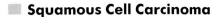

Basal Cell Carcinoma (Rodent Ulcer)

This is the commonest of skin cancers and is most often diagnosed in elderly males, presumably resulting from a lifetime accumulation of solar exposure. These tumours are generally easy to recognize (Fig. 14.9), situated characteristically on the face and around the eyes, with a well-defined, irregular, raised margin, a typical 'pearly' appearance and sometimes a depressed or ulcerated central area. These lesions are usually painless. Variants include the pigmented, cystic, infiltrating and sclerosing forms (Fig. 14.10). Microscopically, the appearance is very distinctive (Fig. 14.11) with uniform cell size, darkly staining nuclei and no evidence of keratinization. The cell of origin is in the undifferentiated basal cell layer of the skin – basal cell cancers are virtually never found in any site other than in the skin. Direct local extension is the most important means of tumour progression with virtually no tendency to metastasize to regional lymph nodes or distant sites, even when the tumour has reached a very large size with local destruction of underlying structures. Even when a tumour is very large it tends to be pain free. Treatment is discussed below.

Squamous Cell Carcinoma

This is a less common tumour, although there are many similarities in aetiology, treatment and relative frequencies at different primary sites. Although the appearance may be similar (Fig. 14.12), the histology is quite different (Fig. 14.13), with typical keratin pearls and other features of squamous carcinoma. Other characteristics which differ from those of basal cell carcinomas include a tendency to spread by local lymph node metastasis (Fig. 14.14) and, occasionally, dissemination to other parts of the body. Local invasiveness is also important, but these tumours do not characteristically have the deep destructiveness of basal cell carcinomas. Apart from the face, typical sites include the dorsum of the hands, the scalp, and pinna. The visual differences from a basal cell carcinoma often include a more crusty, ulcerated appearance, fungation and central necrosis, a less distinct margin and local lymphadenopathy. Since squamous carcinoma of the skin may occur at more widespread anatomical sites than basal cell carcinoma, a superficial non-pigmented skin tumour at an unusual site is more likely to be squamous than basal cell cancer. Squamous cell

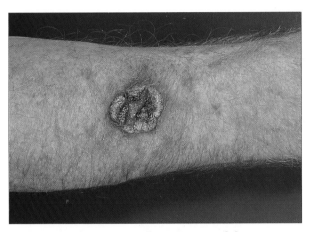

Fig. 14.12 Squamous cell carcinoma of the forearm. In this site, squamous carcinomas are more common than basal carcinomas, though the appearance in this case is similar to that of a rodent ulcer. This tumour required surgical excision.

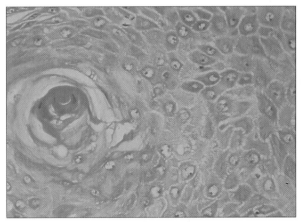

Fig. 14.13 Well differentiated squamous cell carcinoma. In this high power view, intercellular bridges (prickles) are conspicuous. Courtesy of Dr A. du Vivier.

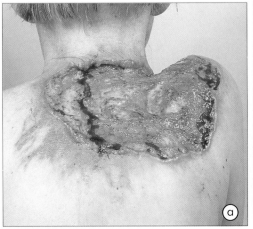

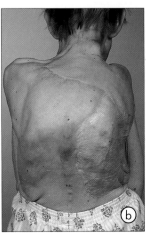

Fig. 14.14 Squamous cell carcinoma and lymph node metastasis. (a) Large destructive squamous cell carcinoma with obvious extension well beyond the initially ulcerated lesion. (b) Two years following successful resection and grafting, the patient presented again with an occipital lymph node. Aspiration cytology confirmed squamous cell carcinoma, and this was then treated successfully by radiotherapy.

carcinomas can reach a large size, particularly if arising on an area of the body which the patient cannot frequently see, and can spread with direct skin infiltration far beyond the confines of the visible tumour.

Benign skin disorders which can be confused with basal or squamous cell carcinomas include solar keratoses (Fig. 14.15), which are typically pigmented and crusty with a well demarcated margin. They are

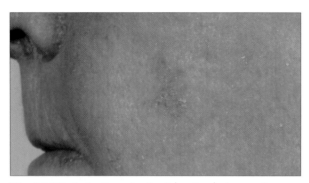

Fig. 14.15 Solar keratosis. A benign but sometimes premalignant tumour, chiefly occurring on the face and dorsal surface of the hands. Other changes due to prolonged exposure to sunlight are also present, including atrophy, pigmentation and other dysplastic changes. Courtesy of Dr A. du Vivier.

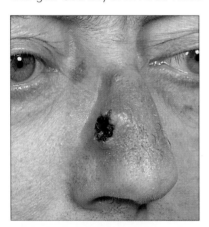

Fig. 14.16 Kerato-acanthoma. The nose is a fairly typical site and although the lesion looks dramatic, the central keratin plug and sharp edge are characteristic.

usually thickened flat lesions occurring on the head and face of elderly people. Although benign, there is sufficiently high incidence of malignant change to warrant the excision of large tumours. Papillomas and skin tags can occasionally mimic a skin cancer, but the most difficult benign lesion to distinguish from squamous cell skin cancer is the kerato-acanthoma, typically a well-demarcated raised lesion with a central keratin plug, often of similar size to a squamous carcinoma (Fig. 14.16). Chronic ulceration, particularly on the leg, may undergo malignant transformation ('Marjolin's ulcer'), a change which is typically insidious and easily missed. Treatment is discussed below.

Malignant Melanoma

This is the most feared of all skin cancers, with a far more aggressive and unpredictable pattern of behaviour than the other tumours, and a much higher mortality. Though much less common it has been increasing in incidence for the past several decades, probably because it is closely related to ultraviolet light exposure. Our predilection for exposing ourselves to the sun, combined with the reducing protective effect of the ozone layer, has begun to take

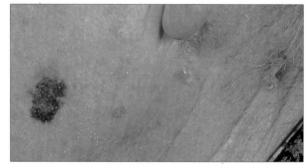

Fig. 14.17 Lentigo maligna. Typical localized 'early' malignant melanoma occurring in a sun-exposed site. Courtesy of Dr A. du Vivier.

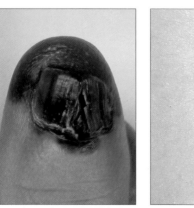

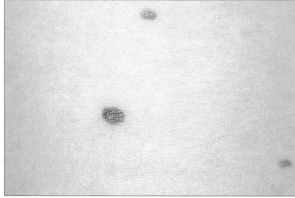

Fig. 14.18 Subungual melanoma of the nailbed. The lesion has an irregular outline and its colours vary from black to grey and blue. As it invades, the lesion distorts and splits the nailplate. Such lesions are not usually so grossly abnormal. Courtesy of Dr A.C. Pembroke.

Fig. 14.19 Junctional naevus. The nodule is quite dark but the pigment is distributed evenly and there is no indentation or notching in the outline. Courtesy of Dr A. du Vivier.

effect. At present malignant melanoma forms 3% of all skin tumours in Britain, but is much more common in Australia and New Zealand. Unlike the other major types of skin cancer, it is more frequent in younger and middle-aged people than in the elderly. It is also more common in females, suggesting a possible hormone relationship – a possibility further supported by the occasional case report of spontaneous regression, even of advanced tumours, during or following a pregnancy. Once again, these tumours are found principally, but not exclusively, on sun-exposed parts of the body (Fig. 14.17).

The tumour arises in four main clinical settings:
- Enlargement of a pre-existing benign naevus is found to be part of the clinical history in at least a third of all patients. All of us have benign naevi or moles scattered over the body, and the risk of malignant change of any one of them is extremely small. However, any change in appearance, particularly if it includes pigmentation, bleeding, ulceration or local pain, should be taken seriously, particularly if the lesion is situated on the palm of the hand, sole of the foot or subungual areas (Fig. 14.18). Dermatologists recognise several types of naevus. Junctional naevi (Fig. 14.19) are small, flat, pigmented lesions arising at the junction of

the dermis and epidermis. Compound naevi are larger than the junctional type and show more penetration of the dermis. In the intradermal naevus, the pigmented cells (melanocytes) have lost all contact with the epidermis (Fig. 14.20). Although these lesions may be difficult to distinguish from malignant melanoma, it is the clinical history of a change in appearance that is the most reliable guide to malignant transformation. There are at least twenty other documented types of naevus!

- Lentigo maligna (Hutchinson's melanotic freckle) is an epidermal pigmented type of melanoma commonest over the face and neck. It begins as a flat, irregular tumour, enlarging and changing in appearance gradually over the years (Fig. 14.21). It tends to occur in elderly patients.

- Superficial spreading melanoma is a more sharply demarcated lesion, often occurring in middle-aged people and with a typically irregular edge, a paler centre, and a tendency to ulceration or bleeding (Fig. 14.22). The pattern of growth is more rapid than a lentigo maligna, although occasionally a partial regression may occur.

- Nodular melanomas are generally darker and occur initially as a raised nodule with sharply

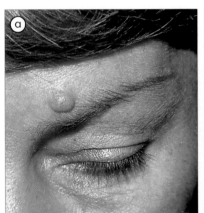

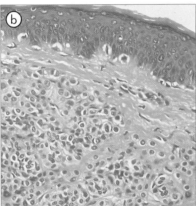

Fig. 14.20 Intradermal naevus.
(a) The lesion is raised, regular in outline and smooth-surfaced.
(b) The epidermis is flattened over the surface of the lesion. Scattered melanocytes are seen but there is no evidence of junctional activity. In the dermis there are collections of non-pigmented melanocytes, many of which have rather hyperchromatic nuclei. Courtesy of Dr A. du Vivier.

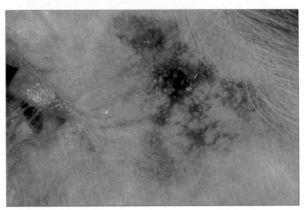

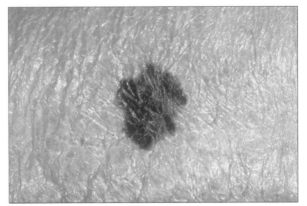

Fig. 14.21 Lentigo maligna. Here occurring in a typical site as a flat, irregular, slowly-enlarging tumour. Courtesy of Dr A. du Vivier.

Fig. 14.22 Superficial spreading melanoma. A more sharply demarcated lesion. Courtesy of Dr A. du Vivier.

defined edges. This form of melanoma may progress extremely quickly, even though initially small in size (Fig. 14.23) with rapid penetration to deeper tissues.

In about 10% of cases, disseminated melanoma occurs without any obvious primary site. Important occult primary sites include the nail bed (subungual melanoma) and head and neck primary sites such as the nasal fossa or paranasal sinuses.

Several other skin lesions, both benign and malignant, can mimic melanomas; these include pigmented basal carcinoma (see Fig. 14.10), the benign blue naevus (Fig. 14.24), simple or epidermal naevi (Fig. 14.25), haematomas, particularly of the nailbed, and Kaposi's sarcoma (KS). KS, previously a rare tumour seen mainly in elderly mediterranean

males (Fig. 14.26), is chiefly seen these days as part of the spectrum of AIDS. In AIDS patients the lesions tend to be multiple and rapidly progressive, only responding to treatment in the short term. It is the multiplicity of KS lesions that usually makes for easy distinction from melanoma, although melanoma itself can also present with widespread skin involvement.

Pigmentation within the oral cavity, particularly on the palate, can be difficult to diagnose accurately. It can occur in Addison's disease as a feature of normal pigmentation of coloured and black patients and as a typical part of Peutz–Jeghers syndrome (multiple gastrointestinal polyposis with melanin pigmentation in the mouth, lips and on the fingers – Fig. 14.27).

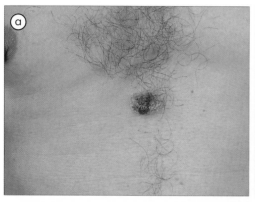
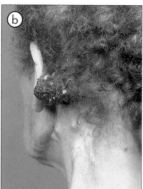

Fig. 14.23 Nodular melanoma. (a) Presenting as a raised nodule with sharply defined edges and rapid tumour growth. (b) Large nodular melanoma over the mastoid area, with several skin nodules visible beneath the primary site.

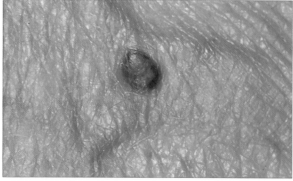
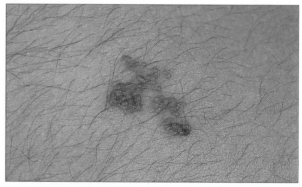

Fig. 14.24 Blue naevus. The lesion is raised and appears blue in colour. The naevus cells are deep in the lower dermis and incident light refracts blue. Courtesy of Dr A. du Vivier.

Fig. 14.25 Epidermal naevus. Sometimes epidermal naevi are arranged in a linear manner. Courtesy of Dr A. du Vivier.

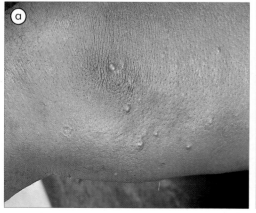
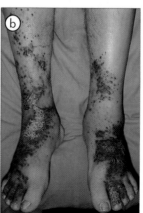

Fig. 14.26 Kaposi's sarcoma. (a) This case was not AIDS-related, presenting as small raised nodules in a patient from West Africa. (b) Widespread bilateral Kaposi's sarcoma in an elderly mediterranean male. AIDS-related cases tend to evolve more rapidly. Both types are partially responsive to radiotherapy.

Spread of melanoma occurs via the three major routes; local extension, lymphatic involvement and blood-borne metastases. It is one of a small group of cancers that can present with metastatic disease many years after its initial appearance, involving such distant sites as lungs, liver, distant areas of skin, and brain (see Figs 2.3 and 3.1). It may also metastasize to sites rarely involved by secondary tumours, such as the spleen and bowel wall. Locally, the tumour is not normally as destructive to deeper tissues as a basal cell carcinoma, though local skin satellite nodules are very characteristic (see Fig. 14.23). Metastasis to local lymph nodes is common (Fig. 14.28).

The depth of tumour invasion is an extremely important prognostic feature (Fig. 14.29). The staging system devised by Clark and colleagues has been widely used. The Breslow grading (depth of invasion in millimetres) is also a clear guide to prognosis. Thicker lesions carry a much higher risk of wide

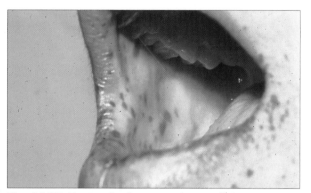

Fig. 14.27 Peutz–Jeghers syndrome. This case shows typical intra-oral and other skin lesions. These patients also have a raised incidence of small bowel carcinomas. Courtesy of Dr B. Leppard.

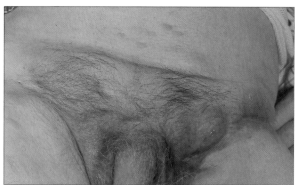

Fig. 14.28 Melanoma and metastasis. Local groin involvement (left inguinal region) together with multiple skin metastases in a case of amelanotic melanoma (primary situated on inner thigh and resected two years previously).

PROGNOSIS IN MELANOMA

LEVELS OF PENETRATION IN MELANOMA

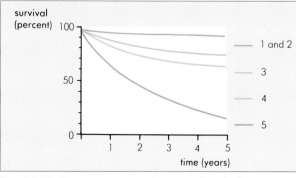

CLARK'S LEVELS

Level	Depth of infiltration of the dermis
1	Confined to the epidermis (*in situ*)
2	Infiltration of the papillary dermis
3	Infiltration to the junction of the papillary with the reticular dermis
4	Infiltration of the reticular dermis
5	Infiltration of the subcutaneous fat

PROGNOSIS RELATED TO CLARK'S LEVELS

FIVE YEAR SURVIVAL RELATED TO BRESLOW THICKNESS

Breslow thickness (mm)	5-year survival rate (%)
<1.5	93
1.5–3.5	67
>3.5	37

Fig. 14.29 Prognosis in melanoma. Level of penetration (Clark's system) is a powerful determinant of outcome. The Breslow grading system relates prognosis to depth of invasion and is equally predictive.

dissemination and early mortality; the presence of local nodal involvement is also an adverse feature, with few patients surviving five years.

Investigations to stage skin tumours are not generally useful for squamous or basal carcinomas. In patients with these conditions, no further studies are required prior to treatment. For patients with a malignant melanoma, a full clinical examination is mandatory and liver function tests and chest x-ray essential. A careful neurological history is worth taking, since these patients have a very high incidence of occult brain metastases.

Miscellaneous Skin Tumours

These include a variety of conditions which are shown in Fig. 14.30.

Management of Skin Tumours

Ideally all skin tumours should be biopsied, though this rule is sometimes ignored in elderly or infirm patients with very typical rodent ulcers. In general, however, biopsy is very important and surprises may occur – for example, a pigmented basal cell

carcinoma may prove to be a malignant melanoma. Almost all basal and squamous cell carcinomas can be cured by appropriate use of cryosurgery, topical chemotherapy, electrocautery, curettage, local surgical excision and/or radiotherapy.

All these methods are effective for small tumours, though once the lesion has reached half a centimetre or more most would agree that surgical excision or radiotherapy are the treatments of choice. Surgery has the advantage of speed (often undertaken under local anaesthetic), a good cosmetic result and a high likelihood of cure. On the other hand, radiation is preferred by many patients who wish to avoid surgery, especially on the face, where a surgical scar might be thought disfiguring. The cosmetic result following radiotherapy is usually very good (see Fig. 6.30), though it can be marred by telangiectasia or depigmentation. Tumours around the eye, a very common site for rodent ulcers, are generally dealt with by radiotherapy to avoid distortion of skin and lower eyelid and occlusion of the nasolacrimal duct with consequent epiphora.

For larger tumours it can be extremely difficult, particularly with basal cell carcinomas, to achieve control, even with the use of wide surgical excision,

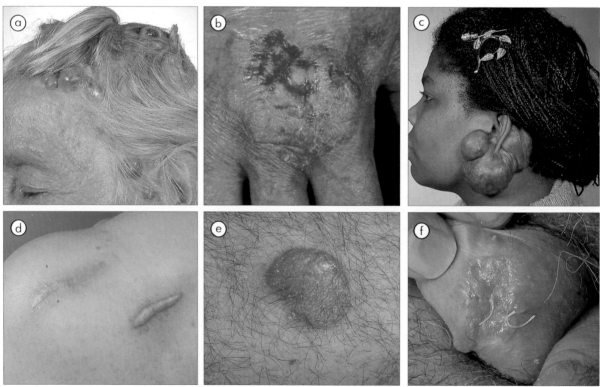

Fig. 14.30 Miscellaneous skin tumours. (a) Multiple cylindromas of the scalp ('turban tumour'). Histologically, these are similar to adenoid cystic carcinomas. (b) Bowen's disease (intradermal squamous cell carcinoma *in situ*). This lesion is generally found on the trunk and limbs and characteristically spreads laterally within the cutis. It may be indicative of a deep-seated malignancy. Courtesy of Dr A. du Vivier. (c) Huge keloid of the left earlobe following an attempted ear-piercing. The lesion was removed and treated with postoperative radiotherapy. No recurrence at three years. (d) Hypertrophic keloid change following ritual scarring in West Africa. The upper lesion has been excised and irradiated, the lower is untreated. (e) Well demarcated, solitary T cell skin lymphoma. This was completely cured with local radiotherapy, but the patient developed three more lesions in the subsequent ten years. (f) Erythroplasia of Queyrat, essentially an intraepidermal lesion situated on the penis, presenting as a persistent red papule or plaque.

grafting and postoperative radiotherapy. These tumours can prove relentlessly recurrent and destructive and may even, eventually, prove fatal. Such patients often have multiple tumours appearing in areas of dysplastic skin; the scalp is a particularly troublesome site for this type of rodent ulcer (Fig. 14.31).

Surgical excision of squamous cell carcinoma should be more generous than with rodent ulcers because of the occult lateral intraepithelial spread that commonly occurs. Where local lymphadenopathy is present a block dissection of these nodes is generally the treatment of choice, and can often be undertaken in continuity with the primary tumour resection. For malignant melanoma, wide surgical excision is the cornerstone of adequate treatment. The tumour should be removed with a generous margin of normal tissue, both in the lateral and deep directions. Although this may prove disfiguring, with skin grafting often required, this type of surgery can be life-saving. Melanoma is far less responsive to radiotherapy than basal and squamous cell carcinomas and wide surgical removal is correspondingly more important (Fig. 14.32). For patients with obvious lymphadenopathy a block dissection should be undertaken – sadly, the overall cure rate is still low. The surgical resection in this type of case is performed to avoid fungation through the skin with highly offensive local ulceration.

Radiotherapy is widely used in the management of primary skin cancer and is given in a variety of ways. For basal and squamous cell carcinoma it is generally given over a 1–3 week period using a low-voltage, relatively non-penetrating beam to avoid unwanted irradiation of deeper tissues. The eye and mouth can easily be shielded where necessary. Although cosmetic results are usually very good, patients should be warned to expect a fierce crusting skin reaction for a few weeks while the new skin regenerates.

In malignant melanoma few primary lesions are so large that surgical resection is not possible, especially since the advent of vascularized myocutaneous grafts which provide cover even for very large defects. For large or recurrent melanoma, a combination of surgical resection and interstitial irradiation may offer the best chance of local control (see Fig. 14.32).

Radiotherapy also has an important role in the management of secondary deposits from melanoma and squamous carcinomas of the skin. Because of the relative radioresistance of melanoma, large dose fractions of radiation, given at approximately weekly intervals, may give better control of, for example, symptomatic brain metastases. With lymph node involvement from either of these conditions, postoperative radiotherapy is often used following block dissection to try to prevent local fungation. Skin deposits from melanoma can also be treated primarily with radiotherapy in this way.

Chemotherapy is not used for basal cell carcinomas of the skin. There are however one or two anecdotal reports of its value in very troublesome cases which are incurable by surgery or radiotherapy. For squamous carcinomas chemotherapy is hardly ever used, though response rates are probably similar to those for squamous cancers at other sites. Chemotherapy is very occasionally worth considering in order to reduce the size of the tumour prior to local irradiation or surgery, though such cases are few and far between.

In malignant melanoma chemotherapy has been extensively tested, since the problem is so frequently beyond any possibility of surgical cure. A number of agents do show activity, notably vindesine, a mitotic spindle poison which has a response rate in melanoma of at least 20% and few adverse effects, dacarbazine, a highly toxic drug with a similar response rate to vindesine in melanoma, doxorubicin and cyclophosphamide (see Fig. 3.14). Despite substantial toxicity from the drugs, whether alone or in combination, useful responses are sometimes seen, although they tend to be short-lived – many

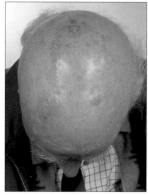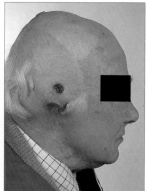

Fig. 14.31 Multiple basal cell carcinomas within dysplastic skin. Despite mutilating surgery and major reconstruction, this patient still has persistent disease at the area of the right external auditory canal. Eventually the disease recurred despite further surgery and radiotherapy and the patient died of meningitis as a result of inadequate skin coverage and sepsis.

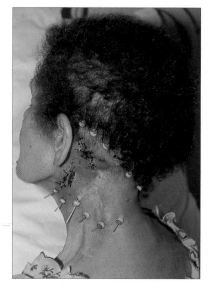

Fig. 14.32 Combined surgical and radiotherapeutic approach. This shows an iridium wire implant in the patient shown in Fig. 14.23. Neither radiotherapy nor surgery alone would have been sufficient for this large nodular melanoma.

doubt the value of chemotherapy in disseminated melanoma.

Some years ago, it became popular to offer direct intralesional treatment with immunotherapy using BCG, but the technique has largely been discontinued because most of the responses were insufficiently durable. A more recent immunological method of treatment is with interleukin-2 and other biological growth modifiers but these are not yet established for routine use.

Outcome of Treatment

Most basal and squamous cell carcinomas are cured by surgery or radiotherapy. In the 10% of patients who are not so cured, a wider surgical excision and/or radiotherapy is usually effective (see Fig. 14.12), though a small minority of cases progress and eventually prove fatal (see Fig. 14.31). In malignant melanoma, prognosis is much more uncertain. In patients with Stage I tumours, confined to superficial layers of the skin, about 70% of patients will be alive and well in five years. However, late recurrences in melanoma are well recognized so this is not a true cure rate. About a quarter of melanoma patients have evidence of lymph node involvement from the outset (Stage II disease) and the majority of these patients develop further evidence of dissemination, with an overall survival of less than 30%.

On the whole, female patients do rather better than males, with better results in patients with primary limb sites (60% overall survival at five years) than in melanomas of the head and neck or trunk (40–50% at five years).

Because of these poor figures in melanoma, early detection is extremely important. With vigorous application of an early diagnostic checklist (Fig. 14.33) it may be possible to improve the overall survival rate.

EARLY DETECTION OF MELANOMA
1 Slight altered skin sensation or mild itch
2 Size – maximum diameter greater than 1 cm
3 Increasing size
4 Shape – an irregular or geographical lateral margin
5 Colour variation – multiple shades of brown black, and even red and blue in the lesion
6 Inflammation
7 Bleeding or crusting from the lesion

Fig. 14.33 Seven point checklist for early detection of melanoma. An aid to clinical distinction of melanoma and non-melanomatous pigmented skin lesions.

Bone and Soft Tissue Sarcoma

Introduction

These uncommon mesenchymal tumours fall into two distinct groups, one arising from bone and cartilage, the other from soft tissues (Fig. 15.1). Primary bone tumours are among the more common tumours of young adult life and therefore form the bulk of cases at adolescent cancer centres. Soft tissue sarcomas, however, are typically adult tumours, though childhood varieties also occur (see chapter 16).

Little is known of the aetiology of these disorders. In adult life, osteosarcoma (and occasionally other sarcomatous tumours) may occur as a consequence of Paget's disease (Fig. 15.2), and childhood osteosarcoma is an occasional complication of treated retinoblastoma, both within and outside the irradiated area (see chapter 16). There are case reports of both bone and cartilaginous sarcoma tumours arising

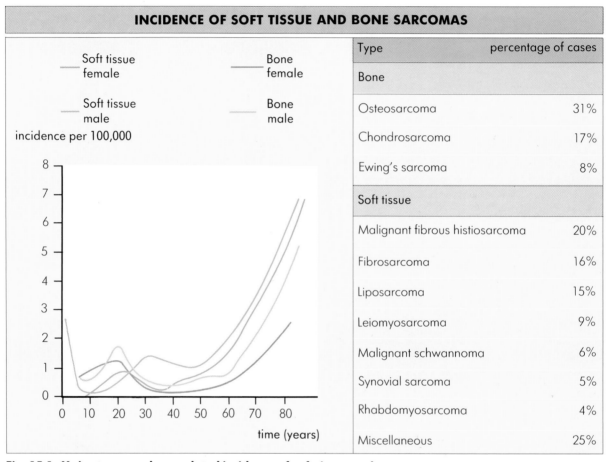

INCIDENCE OF SOFT TISSUE AND BONE SARCOMAS

Soft tissue female

Bone female

Soft tissue male

Bone male

incidence per 100,000

Type	percentage of cases
Bone	
Osteosarcoma	31%
Chondrosarcoma	17%
Ewing's sarcoma	8%
Soft tissue	
Malignant fibrous histiosarcoma	20%
Fibrosarcoma	16%
Liposarcoma	15%
Leiomyosarcoma	9%
Malignant schwannoma	6%
Synovial sarcoma	5%
Rhabdomyosarcoma	4%
Miscellaneous	25%

Fig. 15.1 Major types and age related incidence of soft tissue and bone sarcoma.

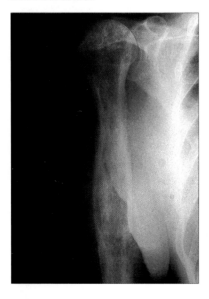

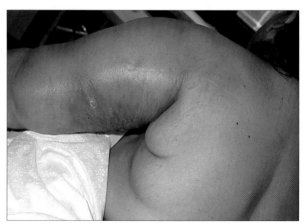

Fig. 15.2 Osteosarcoma of humerus in Paget's disease. The radiological findings include features of both of these conditions.

Fig. 15.3 Lymphangiosarcoma of Stewart and Treves. This patient was previously treated by mastectomy and postoperative radiotherapy for carcinoma of the breast.

in irradiated sites following treatment of adult cancer, for instance chondrosarcoma of the chest wall following treatment for carcinoma of the breast. A specific type of adult soft tissue sarcoma, the lymphangiosarcoma of Stewart and Treves, occurs very rarely as a complication of radiation and surgery for breast cancer, leading to a chronically lymph-oedematous and cellulitic arm (Fig. 15.3). Other bone or soft tissue sarcomas, chiefly malignant fibrous histiocytoma, can also occur, though rarely, as a late complication of radiation therapy (Fig. 15.4), typically with a lag delay period of 10–20 years. In cases of Ewing's sarcoma of bone, some patients have a history of a previous tumour or even fracture at the site of the lesion, though it is generally felt that this relationship is no more than spurious.

A few inherited conditions are complicated by sarcoma, for instance malignant transformation to neurofibrosarcoma in patients with von Reckling-hausen's disease (see chapter 14) and Gardner's syndrome with polyposis coli, which undoubtedly predisposes to development of desmoid tumours. Clearly, oncogene expression is detectable in many human sarcomas including the *ras* and *myc* genes (osteosarcoma, rhabdomyosarcoma, fibrosarcoma).

Primary Sarcoma of Bone

Primary bone tumours are uncommon but are none-theless an extremely important group of tumours since they chiefly occur in young adult life, and require expert and complex management. With the appropriate resources they can often be cured, with surprisingly little long-term damage to the patient.

The most frequent varieties are osteosarcoma and Ewing's sarcoma. Both occur most frequently in

the adolescent period and osteosarcoma is approximately three times more common. Although some 60% of osteosarcomas occur around the knee (i.e. arising from the lower femur or upper tibia), the common sites in Ewing's sarcoma are more widespread (Fig. 15.5). Clinically, osteosarcoma is characterized by a short history, usually less than 6 months, of a gradually enlarging tender mass (see Fig. 15.6). It is very unusual for the skin to ulcerate, and the rest of the clinical examination is generally normal. The commonest mode of dissemination is by local extension and haematogenous spread to the lungs, producing typically rounded 'cannonball' metastases ranging in size from a few millimetres, detectable only by CT scanning, to very large lesions measuring several centimetres across, with features similar to those seen in Fig. 2.12. Histologically, the

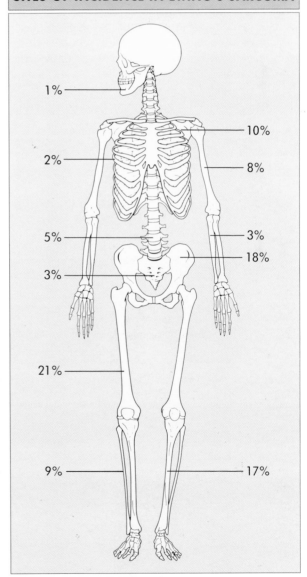

SITES OF INCIDENCE IN EWING'S SARCOMA

1%
2%
5%
3%
21%
9%
10%
8%
3%
18%
17%

Fig. 15.5 Main sites of incidence in Ewing's sarcoma.

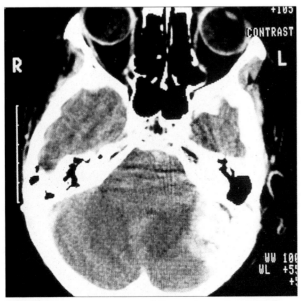

Fig. 15.4 Osteosarcoma of the petrous temporal bone. This tumour developed within the irradiated volume following treatment for a brain stem glioma five years previously.

tumour consists of osteoid-forming cells which are generally distinct, though the tumour may be pleomorphic and a number of characteristic variants have been described (Fig. 15.7). Important varieties include both the parosteal and periosteal types of osteosarcoma, which arise from the outer table of the affected bone and exhibit both a lower propensity for metastatic spread and a much improved prognosis compared with the more common 'classical' type (see below).

Radiologically, osteosarcomas usually display typical features both on plain X-ray, and on CT, MRI and isotope uptake scanning. The plain radiograph generally shows obvious new bone formation well outside the affected bone, often with a Codman's triangle caused by periosteal elevation (Fig. 15.8). A large soft tissue component is often also apparent. Ideally, all three types of scan should be undertaken in each case, since this will provide the maximum anatomical information for the surgeon, often a critical factor in the decision as to whether the individual case is suitable for internal prosthetic replacement without amputation (see below). In particular, isotope and MRI scanning often demonstrate the lesion extending well beyond the limits identified by the plain radiograph. In view of the common route of dissemination, CT lung scanning is also mandatory

in each case. Occasionally, the isotope uptake scan shows evidence of bone metastasis from osteosarcoma at a distant site though this is extremely unusual.

On purely clinical grounds, Ewing's sarcoma is often indistinguishable from osteosarcoma, generally occuring with a similar history though with a slightly earlier peak age of onset and a different pattern of predominant sites (see Fig. 15.5). Histologically, however, the tumour is quite different, typically characterized by small, malignant, densely blue-staining cells, with large nuclei and little cytoplasm, and without osteoid formation. The tumour can be difficult to distinguish histologically from other small blue round-cell tumours which include neuroblastoma, non-Hodgkin's lymphoma and others. Occasionally a lesion of this type may be unclassifiable even with the most sophisticated immunohistochemical stains.

Radiologically, Ewing's tumours are often easily distinguishable from osteosarcoma (Fig. 15.9). Although both lesions show areas of bone erosion at the primary site, Ewing's sarcomas sometimes demonstrate an 'onion skin' effect with layering of the cortex, though diffuse erosion of the bone is the cardinal feature. CT, MRI and isotope uptake scans should be carried out, to give detailed definition of

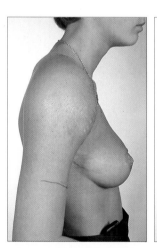
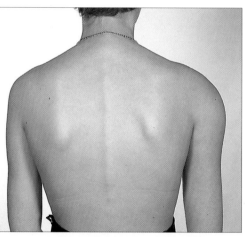

Fig. 15.6 Osteosarcoma. Typical clinical features, showing a firm smooth swelling at the site of the tumour (see also Fig. 15.8).

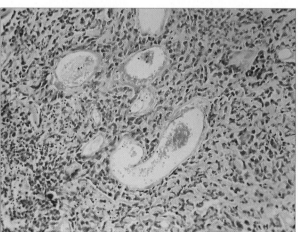
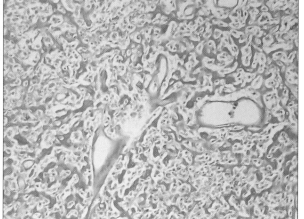

Fig. 15.7 Histological features of osteosarcoma showing osteoid-forming malignant osteoblasts. (H&E and HVG). Courtesy of Dr J. Geddes.

local anatomy (Figs 15.10 & 2.9). Once again a CT lung scan should be a routine part of investigation.

Local extension occurs, as with osteosarcoma, both along the cortex of the affected bone, internally to the medullary cavity and externally towards the skin surface. Unlike osteosarcoma, local or regional lymph node involvement may occur (Fig. 15.11), though this is unusual even in Ewing's sarcoma.

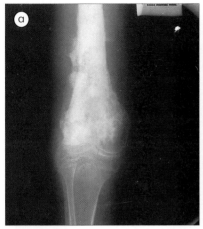
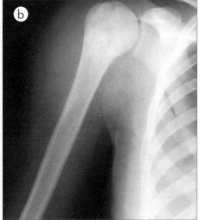

Fig. 15.8 Radiological features of osteosarcoma.
(a) Osteosarcoma of lower tibia showing massive new bone formation together with destructive change and soft tissue swelling.
(b) Osteosarcoma of upper humerus showing major soft tissue involvement, periosteal elevation of the lateral aspect, and new bone formation of the upper humerus (same case as in Fig. 15.6).

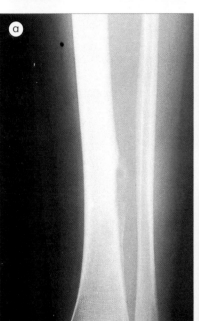
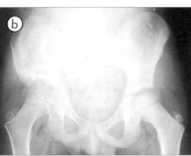
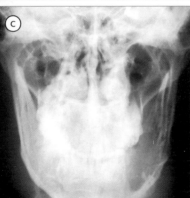

Fig. 15.9 Ewing's sarcoma. (a) In this lesion of the lower tibia, there is major periosteal elevation and 'saucerization' of the affected bone.
(b) Ewing's sarcoma of the right ileum, with bone expansion and destruction of the acetabulum.
(c) Left mandible with massive destruction of the whole of the upper table and normal appearances on the right side.

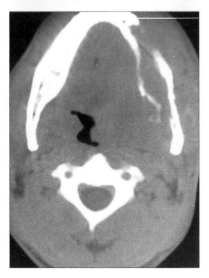

Fig. 15.10 Ewing's sarcoma of the mandible. CT-scan showing major soft tissue swelling and complete destruction of the outer table (same patient as in Fig. 15.9c). Clinical features in this case are shown in Fig. 15.20a.

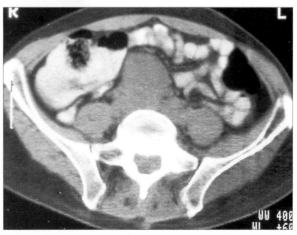

Fig. 15.11 Ewing's tumour of the pelvis. CT-scan showing massive para-aortic nodal disease.

Haematogenous spread occurs to distant sites chiefly the lung, but also occasionally, to liver, bone (Fig. 15.12) and brain.

Other types of primary bone tumour are less common. Osteoclastoma (giant cell tumour) generally occurs at a diffusively expansile lesion arising in long bones (Fig. 15.13), often in sites around the wrist and knee but sometimes also affecting the upper limb. It has a characteristic histological appearance, though the differential diagnosis from osteoclast-rich osteosarcoma can be difficult. Occasionally, the osteoclastoma can arise as a complication of Paget's disease.

Aneurysmal bone cysts also occur as expanding bone lesions in young people, and although not strictly malignant, are often grouped with primary bone tumours since they can be persistently locally recurrent and may require similar treatment, with surgical resection and/or radiotherapy (see below). Radiologically they are often extremely destructive and often have a characteristic 'soap-bubble' appearance (Fig. 15.14).

Malignant fibrous histiocytoma (MFH), though generally a soft tissue sarcoma, is increasingly recognized as an occasional primary bone lesion. Its histological and clinical features are described below. It is histologically identical to soft tissue MFH, though its response to treatment may be different to that of its soft tissue counterpart; in particular, it shows an apparently greater sensitivity to chemotherapy if the primary MFH has arisen from a bony site.

Of the cartilaginous tumours, chrondrosarcoma is by far the most common. It generally arises as a slowly enlarging, often painless mass, with a history sometimes stretching back several years (Fig. 15.15). Its distinct histological features usually make pathological diagnosis straightforward. It may occur as a malignant transformation of a benign enchondroma of bone, or in patients with multiple enchondromatous lesions (Ollier's disease). Apart from the

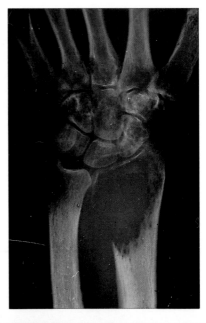

Fig. 15.13 Osteoclastoma of distal radius showing massive erosion and diffuse expansion.

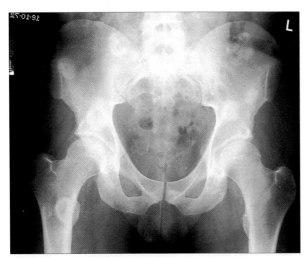

Fig. 15.12 Involvement of bone in Ewing's sarcoma. Secondary bone deposits scattered widely throughout the pelvis and right femur. The primary site is not shown.

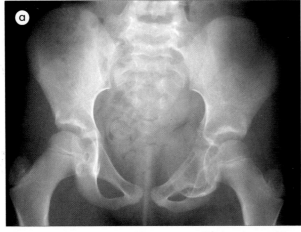

Fig. 15.14 Aneurysmal bone cyst of superior pubic ramus.
(a) Appearance prior to treatment with typical 'soap bubble' appearance.
(b) Appearance after radiotherapy. This film was taken six months later. Massive healing with sclerosis is already evident.

local extension into adjacent tissues, characteristic of low-grade tumours, haematogenous dissemination to lung may also occur. It is often a tumour of the elderly with a peak age incidence of 50–60 years.

Primary lymphoma of bone is discussed in chapter 12.

Management of Malignant Bone Tumours

These tumours should, wherever possible, be treated at specialist centres where the many skills and resources for optimal treatment are readily available. Management of bone sarcomas has been revolutionized over the past 20 years by advances in both chemotherapy and conservative surgery, dramatically reducing the need for limb amputation, previously often necessary as a curative procedure.

Several studies published in the mid-1970's confirmed that recurrent osteosarcoma was occasionally

responsive, at least in the short term, to chemotherapy; more importantly, chemotherapy given as an adjuvant following limb amputation (then the standard treatment) was seen to give superior results to treatment by surgery alone. Although these early series were flawed by use of historic controls and variation in tumour types, later more rigorous studies confirmed the early findings.

Chemotherapy has therefore become firmly established as a treatment for this disease. Indeed the best results have been obtained when chemotherapy is given as the primary therapeutic manoeuvre even before surgery. The logic of this approach lies in the distinction between the chemoresponsive and non-chemoresponsive tumours, a feature determined by comparing the histology of the tumour specimen removed after primary chemotherapy with that of the initial biopsy specimen. This then allows for a more tailor-made approach after surgical resection, depending on the degree of responsiveness.

Although chemotherapy is now an essential part of management for every case of classical osteosarcoma, it is not generally recommended for periosteal or parosteal lesions in view of the much reduced propensity for distant spread.

Details and schedules of chemotherapy vary widely, most groups employing combinations rather than single agent treatment. The agents most frequently used include cisplatin, doxorubicin, methotrexate and isofamide. Most European and American studies are currently randomizing between different intensities and combinations of chemotherapy since the optimal choice and schedules have yet to be determined.

Wherever possible, surgical treatment should consist of a conservative limb-sparing resection, with internal replacement using a tailor made prosthesis (Fig. 15.16). It may be necessary to replace the knee, hip, shoulder or other joint as well as part or all of the shaft, depending on the site of the primary.

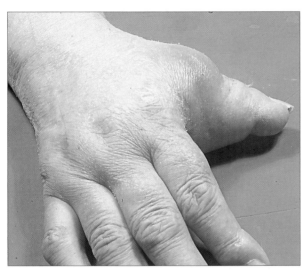

Fig. 15.15 Chondrosarcoma of the base of the thumb. Typically, this was an elderly patient with a three year history of a slowly enlarging mass.

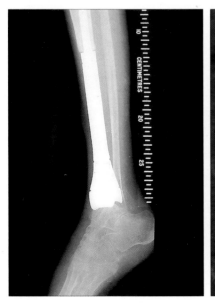
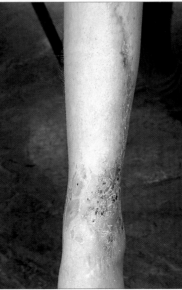

Fig. 15.16 Prosthetic replacement of lower tibia in Ewing's sarcoma. (Same case as in Fig. 15.9a.)

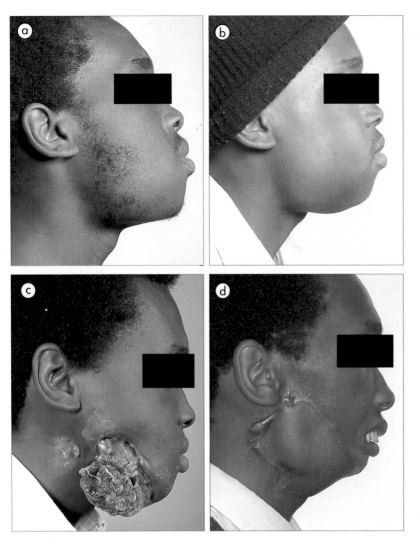

Fig. 15.17 Unresectable osteosarcoma of the mandible. (a) Appearance at presentation. (b) After three months chemotherapy with apparent progression of disease. The patient was then irradiated. (c) Two years later, with major necrosis of the tumour and extrusion through the skin. This was resected and no viable tumour found. (d) Final appearance four years later after reconstructive surgery.

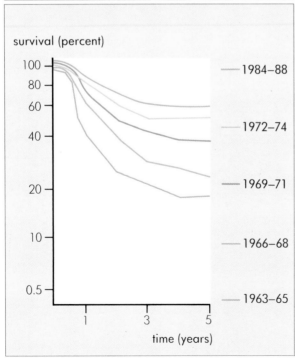

SURVIVAL IN OSTEOSARCOMA

survival (percent)

- 1984–88
- 1972–74
- 1969–71
- 1966–68
- 1963–65

time (years)

Fig. 15.18 Overall survival after therapy in osteosarcoma showing progressive improvement.

The past decade has seen a dramatic rise in the number of patients treated in this way, an approach that would probably have been impossible without advances not only in bio-engineering techniques but also in effective chemotherapy to deal with micrometastatic or residual disease. Although there was considerable concern over the possibility of local recurrence, this has not been a major problem in most series, even in those in which a substantial soft tissue component was present, and removed together with the affected bone. Naturally the degree of resection of the primary tumour is guided more by CT and other scanning techniques than by the plain radiograph since these give greater accuracy. Frozen section analysis of the host residual margin should also be undertaken before the surgeon is satisfied that the resection has been adequate. Postoperative radiotherapy is not recommended in such cases, though it may be used in the occasional patient with a completely non-responsive or unresectable osteosarcoma (Fig. 15.17). Advances in reconstructive surgery, for example of the mandible using fibula or other grafts, have restricted the use of non-surgical treatment.

For patients with recurrent disease, further chemotherapy is often employed. Radiotherapy

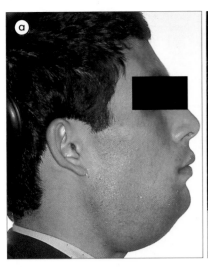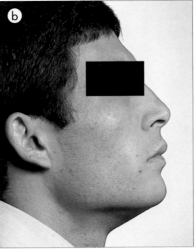

Fig. 15.19 Chemotherapy responsiveness of Ewing's sarcoma. (a) Tumour at presentation. (b) Tumour after one course of combination chemotherapy (photograph taken only one month later). (Same case as in Figs 15.9c and 15.10.)

SURVIVAL IN EWING'S SARCOMA

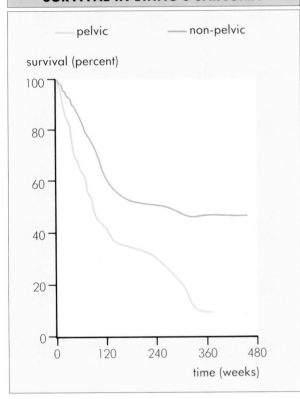

Fig. 15.20 Survival in Ewing's sarcoma. The outlook is clearly site dependant, with pelvic tumours having a far worse prognosis.

may also be useful, though the lung is much the commonest site of metastatic spread, therefore limiting the value of radiotherapy. A few patients present with late onset lung metastases, and may be suitable for metastatectomy particularly if the recurrence is confined to one or two metastatic lesions. Although opinions are divided as to the appropriateness of this type of surgery, some patients have successfully undergone repeated operations, including bilateral thoracotomy with removal of multiple lesions, and a few have enjoyed long-term survival, even possible cure. Careful patient selection is the key to success.

The outlook for patients with osteosarcoma has improved greatly over the past 20 years (Fig. 15.18) both in life expectancy and quality of life. Although this is partly due to improved adjuvant chemotherapy regimens, other factors are also involved. For example, conservative limb resection generally gives a very satisfactory cosmetic and functional result, particularly in the lower limb.

Ewing's sarcoma is now managed in a very similar fashion, with preoperative chemotherapy, surgery by conservative resection wherever possible, and postoperative chemotherapy with cytotoxic combinations. Ewing's sarcomas are both more chemosensitive and radiosensitive than osteosarcomas, and major reduction in tumour bulk is often seen with dramatic speed (Fig. 15.19). Before conservative surgery became possible, radiation therapy was often used as primary management of these lesions, though long-term late recurrences reduced the overall success rate. Local resection is now generally preferred, though postoperative radiotherapy may be useful. As with osteosarcoma, current international studies in Ewing's tumour are chiefly addressed towards the definition of better and less toxic chemotherapy. Overall survival of sarcoma is clearly better where the primary site is in a limb than for pelvic tumours (Fig. 15.20).

The management of osteoclastoma has always been controversial. Even though the tumour is clearly radiosensitive, most surgeons prefer local resection and/or bone curettage, since frank malignant change has occasionally been reported following radiotherapy for this tumour. However, such changes may simply be related to the selection of the more malignant lesions as suitable for radiotherapy in the first place. Although giant-cell tumours are generally cured by local methods of treatment they can be both destructive and seriously damaging if they arise at a critical site, for example in the cervical spine (see Fig. 15.21). For aneurysmal bone cysts (see Fig. 15.15), surgical removal is usually recommended though again, these lesions are often remarkably radiosensitive, and radiotherapy should be preferred to local resection if serious functional disability would otherwise result. There does not appear to be any risk of malignant change if radiotherapy is used for aneurysmal bone cysts.

Soft Tissue Sarcoma

This is an heterogenous group of tumours, arising from different tissues within the mesenchyme and including those derived from fibrous tissue, smooth and stratified muscle, blood vessels, endothelial cells, fat cells and other sites (see Fig. 15.1).

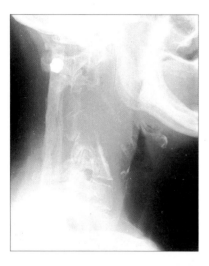

Fig. 15.21 Massive giant cell tumour (osteoclastoma) of the cervical vertebrae. In this patient the neck was stablized by a graft taken from the iliac crest and the patient then treated with radiotherapy.

The uncertain pathogenesis of these diseases has made tumour classification difficult but histologically they are characterized by increasing degrees of tumour cell dedifferentiation and pleomorphism with respect to the parent tissue. Three of the more common types are shown in Fig. 15.22.

Malignant fibrous histiocytoma (MFH), the commonest soft tissue sarcoma, is probably derived from supportive cells, though often characterized by fibrous infiltration which led to many of these lesions being previously misdiagnosed as fibrosarcomas. True fibrosarcoma is much less common.

Clinically, soft tissue sarcomas generally present as a visible swelling at almost any part of the body, most typically painless and sometimes growing to a large size (Fig. 15.23).

Many of the MFH's and fibrosarcomas are extremely firm on palpation, though liposarcomas tend to be softer in texture. Kaposi's sarcoma, discussed in chapter 14, is the only soft tissue sarcoma specifically related to AIDS. It is now thought to be a sexually transmitted disorder in the large majority of AIDS-related cases, though previously it was a rare disease with a specific geographical incidence and a slowly evolving pattern quite unlike present day AIDS-related cases. Like many bone sarcomas, soft tissue sarcomas spread widely throughout the body by direct extension, nodal involvement and, most

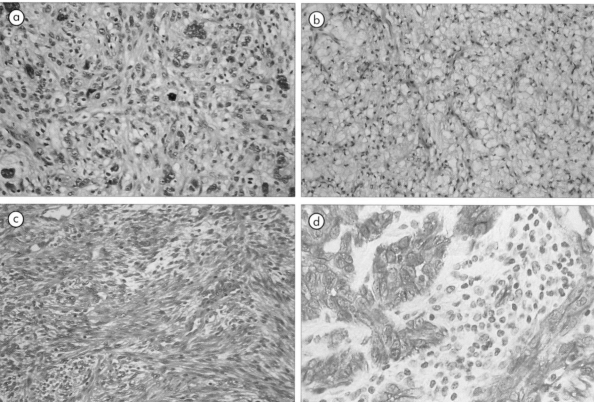

Fig. 15.22 Histological characterization of soft tissue sarcomas. (a) MFH malignant fibrohistiocytoma of storiform pleomorphic type. (b) Mixoid liposarcoma showing characteristic vascular pattern and lipoblasts. (c) Fibrosarcoma showing herring bone-like pattern of spindle cells (H&E ×63). Courtesy of Dr C. Fisher. (d) Invasive, poorly differentiated angiosarcoma (UEA staining). Courtesy of Prof L.D. True.

particularly, haematogenous spread chiefly to the lungs. In the case shown in Fig. 15.23, the patient presented at the outset with an abdominopelvic mass, probably through nodal involvement, of similar size to the primary lesion.

Management of soft tissue sarcomas has been far less successful than primary bone sarcomas, chiefly because of the almost complete failure of chemotherapy to make any impact in these diseases (see below).

A system for staging soft tissue sarcomas, devised by the American Joint Staging Committee, is shown in Fig. 15.24.

If chest X-ray, CT lung scan and other investigations have failed to demonstrate evidence of distant spread, the lesion should be surgically removed wherever possible. Most of the soft tissue sarcomas arise in limbs or over the chest wall, and in either case, wide local resection is essential for long-term control. For limb lesions, wide local excision may require compartmentectomy (Fig. 15.25), ideally with complete removal of the effected anatomic part and without exposure of the lesion, which should be removed in its entirety, surrounded by normal tissues. Histological confirmation of malignancy will already have been obtained by atraumatic needle biopsy. Postoperative radiotherapy is essential in all cases, since the results of this conservative surgical resection are otherwise inferior to the long-term result following amputation. Even if adequate removal has been

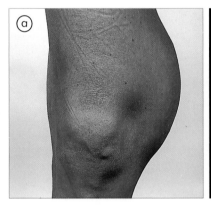
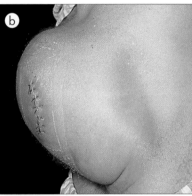

Fig. 15.23 Clinical presentation of soft tissue sarcoma.
(a) Liposarcoma of the knee. The patient only presented when he was no longer able to wear his normal trousers. (b) Fibrosarcoma of the buttock. Surprisingly, this was a painless lesion.

STAGING FOR SOFT TISSUE SARCOMAS

Stage	Criteria
Ia	Low-grade tumour, <5cm in diameter with no regional lymph node or distant metastasis
Ib	Low-grade tumour, >5cm in diameter with no regional lymph node or distant metastasis
IIa	Tumour of moderate differentiation, <5cm in diameter with no regional lymph node or distant metastasis
IIb	Tumour >5cm in diameter with no regional lymph node or distant metastasis
IIIa	High-grade tumour, <5cm in diameter with no regional node or distant metastasis
IIIb	High-grade tumour, >5cm in diameter with no regional lymph node or distant metastasis
IVa	Tumour of any grade or size with regional lymph nodes but no distant metastasis
IVb	Clinically diagnosed distant metastasis

Fig. 15.24 Simplified American Joint Staging Committee staging system for soft tissue sarcoma.

COMPARTMENTECTOMY

anterior superior iliac spine

tensor fasciae latae

adductor longus

sartorius

tumour

vastus medialis

patella

Fig. 15.25 Compartmentectomy. This diagram illustrates the wide surgical excision of soft tissue from the anterior compartment of the thigh.

undertaken by means of compartmentectomy, post-operative radiotherapy should be given at radical doses to eradicate micrometastatic disease, since soft tissue sarcomas are not among the most sensitive of human tumours. It is not unknown for patients to develop local recurrence, i.e. within the irradiated field, even under these most favourable circumstances. Occasionally soft tissue sarcomas will require amputation for adequate control, particularly if situated in the upper part of the arm or leg. In these cases, forequarter or hindquarter amputation may sadly be necessary to secure both local control and any realistic chance of cure. Even after such drastic surgery, there is no guaranteed freedom from local recurrence, and postoperative radiotherapy may have to be considered (Fig. 15.26).

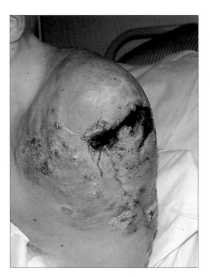

Fig. 15.26 Soft tissue sarcoma of upper humerus treated by disarticulation. The patient developed recurrent local satellite nodules despite the radical surgery.

If amputation is necessary, the level of resection will naturally be determined by the anatomical site of the lesion. It is generally wise to choose a level one joint above the lesion, for instance mid-thigh amputation for a sarcoma situated around the knee. The same is true for primary bone sarcomas which cannot be dealt with by conservative local resection.

Unlike bone sarcomas and most childhood soft tissue sarcomas, there is no proven role for adjuvant chemotherapy following local treatment. Several trials have failed to establish any survival benefit, though further trials of newer agents continue.

Little effective treatment exists for patients with metastatic disease, whether diagnosed at the outset or later in the illness, after apparently successful treatment of the local primary site. Combination chemotherapy has frequently been attempted, with occasional benefits, since there is an overall response rate of approximately 25%. However few durable complete responses are seen and the side effects of such treatment are considerable. Recently, there has been interest in the possible use of isofamide which is probably the most effective single agent.

The outlook in soft tissue sarcoma (Fig. 15.27) relates both to the position of the primary site, to its resectability and most importantly the presence of distant metastases. As with most other adult solid tumours, metastatic disease is almost always fatal, though palliative chemotherapy and radiotherapy may be helpful in the short term.

There is no clear evidence of major differences in outlook in the main histological subtypes, though some of the less common varieties, notably alveolar

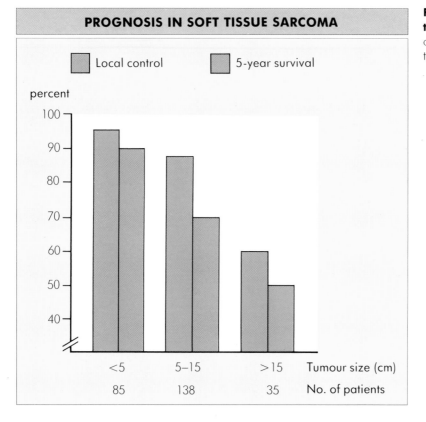

Fig. 15.27 Prognosis in soft tissue sarcoma. The results depend on the initial size (bulk) of the tumour.

PROGNOSIS IN SOFT TISSUE SARCOMA

Local control   5-year survival

Tumour size (cm)	No. of patients
<5	85
5–15	138
>15	35

soft part sarcoma and angiosarcoma, do seem particularly adverse. One possible exception is the Askin's tumour, a recently described entity with histological features and chemosensitivity similar to that of Ewing's and other 'small-round-cell' malignant sarcomas. This is a lesion which generally arises in the upper chest or chest wall, appears to have a relatively low propensity for metastatic extrathoracic spread, and can be chemosensitive even when initially bulky (Fig. 15.28).

Unlike bone sarcomas, there is little or no need for metastatectomy in the treatment of soft tissue sarcomas, since solitary late metastases are even less common in these conditions than in the bone sarcoma group. The prognosis for limb tumour appears better than for lesions on the trunk, possibly due to greater ease of adequate wide surgical resection at the limb sites. However, wide excision of chest wall lesions, with removal of several ribs and substantial portions of the chest wall are often possible and should always be considered since surgery is much the most important part of management. Particular care must be taken to stage the patient adequately before major surgical resection is undertaken, as demonstration of microscopic lung deposits, for example, would make such surgery unsuitable. An operation may still be required, however, simply to achieve adequate local control and to avoid painful and unpleasant fungation at the primary site.

Desmoid tumours are curious borderline low-grade tumours thought to arise from fibroblasts or their precursor cells. Although of low grade, non-metastasizing and often not considered as malignant, they can be multiple, progressive and ultimately fatal because of pressure on vital local structures. Surgical removal is the cornerstone of treatment, though they can sometimes be unresponsive to radiotherapy. One exciting new advance in the management of these tumours is the use of the tamoxifen derivative drug toremifene, which has resulted in apparent liquefaction of these lesions, so far only reported anecdotally in a number of 'endstage' cases.

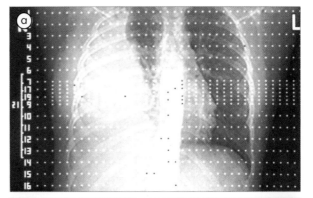
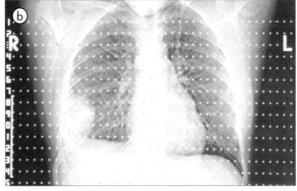
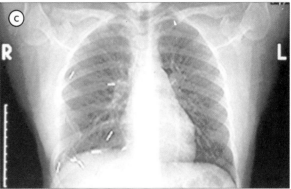

Fig. 15.28 Askin's tumour. (a) X-ray showing massive thoracic tumour arising from the right chest wall. (b) Substantial volume reduction following treatment with combination chemotherapy. (c) Normal chest X-ray following surgical removal of residual tumour. Courtesy of Prof R.L. Souhami and Dr J.N. Godlee.

Childhood Tumours

16

Introduction

Although cancer in childhood is the most common natural cause of death between infancy and adolescence (second only to accidental death), childhood cancers are, fortunately, very uncommon. A family doctor is unlikely to see more than one or two cases during a working lifetime; specialists of course develop a distorted view of the frequency. Some units may see a new childhood brain tumour almost every week, but this represents a substantial proportion of all childhood brain tumours occurring within the area covered by the unit.

The diagnosis of a childhood cancer is always a devastating event, imposing exceptional difficulties for the child, the family, the family doctor and the specialists involved. Other professional colleagues, both medical and non-medical, also play an important role, as well as the school, the local community and, in some cases, specialists in terminal care. Good communication is essential, both between the doctor and the patient and family, and also between the doctor and other specialists. For this particular form of cancer, it is essential that a single specialist remains in the driving seat throughout the whole of the child's care, although invariably he will need the

skills of others. The importance of communication and adequate support is heightened further by the fact that many children are referred to specialist centres long distances from home in order to gain the best possible care. This may lead to the undesirable but inevitable exclusion, at least to some extent, of the local hospital and paediatric services. They may be required only at the end of the day when treatment may have been unsuccessful, and the child is in need of skilled supportive and terminal care which the specialist hospital cannot easily provide, particularly at such a distance from home. Even where treatment has been successful, children need tremendous support whilst undergoing unpleasant chemotherapy and other treatments, particularly since alopecia and steroidal facial change are all too apparent to school friends.

Despite these difficulties, over half of all childhood cancers are now curable. This applies particularly to childhood leukaemia, retinoblastoma and Wilms' tumour. These advances have come about by improvements in staging, surgery and radiotherapy, but above all as a result of the astonishing impact of chemotherapy. Childhood tumours are one of the

INCIDENCE OF CHILDHOOD TUMOURS BY SITE		
Site	Incidence per 100,000	Proportion of childhood cancer (%)
Leukaemia	3.4	30
Central nervous system	2.1	19
Lymphomas	1.5	14
Sympathetic nervous system	0.9	8
Soft tissue	0.7	7
Kidney	0.6	7
Bone	0.5	5
Retinoblastoma	0.3	3
Liver	0.1	1
Others	0.6	6

Fig. 16.1 Incidence of childhood tumours by site.

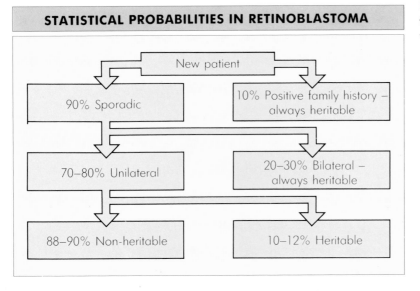

STATISTICAL PROBABILITIES IN RETINOBLASTOMA

Fig. 16.2 Statistical probabilities for a newly diagnosed patient with retinoblastoma.

great success stories for anti-cancer chemotherapy, a story which began only in the late 1940's with the discovery of methotrexate by Sidney Farber and the identification of nitrogen mustard as a useful cytotoxic agent. They were rapidly introduced as the first effective drugs for childhood leukaemia. Increasing intensity and complexity of drug regimes has been made possible by improved supportive care (better antibiotics, more widespread platelet transfusion, routine use of long-term intravenous catheters, and so on), which in turn has led to higher response rates. We are still learning how to use combinations of chemotherapy, surgery and radiotherapy to best effect, and attention is turning increasingly towards the avoidance or, at second best, treatment, of long-term side effects such as interruption of growth.

Aetiology

The relative frequency of the commoner types of childhood cancer are shown in Fig. 16.1. Childhood leukaemia is discussed in chapter 13, childhood brain tumours in chapter 5. The other types of childhood cancer, often referred to as the solid childhood tumours, are described here. Very little is known about their aetiology though, as with adult cancers, there are considerable geographical variations in incidence. For example, primary hepatoblastoma, a very unusual paediatric liver tumour in the UK, is relatively frequent in the Far East; but possibly the best example is Burkitt's lymphoma which is relatively common in children in certain parts of Africa, but virtually never encountered in European children.

Genetic factors are important in a number of childhood tumours. First, retinoblastoma, much the commonest of childhood eye tumours, has a marked familial incidence (Fig. 16.2) especially when it is bilateral, so that half of the children of surviving patients will themselves be affected. In von Recklinghausen's syndrome there is an increased incidence of cerebral tumours and, usually in later life, neurosarcomatous change. In tuberous sclerosis there also appears to be an increased incidence of brain tumours, often of higher grade than would generally be encountered in childhood. There is even some evidence for childhood cancer families where more siblings are affected than can possibly be explained by chance. The highest risk is probably for childhood leukaemia, especially if the affected child is an identical twin, in which case the risk to the twin is very high. All these points clearly have implications for counselling of families. Parents are of course anxious for reassurance that their other children will not be affected by the cancer. In general, this can be given, though as discussed above, there are a number of familial syndromes associated with childhood cancer (Fig. 16.3). The genetic alterations in some of these syndromes are known (see Fig. 16.4). The vast

CHILDHOOD CANCERS ASSOCIATED WITH CONGENITAL SYNDROMES OR MALFORMATIONS

Syndrome or Anomaly	Tumour
Aniridia	Wilms' tumour
Hemihypertrophy	Wilms' tumour, hepatoblastoma, adrenocortical carcinoma
Genito-urinary abnormalities (including testicle maldescent)	Wilms' tumour, Ewing's sarcoma, nephroblastoma, testicular carcinoma
Beckwith–Wiedmann syndrome	Wilms' tumour, neuroblastoma, adrenocortical carcinoma
Dysplastic naevus syndrome	Melanoma
Nevoid basal cell carcinoma syndrome	Basal cell carcinoma, medulloblastoma, rhabdomyosarcoma
Poland's syndrome	Leukaemia
Trisomy-21 (Down's syndrome)	Leukaemia, retinoblastoma
Bloom's syndrome	Leukaemia, gastrointestinal carcinoma
Severe combined immune deficiency disease	EBV-associated B-lymphocyte lymphoma/leukaemia
Wiscott–Aldridge syndrome	EBV-associated B-lymphocyte lymphoma
Ataxia telangiectasia	EBV-associated B-lymphocyte lymphoma, gastric carcinoma
Retinoblastoma	Wilms' tumour, osteosarcoma, Ewing's sarcoma
Fanconi's anaemia	Leukaemia, squamous cell carcinoma
Multiple endocrine neoplasia syndromes (MEN I, II, III)	Adenomas of islet cells, pituitary, parathyroids, and adrenal glands Submucosal neuromas of the tongue, lips, eyelids Pheochromocytomas, medullary carcinoma of the thyroid, malignant schwannoma, non-appendiceal carcinoid
Neurofibromatosis (von Recklinghausen's syndrome)	Rhabdomyosarcoma, fibrosarcoma, pheochromocytomas, optic glioma, meningioma

Fig. 16.3 Childhood cancers associated with congenital syndromes or malformations. [Adapted from DeVita, Hellmann and Rosenberg (eds) (1989) *Cancer: Principles and Practice of Oncology.* J.B. Lippincott Co., Philadelphia.]

CHROMOSOMAL ALTERATIONS IN PAEDIATRIC MALIGNANCIES	
Tumour	Chromosomal Alterations
Retinoblastoma	13q14
Osteosarcoma	13q14
Wilms' tumour	11p13
Embryonal tumours of Beckwith–Wiedermann syndrome	11p
Acoustic neuroma and meningioma	22
Meningioma	22

Fig. 16.4 Paediatric malignancies with recognized recessive genetic alterations.

PRIMARY SITES AND METASTASIS IN NEUROBLASTOMA

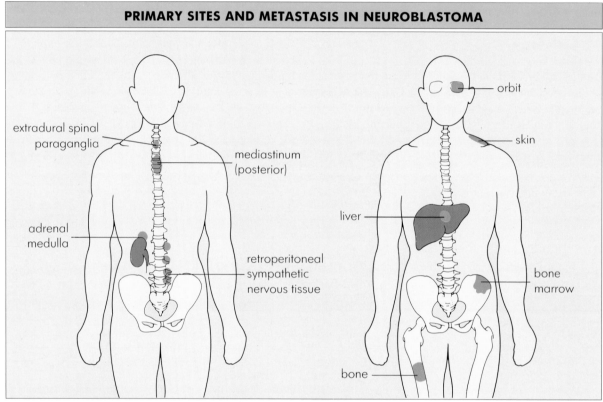

Fig. 16.5 Primary sites for the development of neuroblastoma and common sites of metastasis.

majority of childhood cancers are, however, sporadic and neither present nor future offspring are likely to be affected. Some parents even need to be reassured that the disease is in no way infectious.

Neuroblastoma

This is the commonest solid childhood cancer. It affects very young children, three-quarters of all patients being between the ages of 0 and 4 years. The tumour arises from malignant change within neural tissue, chiefly the adrenal medulla and ganglia of sympathetic nerves. These tumours are commonly situated in the adrenal medulla itself or in mid-line structures such as the posterior mediastinum or retroperitoneal sites, mirroring the embryological

development of neural crest tissue (Fig. 16.5). The primary tumour can sometimes reach a very large size, and histologically the appearance is rather characteristic, with the small malignant cells often arranged as rosettes. They are highly malignant tumours, often spreading widely by blood-borne dissemination, particularly to bone marrow, liver and bone (Fig. 16.6), though less commonly to the lung.

Diagnosis
The presenting clinical features vary widely because of the variety of primary sites, but many children will have weeks or months of malaise and lassitude, together with loss of appetite and weight, and anaemia, as common features. The tumour may also

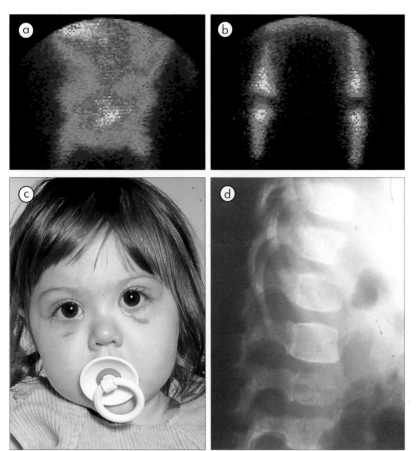

Fig. 16.6 Metastatic neuroblastoma. (a) ^{131}-I-meta-iodobenzylguanidine (MIBG) image showing tumour uptake in the liver and in an adrenal neuroblastoma. (b) MIBG image in the same child showing uptake in bone marrow of the legs involved with neuroblastoma. (c) Ten-month-old baby girl with typical 'bruising' around the orbit due to stage IV neuroblastoma involving the orbit. (d) Involvement of vertebrae with neuroblastoma.

present as a pyrexia of undetermined origin. When the adrenal gland is the primary site, most children present with abdominal pain and a mass (Fig. 16.7); the other classical form of presentation is with spinal cord compression from a posterior mediastinal or paravertebral primary tumour. Spinal cord compression in childhood is particularly difficult to diagnose, so impending paraplegia may have been present for many weeks or months, making the prognosis for return of function guarded. If liver or bone metastases have occurred early the abdominal mass may be hepatic, rather than the palpable primary tumour. Skin, orbit (see Fig. 16.6) and brain are other secondary sites.

The diagnosis can sometimes be made by urine analysis since neuroblastoma almost always secretes catecholamine metabolites, chiefly HVA (homovanillic acid) or VMA (vanillyl mandelic acid). A 24-hour urine collection gives good quantification, and may help to determine progress after treatment. If these metabolites are elevated, the diagnosis is virtually secure but a biopsy should still be obtained, either from the primary site or from an accessible metastasis. X-ray and CT scanning often show typical appearances, with a large soft tissue primary and in metastatic cases, lytic lesions in the bones (see Fig. 16.8). Isotope bone imaging, including MIBG (see Fig. 16.6) and bone marrow investigation are likely to be requested by the paediatric oncologist, and marrow involvement is more common than with any other solid paediatric tumour.

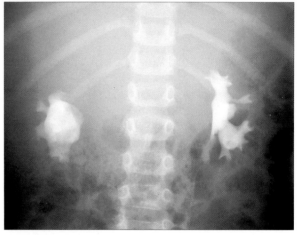

Fig. 16.7 Neuroblastoma presenting as an abdominal mass. There is blunting of the calyces of the right kidney and a large mass occupying much of the upper abdomen, pushing the bowel downwards (same case as in Fig. 16.6a and b).

Despite these characteristic features, the diagnosis is not always easy, particularly where lassitude, loss of appetite and a low-grade fever are the only presenting features. The distinction from other types of childhood cancer is important, since neuroblastoma and Wilms' tumour can present in a very similar way. Likewise, if the primary site is in the posterior mediastinum or paravertebral ganglia, a primary spinal intramedullary tumour such as an ependymoma can present almost identically. Other causes of cord compression in the child include spinal tuberculosis and traumatic haematoma (both now very unusual), and benign tumours such as neurofibroma, as well as primary or secondary spinal tumours including, for example, deposits from a medulloblastoma.

Staging

Clinical staging (Fig. 16.9) is important in neuroblastoma since the degree of tumour spread has considerable bearing on the choice of treatment and outcome. The child with disease confined to the primary site (stage I) has an excellent survival rate following treatment (approximately 90%; Fig. 16.10) whereas with distant spread the cure rate is still very low (10–20%). Survival also correlates with age at diagnosis. Curiously, some children with advanced disease occasionally appear to undergo spontaneous remission, and there is even a stage of advanced tumour (stage IVS; Fig. 16.11) where the tumour is localized to one side of the midline but with evidence of dissemination to marrow, liver or skin, in which the prognosis is substantially better (see Fig. 16.10), and a probability of cure as high as 50%. This stage is usually only seen in very young children. How much of this relates to the well documented feature of occasional spontaneous remission is uncertain.

Abdominal tumours have a worse prognosis than mediastinal disease, even though they may be better encapsulated and more easily resectable. Presumably

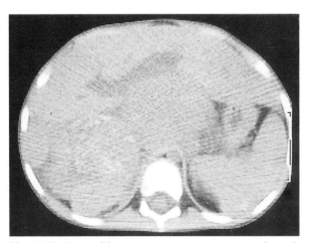

Fig. 16.8 Neuroblastoma presenting as an adrenal mass. CT scan showing a large right adrenal mass with calcification and grossly enlarged para-aortic lymph nodes (same case as in 16.6a and b, and 16.7).

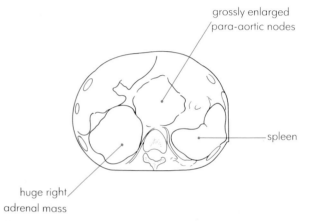

Fig. 16.9 Staging system for neuroblastoma.

STAGING SYSTEM FOR NEUROBLASTOMA	
Stage	**Criteria**
I	Tumour confined to organ or structure of origin
II	Tumour extends in continuity beyond the organ or structure of origin, but does not cross the midline. Homolateral regional lymph nodes may be involved. Tumours arising in the midline structure (such as the organ of Zuckerkandl) penetrating beyond the capsule and involving the lymph nodes on the same side should be considered stage II. Bilateral extension should be considered stage III
III	Tumour extends in continuity beyond the midline. Bilateral regional lymph nodes may be involved
IV	Remote disease involving skeleton, parenchymatous organs, soft tissues or distant lymph node groups
IVS	A special category: stage I or II with remote disease confined to one or more of the following sites: liver, skin or bone marrow without radiological evidence of bone metastases on skeletal survey

this relates to a higher metastatic rate and/or relatively later diagnosis. Pelvic tumours seem to do rather better.

Management

From the point of view of clinical management this tumour remains extremely frustrating, since despite undoubted chemoresponsiveness, curability is much lower than with other types of childhood cancer. Although chemosensitive, the durations of response are often limited, and attempts have been made in recent years to increase the intensity of such treatment. Where the primary tumour is resectable, this certainly should be undertaken, and surgery may even be curative in early stage diseases. If the operation is incomplete, radiotherapy should be considered; where there is evidence of more extensive disease, chemotherapy must always be given. For children with large primary tumours but obvious evidence of metastatic disease, it may be best to give chemotherapy first and consider resection of the primary tumour later, when hopefully it will have shrunk. It would certainly be unwise, in such cases, to ignore the importance of controlling the primary tumour, just because widespread secondary deposits are present.

Standard chemotherapy regimes continue to evolve rapidly, but mostly include vincristine, actinomycin D, cyclophosphamide, doxorubicin and cisplatin. Overall response rates to conventional

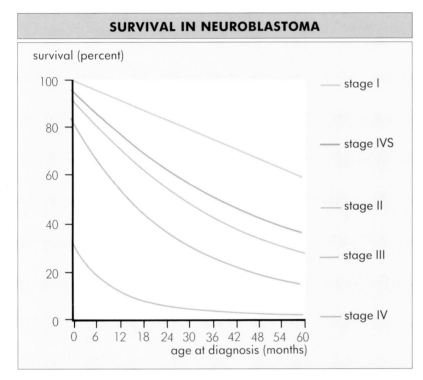

SURVIVAL IN NEUROBLASTOMA

survival (percent)

stage I

stage IVS

stage II

stage III

stage IV

age at diagnosis (months)

Fig. 16.10 Survival by stage and age at dignosis in neuroblastoma. Prognosis worsens with increasing stage, except for patients with stage IVS who show surprisingly good survival.

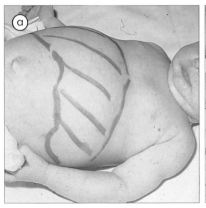
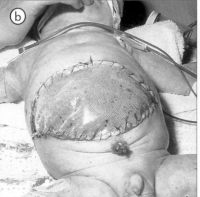
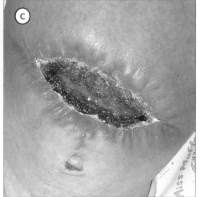

Fig. 16.11 Stage IVS neuroblastoma. (a) Grossly swollen abdomen due to hepatic involvement with stage IVS neuroblastoma in a baby. Note the small area of blue pigmentation close to the left nipple – this is a 'blueberry muffin nodule' of metastatic tumour. This tumour regressed spontaneously. Courtesy of Dr J. Kohler. (b) Infant presenting with gross liver involvement due to stage IVS neuroblastoma. This mass was causing such respiratory difficulties that an abdominal incision with silastic prosthesis was required. (c) Minimal radiotherapy to the liver was given. The adrenal mass and liver regressed and the incision is shown healing. This child is currently well, the abdominal cavity having completely closed. Courtesy of Mr J.D. Atwell.

combination chemotherapy are about 70%, but a much smaller proportion of these remissions are well maintained, and many children will relapse and require additional treatment at a later stage. Intensive chemotherapy has become widely used, often employing high dose melphalan, together with autologous marrow transplantation. The use of magnetic separation of neuroblastoma cells from the bone marrow has been widely publicized but it is not yet certain whether this treatment will prove to have a long lasting impact on cure rates. Because of the extremely rapid clinical evolution of this tumour, a trouble free period of three years from treatment is likely to represent a cure.

Wilms' Tumour

Wilms' tumour or nephroblastoma is the other important intra-abdominal tumour of childhood. It is slightly less common than neuroblastoma but arises only from the kidneys and is therefore slightly more common within the abdomen. Like neuroblastoma, it generally develops sporadically, without a familial history, though occasionally families with a genetic predisposition to this tumour are encountered. Although the cause of this tumour is unknown, some affected children suffer from congenital abnormalities (generally genito-urinary or musculoskeletal malformations) and the importance of genetic factors is underlined by the high frequency with which chromosome abnormalities may be present. Like neuroblastoma, it is chiefly a tumour of younger children of less than 5 years and its incidence is approximately equal in both sexes.

Diagnosis

Wilms' tumour commonly presents with an abdominal mass, generally painless, and sometimes with haematuria (approximately one-third of cases). The constitutional features often associated with neuro-

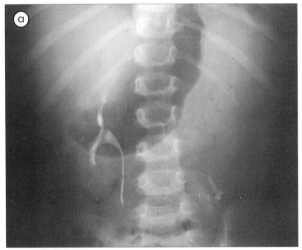
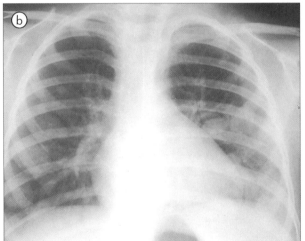

Fig. 16.12 Wilms' tumour. (a) IVU showing a large left-sided Wilms' tumour pushing the stomach to the right, depressing the kidney and distorting the renal pelvis. (b) Chest X-ray showing numerous pulmonary metastases, each measuring several centimetres in diameter.

STAGING SYSTEM FOR WILMS' TUMOUR	
Stage	Criteria
I	Tumour limited to kidney and completely excised
II	Tumour extends beyond the kidney, but is completely excised
III	Residual non-haematogenous tumour confined to abdomen
IV	Haematogenous metastases, i.e. lung, liver, bone and brain
V	Bilateral renal involvement at diagnosis

Fig. 16.13 National Wilms' tumour study group staging system.

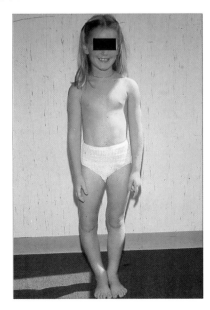

Fig. 16.14 Effects of irradiation on growing bones. This patient has received irradiation to a tumour in the left knee. This has prevented growth of the left leg with resultant shortening compared with the right leg.

blastoma may also be present in Wilms' tumour, and an investigation for hypertension is advised, particularly since it can occasionally produce severe manifestations such as retinopathy. An important distinction from neuroblastoma is the absence of VMA or HVA in the urine, and the non-calcifying nature of the primary tumour on plain radiography. Other important staging investigations include a chest X-ray and CT scan of chest and abdomen (Fig. 16.12) which are particularly important since, unlike neuroblastoma, this tumour metastasizes to the lungs quite frequently. Abdominal CT will not only give details of the degree of renal involvement but also, perhaps more importantly, the degree of local spread and likely prospects for curative surgery. Spread to peri-renal tissues and lymph nodes is common, and sites of blood-borne metastases include lung and bone, though other sites are also common. Unlike neuroblastoma, bone marrow involvement is unusual. Wilms' tumour is sometimes bilateral, without any evidence of disease at non-renal sites, raising the possibility of a bilateral primary ('metachronous') presentation. CT scanning, pelvic ultrasound and IVU may all give useful information on primary tumour anatomy, and MRI scanning may prove even more sensitive.

The renal mass is generally quite well circumscribed but there may be considerable areas of necrosis or haemorrhage, and the whole kidney may be involved in locally advanced cases. As with adult kidney tumours, there may be direct extension outside the renal capsule, and even invasion of the inferior vena cava. The degree of local extension is an important part of tumour staging (Fig. 16.13) and a useful predictor of ultimate prognosis.

Management

Like neuroblastoma, Wilms' tumour is responsive to chemotherapy, with the important difference that responses tend to be more durable, making treatment more successful even where extensive extra-abdominal involvement has occurred. The mainstay of treatment is surgical removal. It is mandatory in patients with stage I and II disease and should be carried out with curative intent in every case. Where the tumour cannot be entirely resected (stage III) additional abdominal irradiation is generally given, though this must be done with considerable caution in young children to avoid undesirable long-term effects on growth, and skeletal and visceral development (Fig. 16.14). Simple adjuvant chemotherapy is given in stage I disease, since the survival is better than with surgery alone, but the importance of chemotherapy clearly increases with advancing stage, and more intensive combination drug regimens are used for patients with stages III and IV. Patients with bilateral tumours (stage VI) form about 5% overall, and adequate surgical resection is usually possible, without complete ablation of all functional renal tissue.

Drug treatment for Wilms' tumour has led to an enormous improvement in survival during the past 20 years (Fig. 16.15). Response rates are high (60–70% for the most active drugs such as vincristine and doxorubicin) but are higher still (over 90%) with drug combinations. Children and families affected by this disease should, therefore, be reassured that the intensive hospital-based drug treatment is generally worthwhile and must be persevered with. Even children with advanced disease can be cured without undue long-term side effects. Apart from curative surgery and chemotherapy, radiation remains important, particularly in the management of stage II disease and also for palliation of brain, spinal, bone and liver metastasis. The prognosis for Wilms' tumour is now better than for any other childhood malignant disease, with overall cure rate of at least 80%. Young children seem to do particularly well.

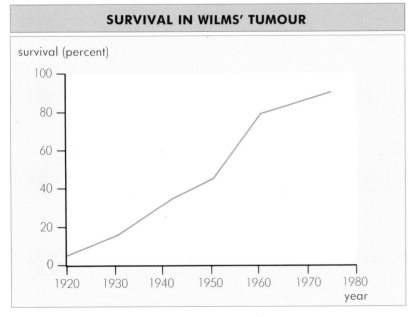

Fig. 16.15 Survival in Wilms' tumour. Two-year survival has improved rapidly since the 1920s. [Modified from D'Angio and Belasco (1981) in *Cancer: Achievements, Challenges and Prospects for the 1980s*. Vol. 2. Grune & Stratton, Orlando.]

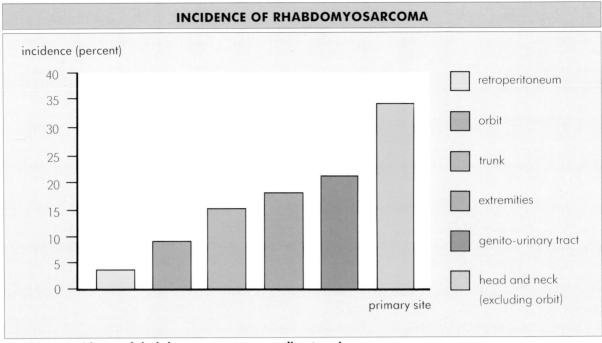

INCIDENCE OF RHABDOMYOSARCOMA

incidence (percent)

retroperitoneum

orbit

trunk

extremities

genito-urinary tract

head and neck (excluding orbit)

primary site

Fig. 16.16 Incidence of rhabdomyosarcoma according to primary site.

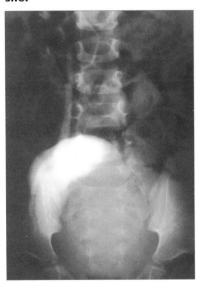

Fig. 16.17 Rhabdomyo-sarcoma of the bladder. This IVU of a child shows an enormous mass in the left side of the bladder and a non-functioning left kidney

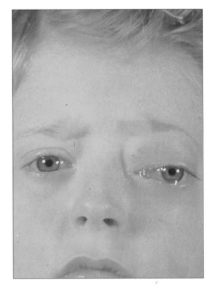

Fig. 16.18 Rhabdomyo-sarcoma of the left orbit.

Soft Tissue Sarcoma

This is a complex group of childhood tumours, with the same variety as the adult group (see chapter 15), but differing in several important respects.

Rhabdomyosarcoma
The commonest type of childhood soft tissue sarcoma is the rhabdomyosarcoma, accounting for over half the total group. This tumour originates from striated muscle and is a highly malignant neoplasm which can present at a variety of sites (Fig. 16.16). Head and neck and genito-urinary presentations (Fig. 16.17) are the commonest, though other sites are important. The orbits are an unusual though characteristic site (Fig. 16.18). Histologically, the tumours are generally of two main types, though other varieties also occur.

These are embryonal, the commonest variety, and the alveolar type. Embryonal rhabdomyosarcoma, often fully differentiated, is generally composed of spindle shaped cells, often irregular in pattern and with a rather characteristic cellular morphology. They are seen particularly in the head and neck or as genito-urinary tumours. Alveolar rhabdomyo-sarcoma, more frequently a limb or trunk tumour, is microscopically different with a less haphazard cellular arrangement of typically round cells, with rather little cytoplasm, and often obvious cross-striations.

With limb and facial primary sites, presentation is usually obvious, but the more deep-seated tumours, for example in pelvic sites, are more difficult to diagnose and consequently present later. These tumours are often associated with lymph node and

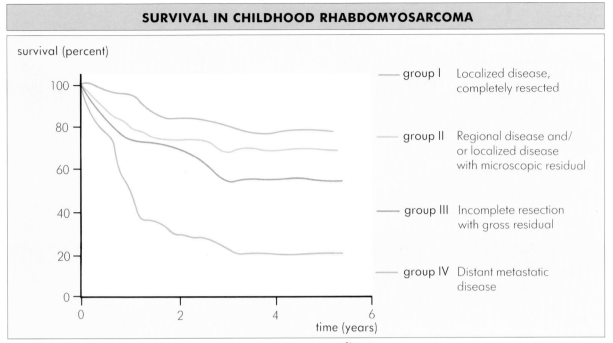

Fig. 16.19 Survival in childhood rhabdomyosarcoma according to stage.

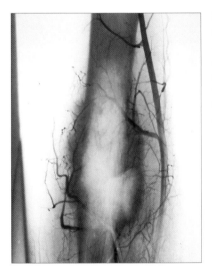

Fig. 16.20 Osteosarcoma. Subtraction angiography showing a large tumour of the femur with extensive new bone formation.

distant metastasis; important metastatic sites include the lungs, bone and liver.

This is another tumour in which chemotherapy has brought real improvements in overall survival. Because of extreme chemoresponsiveness of the tumour, particularly when drug combinations are used, this modality is generally the first approach once diagnosis has been established by biopsy, even before any consideration of local treatments with surgery and/or radiotherapy. Surgery following chemotherapy is often less radical and damaging than was previously the case, and has resulted in many more children undergoing limb-preserving procedures rather than amputation. For the most part such relatively conservative surgical procedures will be followed by radical postoperative irradiation. Good long-term preservation of function is provided

if the growing end of the bone can be shielded from the radiotherapy beam (see Fig. 16.14). It is generally necessary to offer further adjuvant chemotherapy, an approach which has reduced the relapse rate substantially.

In orbital rhabdomyosarcoma one of the aims of treatment is to preserve the eye and its function. This can usually be done by judicious use of chemotherapy and irradiation with careful attention to treatment details such as avoiding irradiation of the lachrymal gland and shielding the lens and cornea. Although high doses of radiotherapy are necessary, long-term side effects are usually quite acceptable. Overall prognosis depends on the tumour stage (Fig. 16.19). Localized resectable tumours have a cure rate of about 80%, which falls to about 50% when there is regional lymph node involvement and incomplete surgery. Children with distant metastasis have a cure rate of about 30%, an astonishing improvement over the results from the pre-chemotherapy era.

Osteosarcoma

Osteosarcomas (as discussed in chapter 15) are most often seen in adolescents. Most start in the diaphysis of bones, the lower limbs being more often involved. About 50% are found in the femur, three-quarters involving the distal end. Presenting features are pain and a palpable mass. X-rays often demonstrate the tumour spreading through the cortex with spicules of new bone being formed (Fig. 16.20). CT may be helpful in assessing the extent of the primary, and isotopic bone imaging may occasionally show metastatic skeletal involvement. Classically metastatic disease affects the lungs.

Although amputation of the affected limb used to be standard, limb conservation is now increasingly attempted (Fig. 16.21). In the past most patients died of metastatic disease, despite amputation for an apparently localized tumour. Because of this, adjuvant chemotherapy was introduced and recent randomized trials have suggested that long-term survival rates have increased from 20% to 40%. Current management often employs immediate chemotherapy (neoadjuvant chemotherapy) to assess tumour responsiveness, followed by limb-sparing surgery and, if the tumour has proven to be responsive, further chemotherapy is then given postoperatively.

Ewing's Sarcoma

Ewing's sarcoma (also discussed in chapter 15) is a rapidly growing malignant non-osseous tumour that usually arises in bone, though it is also seen in soft tissues. It mostly occurs in the first decade. Presentation is with localized pain and swelling. X-ray typically shows a periosteal reaction, with periosteal elevation and sub-periosteal new bone formation – so called 'onion skin' appearance (Fig. 16.22). Investigations should include isotopic bone image, chest X-ray and bone marrow aspirate. The diagnosis should always be confirmed by surgical biopsy. Since this tumour is exquisitely radiosensitive the primary tumour is often treated with radiotherapy whilst combination chemotherapy is given in an attempt to eradicate potential metastasis. Results are good, except when metastases have developed.

Retinoblastoma

Retinoblastoma is a rare tumour of particular importance due to its familial incidence. Although most cases are sporadic (see Fig. 16.2), 30–40% of cases are inherited. Because of this, a close watch must be kept on the contralateral eye in patients with a uni-ocular retinoblastoma. Most children present before 2 years of age with leucocoria (cat's eye reflex; Fig. 16.23). The tumour is typically multifocal within the retina. Spread is forwards into the vitreous humour, and later backwards towards the intracranial space. Extension into the choroid or sclera is generally a late event carrying a poor prognosis. Investigation includes CT imaging, chest X-ray, isotopic bone scanning and, if CNS involvement is suspected, CSF cytology. Treatment depends on tumour extent. Very small tumours may be managed with cryosurgery or photocoagulation, though irradiation is an alternative if the lesion is near the macula. For larger tumours, therapy can either be given by external means, or by the use of radioactive plaques (generally radioactive cobalt) which can be placed very exactly. With single primary tumours greater than 1 cm in size, external irradiation is generally preferred, and surgery is only used for very large tumours, though, in experienced hands, external irradiation may be successful even for the most adverse cases.

Unfortunately, retinoblastoma is a tumour in which there is a high incidence of secondary tumours, sometimes apparently radiation induced. However,

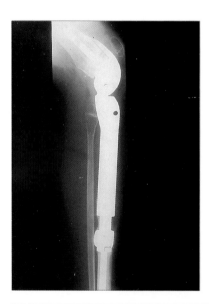

Fig. 16.21 Tibial prosthesis after conservative surgery for an osteosarcoma. As the patient grows the prosthesis is adjusted to give the correct length of leg.

RADIOGRAPHIC CHARACTERISTICS OF OSTEOSARCOMA AND EWING'S SARCOMA

Feature	Osteosarcoma	Ewing's Tumour
Location in bone	Metaphyseal	Diaphyseal
Involvement of long bones	Yes	Yes
Involvement of flat bones	Rare	Yes
Diffuse medullary cavity involvement	Rare	Common ('moth-eaten' or permeative involvement)
New bone formation	Yes	No – only as secondary phenomenon
Periosteal reaction	Yes ('Codman triangle') or spiculation	Yes ('onionskin' appearance)
	Not prominent but may be present	Yes

Fig. 16.22 Typical radiographic characteristics of osteosarcoma and Ewing's sarcoma. [Adapted from DeVita, Hellmann and Rosenberg (eds) (1989) *Cancer: Principles and Practice of Oncology*. J.B. Lippincott Co., Philadelphia.]

the secondary tumour is often well beyond the radiation site, raising the possibility that some other mechanism is responsible. Clearly this cannot be allowed to interfere with the adequacy of the initial attempt at cure.

In advanced cases, chemotherapy also plays a part in management, though its role is much less clear than with Wilms' tumour or rhabdomyosarcoma. Similar drugs are used, often combinations of vincristine, actinomycin D, doxorubicin and cyclophosphamide. Although worthwhile responses are often seen, the results of treatment for advanced disease are dramatically worse than for those with small primary tumours. In contrast to the 90% cure rate with localized disease, the survival with extensive tumours, residual after surgery and extending back to the optic nerve or grossly forwards into the vitreous, is only about 30%.

The family doctor's role in counselling families with children affected by retinoblastoma is particularly important and specialist advice is often helpful. A guide to the likely risks is given in Fig. 16.24.

GENETIC COUNSELLING IN RETINOBLASTOMA

Bilateral disease is almost always familial.

Offspring survivors of hereditary retinoblastoma, or of bilateral sporadic cases, will have a 50% chance of developing the tumour.

Unaffected parents with a child with unilateral disease have a 1–4% chance of having another affected child.

Survivors of unilateral sporadic disease have a 7–10% chance of having an affected child, and are therefore presumed to be silent carriers.

If two or more siblings are affected there is a 50% chance that subsequent siblings will have the tumour.

Unaffected children from retinoblastoma families may occasionally (5%) carry the gene but if they have an affected child the risk in subsequent children is 50% since the parent is then identified as a silent carrier.

Fig. 16.24 Genetic counselling in retinoblastoma.

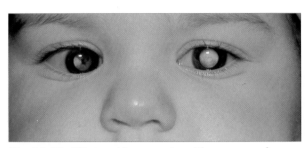

Fig. 16.23 Bilateral leucocoria with gross ocular involvement. Courtesy of Prof D.J. Spalton.

Fig. 16.25 Clinical findings associated with childhood cancer. [Adapted from DeVita, Hellmann and Rosenberg (eds) (1989) *Cancer: Principles and Practise of Oncology.* J.B. Lippincott Co., Philadelphia.]

CLINICAL FINDINGS IN CHILDHOOD CANCER

Clinical Findings	Tumour
Eye or orbit	
Strabismus	Retinoblastoma
Leucocoria ('cat's eye')	Retinoblastoma
Heterochromia – anisocoria and Horner's syndrome	Neuroblastoma
Opsoclonus – myoclonus ('dancing eyes') or acute cerebellar encephalopathy	Neuroblastoma
Proptosis	Neuroblastoma, lymphoma, retinoblastoma, rhabdomyosarcoma
Chronic sinusitis or otitis media	Rhabdomyosarcoma, nasopharyngeal carcinoma
Chronic diarrhoea (Verner–Morrison syndrome)	Neuroblastoma, MEN II
Skin	
'Blueberry muffin' nodules	Neuroblastoma
Seborrhoeic dermatitis	Histiocytosis
Nodular 'blueberry' lips	MEN II
Hypertension	Neuroblastoma, carcinoid, APUD tumours, pheochromocytoma, Wilms' tumour
Virilization	Hepatoblastoma, arrhenoblastoma, adrenal rest tumours, gonadoblastoma
Feminization	Chorioepithelioma, teratoma, hepatoblastoma, adrenal tumour, nongestational choriocarcinoma, embryonal cell carcinoma, granulosa thecal cell tumours

Summary

Childhood cancers represent a wide variety of very rare conditions requiring highly specialized management in paediatric oncology centres. Specific clinical findings, suggestive of particular childhood malignancies, are shown in Fig. 16.25. Sometimes the histological distinction between tumours is difficult and special techniques (cytochemistry, immunohisto-chemistry or tumour markers) may be helpful (Figs 16.26 and 16.27). Despite the devastating nature of the initial diagnosis, treatment of childhood cancer is often extremely gratifying and frequently leads to complete eradication of the tumour. Many skills are required for the optimal management of each individual case, and increased attention is now being paid to the avoidance, as far as possible, of both short- and long-term side effects.

BIOLOGICAL MARKERS IN CHILDHOOD TUMOURS

Tumours	AFP	hCG	Ferritin	CCA	NSE	LDH	Alk. Phos.	Polyamine	Cystathionine	CEA
Germ cell tumour	+	+				+				+
Liver tumour	+	+	+						+	+
Neuroblastoma			+	+	+	+			+	+
Ewing's sarcoma						+				
Osteosarcoma						+	+			
Medulloblastoma					+			+		
Lymphoma						+				

AFP, alpha-1-fetoprotein; hCG, human chorionic gonadotrophin; CCA, catecholamines; NSE, neuron specific enolase; LDH, lactate dehydrogenase; Alk. Phos., alkaline phosphatase; CEA, carcinoembryonic antigen; +, elevated in some or all patients with active disease.

Fig. 16.26 Biological markers in childhood tumours. [Adapted from DeVita, Hellmann and Rosenberg (eds) (1989) *Cancer: Principles and Practice of Oncology.* J.B. Lippincott Co., Philadelphia.]

DIAGNOSTIC TECHNIQUES FOR SMALL ROUND CELL TUMOURS OF CHILDHOOD

Tumours	Electron Microscopy	Immunocytochemistry						
		NSE	LEU 7	HSAN 1.2	Desmin	Mb	Vimentin	CCA
Neuroblastoma	Dense core neurosecretory granules, neural tubules or filaments	+	+	+	–	–	+	–
Lymphoma	Lack of cell attachments, glycogen and dense core granules	–	–/+	–	–	–	+/–	+
Ewing's sarcoma	Cytoplasmic glycogen	–	–	–	–	–	+	–
Peripheral neuroepithelioma	Neurites and dense core granules	+	–	+	–	–	+	–
Rhabdomyosarcoma	Intermediate filaments, fibrillar collagen stroma	+/–	–	–	+	+	+	–

NSE, neuron-specific enolase; Mb, myoglobin; CCA, catecholamines.

Fig. 16.27 Diagnostic techniques to distinguish small round-cell tumours of childhood. [Adapted from DeVita, Hellmann and Rosenberg (eds) (1989) *Cancer: Principles and Practice of Oncology.* J.B. Lippincott Co., Philadelphia.]

Supportive and Terminal Care

17

Introduction

The proper management of cancer- or treatment-related symptoms is one of the most critically important and gratifying aspects of the management of malignant disease. Over the past ten years major advances have been made, with increasing understanding that many patients' lives can be dramatically improved, often by relatively simple means, if careful consideration is given to their needs. Although expert attention is sometimes required, all of us who treat cancer patients should be aware of the essential principles of supportive care, and the simple ways in which management can be dramatically improved.

Pain in Cancer Patients

Most cancer patients suffer pain at some point in their illness, either from the primary lesion, for example a carcinoma of the bronchus eroding the chest wall or a pancreatic carcinoma causing severe abdominal or back pain, or pain from secondary deposits, particularly to bone (Fig. 17.1). The pain is often associated with other symptoms such as constipation consequent to opiate analgesia, or metabolic disorder such as hypercalcaemia, a very potent cause of constipation and widespread discomfort.

Management

With adequate attention to detail, most cancer pain can be greatly reduced by the use of appropriate medication (Fig. 17.2). There are several basic principles for the use of drugs to control cancer pain:

- Analgesics should always, if possible, be given by mouth. Suppositories are second best, and injections or intravenous infusions are painful and intrusive. If the patient is unable to take drugs by mouth or suppository, 24-hour subcutaneous infusion via a syringe driver should be given.
- A patient's treatment can be changed from one preparation to another more potent one until an optimum drug regimen is found. Dosage should be increased until the patient is pain free. A particular drug regimen should be abandoned only when undesirable side-effects occur, or if a stronger drug is clearly needed.
- Drugs of the same class should not be used simultaneously, but drugs with different actions (e.g. opiate and anti-inflammatory for bone pain, or opiate and anti-spasmodic for intestinal obstruction) are effective.
- The patient should be constantly monitored. The physician can decide when symptoms are under control only by consulting the patient. Most patients are able to titrate the dose of analgesics themselves, to obtain maximum pain relief with the minimum of side-effects.
- Response of pain to opiates varies significantly. One patient may need 100 times as much analgesia as another.
- Timing is crucial and treatment must be planned so that the next dose of analgesia is becoming active before the previous dose wears off, thus avoiding peaks and troughs in pain relief (Fig. 17.3).

Fig. 17.1 Secondary bone cancer. False colour bone scintigram of the spine and ribs of a patient suffering from secondary (metastatic) bone cancer affecting the dorsal spine. The tumour appears as the white area. Courtesy of CNRI/Science Photo Library.

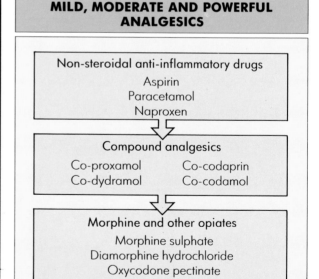

Fig. 17.2 Mild, moderate and powerful analgesics. Patients should be maintained on mild analgesics until the maximum recommended dose fails to control pain. They are then moved onto a moderate analgesic, until once again the maximum recommended dose fails. They then progress to a powerful analgesic.

- Addiction is not a problem when using opiate drugs to treat severe pain. The patient and family should be made aware of this. If the patient requests more pain relief this is because the pain has worsened.
- Pain causes anxiety and depression. If pain control does not relieve these symptoms, they must be treated separately. Factors raising or lowering a patient's pain threshold are shown in Fig. 17.4.
- Some symptoms may be caused by conditions other than cancer. These must be treated separately.

The Use of Morphine to Treat Cancer Pain

Increasingly, middle-order analgesics have been discontinued in favour of early use of morphine given by mouth either in tablet or elixir form, or as long-acting tablets of morphine sulphate (currently available in 10mg, 30mg, 60mg, 100mg and 200mg strength).

The decision to use morphine should not, of course, be undertaken lightly, but on the other hand

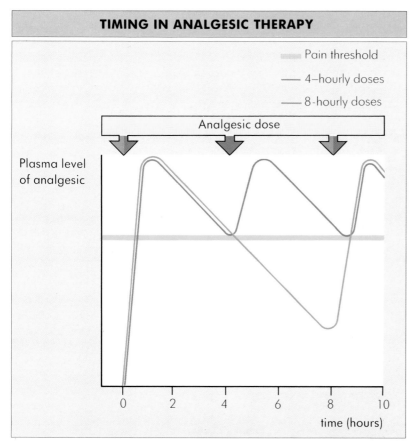

Fig. 17.3 Timing in analgesic therapy. Therapy should be repeated with adequate frequency to maintain the plasma level of the drug above the therapeutic threshold. In this illustration, if morphine is given every 8 hours, the patient is in increasing pain beyond 4 hours as the plasma level falls. Treatment every 4 hours overcomes the problem.

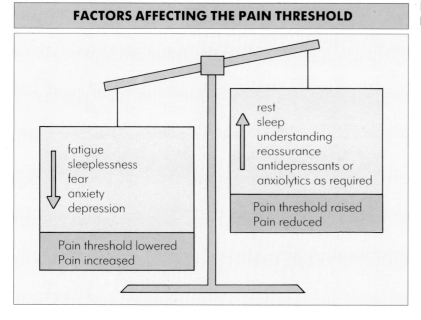

Fig. 17.4 Factors raising or lowering the pain threshold.

should never be delayed unduly; the patient should not have to 'earn their morphine' since low doses (10mg elixir or tablets given every four hours, or 30mg of long acting morphine (MST) given twice daily) often afford rapid relief with few side-effects.

It cannot be over-emphasized that anxieties about morphine addiction, often shared by patient and physician alike, have no relevance to the care of patients with metastatic cancer, and should be laid to rest. An equally important myth is that patients requiring morphine inevitably need rapid increases in dosage to sustain the equivalent effect; this has now been repeatedly demonstrated as false and many patients have their dose reduced once pain control has been achieved. Indeed many patients dying of widespread cancer in hospices or the community require no more than 60mg twice daily of MST until the end of their lives.

From the point of view of effective dosage, morphine is a unique drug within our pharmacopoeia. Unlike all other commonly used agents, patients may benefit from up to a 100-fold difference in dose, some requiring only 10mg elixir every four hours, others requiring several grams of morphine per day to control their pain. However, it is unusual for patients to require more than 600mg morphine daily by mouth. If a patient does require a very high dosage, it is often best to use a syringe driver for constant subcutaneous infusion of morphine, or better still diamorphine since the solubility of the latter is greater and hence the volume of diluent is smaller and less uncomfortable for the patient.

Other routes of administration are rarely necessary, but both rectal, sublinguinal and vaginal routes may be useful in patients who cannot swallow or are so cachectic that even subcutaneous infusions are inappropriate. All patients receiving opiates should be treated prophylactically for constipation, a common side-effect of morphine treatment (see below).

Other Cancer-Related Symptoms

As cancer is a multisystem disorder, it can cause a wide variety of symptoms, as well as pain. The commonest symptoms of a large group of patients with a wide variety of different cancers are shown in Fig. 17.5.

Constipation

This problem is both common and often surprisingly painful. It is particularly frequent in patients with widespread intra-abdominal malignancy, for example ovarian carcinoma. It is very frequent with opiate use, particularly morphine in high dosage, or with use of codeine and its derivatives. Almost all patients on opiates require regular laxatives, which usually give adequate bowel motility if prescribed once daily in the evening.

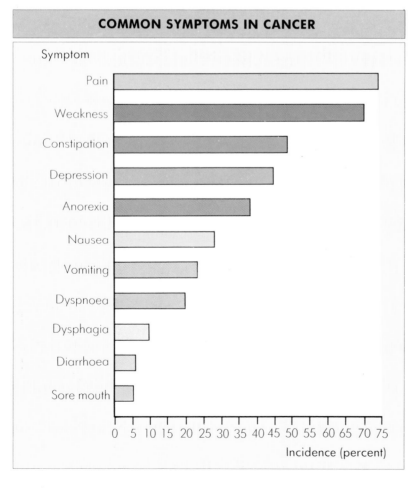

COMMON SYMPTOMS IN CANCER

Symptom

Pain
Weakness
Constipation
Depression
Anorexia
Nausea
Vomiting
Dyspnoea
Dysphagia
Diarrhoea
Sore mouth

0 5 10 15 20 25 30 35 40 45 50 55 60 65 70 75

Incidence (percent)

Fig. 17.5 Common symptoms in 100 consecutive patients with a variety of different cancers. The majority of these problems can be efficiently and rapidly dealt with by intelligent use of the specific supportive measures described in this chapter. Dyspnoea is probably the most difficult and resistant symptom to control effectively, but pain, nausea and constipation usually respond well to modern pharmacological therapy.

Dyspnoea

This relatively common cancer-related problem may limit the patient's normal mobility. There are a variety of causes including pleural effusion, lymphangitis carcinomatosa or major-airway obstruction, particularly with carcinoma of the bronchus. Lung metastases are not usually a cause, unless they are widespread throughout both lungs. If shortness of breath cannot be relieved by specific therapy (Fig. 17.6) such as pleural aspiration or radiotherapy, bronchodilators, steroid therapy and oxygen may be helpful.

Odour from Fungating Tumour

This is usually caused by anaerobic bacteria that are sensitive to the antibiotic metronidazole. Topical metronidazole or charcoal dressing packs may be very helpful and help to restore the patient's morale and dignity.

Anorexia

This is a very common problem, often denoting metastatic disease. It is particularly frequent with gastrointestinal tumours (especially oesophageal and pancreatic carcinoma) and is generally best treated with steroid therapy, often by dexamethasone given at high dose or megestrol acetate. Dietary supplements can also be used, though most are unpalatable to patients. Continued weight loss is often a source of anxiety for patients and relatives, who often equate it with life 'slipping away'.

Cerebral Secondaries

Cerebral secondaries may cause headaches or vomiting, hemiplegia and speech difficulties. High-dose steroids such as dexamethasone which reduce cerebral oedema around the tumour may relieve symptoms temporarily (Fig. 17.7).

Intractable Itching

This is generally caused by jaundice or uraemia, or is related to lymphoma. Itching can be treated with antihistamines, such as chlorpheniramine or terfenadine, or by cholestyramine which aids the retention of bile pigments in the gut. Soothing ointments and creams may also be helpful.

Treatment-Related Problems

Myelosuppression

This is very common, particularly with use of cytotoxic chemotherapy or wide-field irradiation. It generally presents with anaemia, neutropenia, or with a bleeding tendency (including bruising and purpura) as a result of thrombocytopenia.

These complications frequently require intensive treatment with antibiotics and supportive care, but to a large extent can be anticipated, especially where intensive chemotherapy is used. Where necessary, transfusions of blood and platelets can be life-saving, and can be repeated throughout the period of the myelosuppression, which is generally self-limiting. When high-dose chemotherapy is being used, autologous bone marrow transplantation or haemopoietic growth factors may reduce myelosuppression, but such treatments are restricted to specialized units.

Nausea and Vomiting

These problems are particularly common in patients undergoing combination chemotherapy, although wide-field irradiation (particularly total-body irradiation) is also an important cause. Many patients with advanced cancer also suffer these symptoms either as a direct effect of their disease or because of opiate analgesia. Treatment with anti-emetics is essential (Fig. 17.8) and fluid replacement may also be required, sometimes with intravenous rehydration.

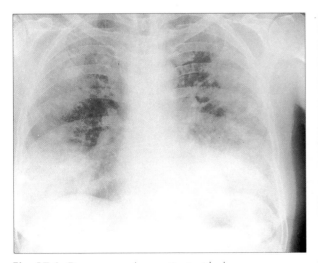

Fig. 17.6 Dyspnoea. Any patient with dyspnoea should be assessed to see if there is a treatable cause. This patient (who incidentally has bilateral breast prostheses) has diffuse lung infiltration caused by *Pneumocystis carinii*. Courtesy of Prof J. Whitehouse.

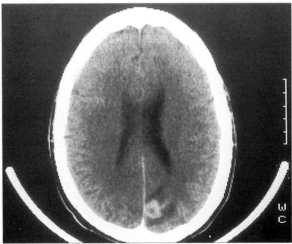

Fig. 17.7 Brain metastasis. The metastasis, enhanced by contrast, is surrounded by oedema. Dexamethasone reduces symptoms by decreasing the oedema. Courtesy of Dr G.M. Mead.

Alopecia

This is a particular problem with certain types of chemotherapy, notably doxorubicin, high-dose cyclophosphamide and etoposide, as well as cerebral irradiation. The alopecia generally occurs after the first or second course of chemotherapy and may be complete. Scalp freezing with a 'cold cap' may be useful with doxorubicin since this agent has a short plasma half-life (less than 30 minutes), but is not generally helpful with other agents. Radiation induced alopecia occurs only with treatment of the scalp (contrary to popular belief) but is much more long-lasting than chemotherapy-related alopecia. Early advice about a wig or hair piece, prior to hair loss, is important and it is usually possible to reassure patients that the alopecia will quickly reverse when chemotherapy has been completed.

Mucositis

This can be a painful and debilitating side-effect of cytotoxic treatment. It may be a particular problem in patients receiving methotrexate, particularly in those with pleural effusions or ascites, which cause a sustained high plasma level of the drug. Methotrexate is a particularly troublesome drug to use when there is renal failure, in which case the drug should be avoided altogether or carefully monitored using methotrexate levels. Folinic acid is often a valuable antidote, even where the methotrexate has been given at 'conventional' doses, and can generally be taken by mouth.

Site Specific Toxicities

Specific chemotherapy-related side-effects that are common when using particular cytotoxic drugs are shown in Fig. 17.8.

Summary

The symptomatic care of cancer patients is of paramount importance at all stages of the disease. For instance, the control of vomiting and other side-effects in a young patient receiving platinum-based chemotherapy for a highly curable testicular teratoma should not be neglected while the physician concentrates on treating the tumour and not the patient.

Likewise, symptomatic care for incurable cancer is a skill that should be developed. In addition to specific treatment of symptoms, it should not be forgotten that emotional and practical support are often as important, and sometimes more important, than pharmaceutical intervention.

MECHANISMS OF NAUSEA AND VOMITING

Cerebral cortex	Raised intracranial pressure
Anxiolytics Relaxation techniques	Dexamethasone

Integrative Vomiting Centres

Vestibular centre	Chemoreceptor trigger zone
Antihistamines e.g. Cyclizine	Antidopaminergic e.g. Metoclopramide or a phenothiazine e.g. Chlorpromazine, Prochlorperazine Cannabinoid e.g. Nabilone

Gut (sympathetic and parasympathetic)

$5HT_3$ antagonist e.g. Ondansetron
Anticholinergic e.g. Hyosine

Fig. 17.8 Mechanisms of nausea and vomiting and effective drugs.

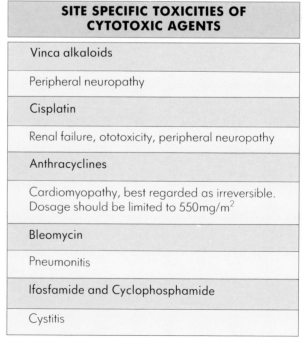

SITE SPECIFIC TOXICITIES OF CYTOTOXIC AGENTS
Vinca alkaloids
Peripheral neuropathy
Cisplatin
Renal failure, ototoxicity, peripheral neuropathy
Anthracyclines
Cardiomyopathy, best regarded as irreversible. Dosage should be limited to 550mg/m^2
Bleomycin
Pneumonitis
Ifosfamide and Cyclophosphamide
Cystitis

Fig. 17.9 Site-specific toxicities of individual cytotoxic agents.

Index

3